ENCOUNTERS WITH **WILD CHILDREN**

ENCOUNTERS WITH **Wild Children**

Temptation and Disappointment in the
Study of Human Nature

ADRIANA S. BENZAQUÉN

McGill-Queen's University Press
Montreal & Kingston · London · Ithaca

© McGill-Queen's University Press
ISBN 13: 978-0-7735-2972-4   ISBN 10: 0-7735-2972-1

Legal deposit first quarter 2006
Bibliothèque nationale du Québec

Printed in Canada on acid-free paper that is 100% ancient forest free
(100% post-consumer recycled), processed chlorine free

This book has been published with the help of a grant from the Canadian Federation for the Humanities and Social Sciences, through the
Aid to Scholarly Publications Programme, using funds provided by
the Social Sciences and Humanities Research Council of Canada.

McGill-Queen's University Press acknowledges the support of the
Canada Council for the Arts for our publishing program. We also
acknowledge the financial support of the Government of Canada
through the Book Publishing Industry Development Program (BPIDP)
for our publishing activities.

LIBRARY AND ARCHIVES CANADA
CATALOGUING IN PUBLICATION

Benzaquén, Adriana Silvia
Encounters with wild children : temptation and disappointment
in the study of human nature / Adriana S. Benzaquén.
Includes bibliographical references and index.
ISBN 13: 978-0-7735-2972-4   ISBN 10: 0-7735-2972-1
1. Feral children. I. Title.
GN372.B45 2006   155.45'67   c2005-905596-0

Set in 10.6/14 Minion Pro with Myriad Pro
Book design and typesetting by zijn digital

Contents

PART FOUR
Variations on a Theme: Brutalization, Abuse, and Freedom

ENCOUNTERS WITH **WILD CHILDREN**

Introduction

1344: A boy was captured in Hesse. As was later known and as he himself said, he was taken at the age of three years by wolves and raised by them in a marvellous way. The wolves offered him the better part of their plunder for food, made him a hole in winter and covered it with leaves to protect the boy from the bitter cold. They urged him to go on all fours, until by exercising he had acquired their speed and was able to make the biggest jumps. After his capture he was set upright and urged to go about in a human fashion by putting splints on his legs to stiffen them. The boy often said that he would have preferred association with the wolves rather than with human beings. He was taken to the court of Henry, the prince of Hesse, as a curiosity and spectacle. The like case happened in Wetterau, near the Echtzel estate, where a boy was captured who had lived for twelve years among wolves, in a dense wood which the people used to call the Hart. He was captured by nobles who used to resort there for hunting. The boy lived until about eighty years of age. His capture occurred in 1344, in winter, in the snow.

Last April, we heard about Djuma, who had been hospitalised in Soviet Central Asia for nearly 30 years. He had been raised by wolves until the age of seven, and even now will eat only raw meat, bites when he is angry and crawls on all fours. Dr Rufat Kazirbaev, chief of psychiatric research in the Turkmenistan hospital where Djuma was looked after, doubted if he would ever lose his wolf ways.

Djuma was found by geologists in a bleak desert region in 1962, running with a wolf pack. The men threw a net over the boy, but the wolves rushed to protect him, tearing at the net. In the end, all the wolves were killed. It was four years before the boy was taught to utter a few words. He told anthropologists how he rode on the back of his wolf mother when the pack hunted, and later learned to run on all fours. It was years before he got used to sleeping in a bed.

THESE TWO ACCOUNTS, one from 1344 (but printed in the late sixteenth century) and the other from 1962 (but reported in the early 1990s), tell stories of encounters with strange children in unusual circumstances and of the responses the children elicited in the adults who saw and took charge of them.[1] The events are separated by more than six hundred years, and yet the two accounts, like the many other stories of "wild children," are intriguingly similar – and enduringly fascinating. For more than four hundred years such stories have been recorded, circulated and reproduced, mainly (but not exclusively) in Europe and North America, not simply as myths, legends, or good tabloid copy but as occurrences deserving of serious scrutiny by scholars and scientists of diverse persuasions and fields of expertise. This book argues that wild children have had a privileged role as objects of knowledge in Western human science and shows how the knowledge produced about them in different disciplines (anthropology, psychiatry, sociology, psychology, pedagogy, linguistics) has contributed to the shaping and reshaping of the modern understanding of childhood and affected the social and institutional practices directed at all children.

The literature on wild children comprises a wide variety of accounts, debates and representations. Through detailed readings of these documents, I restage the encounters with wild children not to find out, once and for all, the truth about wild children and their stories but to explain why, despite having invariably ended in disappointment, the search for the truth about wild children (and the truth *in* wild children) has been a recurring pursuit for several centuries. The wild children were located at the centre of concentric circles of curiosity and intervention: personal, communal, social, transnational. By restaging the encounters with wild children I also seek to encounter those who encountered them, who used them to think, who entangled them in their theories, questions, and projects. What does the persistent interest in wild children tell us about the goals and methods of human science in Western modernity? What does it tell us about how modern adults conceive of, relate to, and fantasize about children? What is the relation between wild children and children in general? How do notions of wildness, civilization, and discovery impinge on shifting approaches to childhood? Whereas most studies of wild children have interpreted their stories from the perspective of a specific discipline or profession and used them to advance a particular theoretical position within it, I want to explore what was (and is) at stake for the human sciences in general in their ongoing involvement with wild children and propose that only by considering each story or debate in relation to the others can we fully understand its significance.[2]

Carlo Ginzburg has observed three approaches to the relation between evidence and historical reality. Positivist historians analyze the available evidence as evidence of something else (assumed to be the proper object of study). As "an open window that gives us direct access to reality," the evidence may be more or less reliable, and is correspondingly to be accepted or discarded, but it is never interesting or valuable in itself. In contrast, for some contemporary historians the evidence is opaque, "a wall, which by definition precludes any access to reality." But, as Ginzburg argues, the theoretically naive positivists and the theoretically sophisticated sceptics, despite their apparent opposition, share a similar fixed understanding of the evidence: it is always a window or a wall. The alternative is to think of the relation between the evidence and the historical reality it is supposed to be evidence of not as a given but as something that must be worked out in each particular case.[3] In this study, which is closer to microhistory than to biography, I exploit the richness of the historical record, made up of complex and conflicting accounts that bring together different genres, voices, subjects, and desires. I scrutinize the evidence not only for what it tells us about wild children themselves (as a matter of fact, it usually tells us very little about them) but to learn something from the very way the accounts were put together. Two dimensions of the relation between evidence and historical reality strike the student of these stories: first, the inextricable relation between the production of historical accounts and the fabrication or invention of fictional narrative, between history and stories; second, the difficulties intrinsic to the search for evidential proof of an event, especially an improbable event that challenges habits or expectations. When can an account or a document be deemed valid, reliable, incontrovertible, or merely sufficient proof that something indeed happened? Whose words count as authentic testimony of the occurrence of an event, and whose need further confirmation? The accounts of wild children, while fragmentary and incomplete, are a rich source of information about other lives, experiences, ideas, and knowledge. Reading this evidence requires that the historian acknowledge both the many voices inscribed therein and the near-complete absence from the record of the voices of wild children themselves.

There is another way in which this study approaches the method of Ginzburg and the microhistorians. In "The Name and the Game" (1991), Ginzburg and Carlo Poni expressed dissatisfaction with the specialization fostered by the "one-sidedness" and fragmentary nature of the archival sources used by historians, as opposed to the anthropologist's reconstruction, through fieldwork, of a complexity of social relationships. To appreciate the complexity of relations linking an individual and a society, they suggest, the historian must circumscribe the area of research so that "the individual documentary series can transcend time and space in a way that permits us to find the same individual or group of individuals in different social contexts. The thread of Ariadne that leads the researcher through the archival labyrinth is the same thread that distinguishes one individual from another in all societies known to us: the name."[4] My purpose is to understand the formation of a type of knowledge and its impact on the lives and experiences of people rather than to reconstruct a web of social relationships; but as I collected and analyzed a series of texts exclusively on the basis of their reference to wild children, I was also following "names": both those given to the individual wild children and, more generally, the label "wild child." As the two brief accounts I juxtaposed at the beginning of this introduction show, the stories of wild children have enough in common to permit a wide-scope comparison bridging disparate times and cultures. When we read them against each other, we notice striking parallels between the stories of the boys captured in Hesse and in Wetterau and Djuma, but also no less striking differences: the first story mentions a court and a prince; the second a hospital, a psychiatrist, geologists, and anthropologists. The wild children unfailingly attracted curiosity and concern, but the meanings they were given and the responses they evoked varied greatly. Close examination of these meanings and responses can teach us a great deal about the people, the communities, the societies (and groups within a society) that came in contact with each wild child. As a corpus, the stories of wild children exhibit both unity and multiplicity; they are homogeneous and heterogeneous at the same time. The area of research is large enough to make visible historical shifts that are obscured in more narrowly conceived studies and focused enough to make the project manageable.

In that sense, this is a study of texts connected by the fact that they are (explicitly) about wild children. Is it then possible to speak of a "discourse" on wild children? In *The Archaeology of Knowledge* (1972) Michel Foucault defined *discourse* as a limited number of statements belonging to a single system of formation (that is, for which certain conditions of existence can be determined), *discursive formation* as the principle of dispersion and redistribution of statements, encompassing a set of rules that govern their objects, enunciations (or subject positions), concepts, and theoretical choices, and *discursive practice* as the "anonymous, historical rules, always determined in the time and space that have defined a given period, and for a given social, economic, geographical, or linguistic area, the conditions of operation of the enunciative function."[5] These terms may only be applied very loosely to the texts (or statements) on wild children, which are not clearly delimited or circumscribed to a single period or area. My goal is different from Foucault's: I do not seek to characterize a single discursive formation or trace the space of dispersion and change within a single discourse but to trace the scattered appearances and uses, incarnations and transformations of a single "discursive element" – the "wild child" – which is neither exactly an object nor a concept. I pursue the wild child's appearances and functions in several discourses to ascertain the role of wild children in the formation of a body of knowledge about "the child" and its eventual transformation into a science of children.

In another sense, the documentary evidence on wild children is a series of "case studies." Foucault explored the value of studying a particular "case" in his work on Pierre Rivière. For Foucault, the case lies at the intersection of impersonal discourse and individual biography, at the point where *subjectivity* invades discourse. The case, moreover, connects the historical and the everyday: in the case of Rivière, we see an instance of the ordinary (a poor, unremarkable peasant) entering the realm of the historical by becoming the *extra*ordinary (the murderer of mother, sister, and brother); in the cases of wild children, we see the extraordinary (the wild child) becoming confused with the ordinary (the child). The wild child becomes a figure for understanding and imagining "the child" through its inscription (and multiple reinscriptions) in discourse. Historians of childhood have often deplored the paucity of sources on children. The evidence on wild children, however, is substantial. Until quite recently, exceptionality may have been the surest, sometimes the only, way for subordinate subjects to break into the historical record and thus conquer anonymity and oblivion. Ginzburg and Foucault, among others, have taken advantage of the exceptional production of documentary evidence (for example, inquisitorial, judicial, and medical records) about people who found themselves in conflict with the law (for example, Menocchio and Rivière). Here I take advantage of the fact that, unlike the majority of ordinary, or "normal," children, wild children left more traces of their existence due to the inordinate interest they provoked.[6]

There are nevertheless in this record persistent gaps and silences that no amount of rigour or dedication on the part of the historian could completely eliminate. But these contradictions, conflicts, gaps, and silences in the sources are meaningful in themselves. They interest me because they not only call for more perceptive interpretive strategies but also remind us that there is always something about the lives and experiences of others that remains beyond the researcher's grasp – and that this unreachable part may be the most important, the most valuable, that which makes us human. Referring to Dostoevsky's heroes, Mikhail Bakhtin wrote: "a living human being cannot be turned into the voiceless object of some secondhand, finalizing cognitive process. *In a human being there is always something that only he himself can reveal, in a free act of self-consciousness and discourse, something that does not submit to an externalizing secondhand definition.*"[7] The historian's approach to her objects of study is necessarily indirect, but, Bakhtin suggests, it has advantages as well. Historical writing is a form of what he called "exotopy": it is produced from a position of outsidedness, or exteriority, in relation to the events it recounts and the people it portrays. Outsidedness is a condition for *creative understanding*: "In order to understand, it is immensely important for the person who understands to be *located outside* the object of his or her creative understanding – in time, in space, in culture. For one cannot even really see one's own exterior and comprehend it as a whole, and no mirrors or photographs can help; our real exterior can be seen and understood only by other people, because they are located outside us in space and because they are *others*."[8] In my investigation of the wild children and their interlocutors, benefactors, and tormentors I have aimed for this kind of creative understanding that is grounded in the external and exotopical position of the subject of knowledge but does not proffer a finalizing definition of the other.

In writing history we temporarily attain a position of outsidedness in relation to our own time and culture as well. We look at the past with the eyes of the present, but we may also reverse the gaze and look at the present from the point(s) of view of the past. In exploring the past, the historian also *questions* the present as something in need of explanation, defence, condemnation, or transformation.[9] Tzvetan Todorov's concept of exemplarity has helped me conceptualize the relation between the closed and individualized discursive space of the "case" and the larger sociohistorical universe in which it is embedded, between the microscopic and macroscopic levels of historical analysis, and between past and present. Todorov distinguishes two forms of remembering, recounting, and interpreting past events: *literal* and *exemplary*. When a past event is interpreted literally, it remains an intransitive fact with no significance beyond itself. When it is interpreted as an example, the event's singularity and specificity are not denied, but it is nonetheless comprehended as an instance among others of a more general category, as an *exemplum* from which a lesson may be derived. Todorov believes that the literal use of history is dangerous, especially when pushed to extremes, because it isolates past events and subordinates the present to the past. The exemplary interpretation of history is potentially liberating because it uses the past as a model to understand new situations involving different agents and as a principle for action in the present. Exemplary history "allows us to profit from the lessons of injustices suffered in the past to fight those that are committed in the present, to leave the self and move towards the other."[10]

What lessons can be learned from an exemplary history of wild children? I focus on three areas of historical and philosophical debate. First, I explore the many relations established between individual adults and wild children in the past as different forms of the relation between self and other and as examples that may be read alongside and against the forms taken by adult-child relations in the present. The writings on and responses to wild children both display and put into perspective the many forms of that most universal, most ordinary, of human experiences – an adult facing a child. I attend to the particularity of each story, of the relation between *an* adult and *a* child as historical actors in specific historical circumstances. I also consider the adult-child relation in general as a microstructure, a microcosm representing the many ways in which a community relates to someone who does not quite, or does not yet, belong to it, someone outside it or someone resisting it, and the many ways in which the community strives to understand, know, classify, and transform the unknown being into a member or an outcast. What interests me is not retrospective judgment but the possible uses of the stories of wild children, in all their complexity, as examples to think through the moral issues raised by the relation between adult and child.[11] Second, I deploy the stories of wild children to elucidate the process of knowing others, by which I mean how we put perceptions and ideas together in statements that entitle us to claim to have knowledge about other people, how we seek and produce certainty in constituting this knowledge, how we build up and validate accounts, theories, and disciplines, how we rely on knowledge to mediate our relations with others, and how we act and create institutions based on this knowledge. The stories of wild children exemplify the entanglement of knowledge and the lives of people: knowledge facilitates or precludes, sanctions or disqualifies relations between people, while the relations themselves give rise to knowledge of various kinds, whether certain, positive, true knowledge or rumours, stories, tales, fictions, lies. Only in some forms does knowledge count, and only some subjects are deemed to possess (and are able to produce) knowledge that counts, while others are rendered or perceived as silent. I am not looking for a general theory of knowledge about people; my epistemology is concrete and contingent: a historical epistemology.[12] Finally, an exemplary interpretation of the stories of wild children may contribute to the current problematization of humanism. These stories vividly expose the ways we include others within, or exclude them from, our definitions of the human. For this reason, they may induce us both to reconsider narrow conceptions of the human and of humanism dependent on a universal or normal subject and to decline antihumanist positions whose ultimate effect is to perpetuate the argument that wild children were somehow *in*human.[13]

Thus, of the many meanings and uses of wild children in thought and in practice, this study highlights a few: how wild children were always positioned outside the norm, though their stories have become props of normative discourses; how the response to the wild child furnishes a test case of a community's capacity to care and a society's ability to tolerate or accept the different; how wild children expose the limitations of our notion of the human; and how the jigsaw puzzle made up of all the stories lets another figure be glimpsed: "the child" emerging at a certain point in time as a new object of scientific knowledge and intervention.

In part one I analyze the epistemological and narrative processes through which the "wild child" was constituted as a class or kind: how the accounts of wild children were put together and reproduced, how they were integrated into emerging taxonomies and classifications, how they gave rise to a *list* of cases and a *story*-form, how wild children were defined and characterized, and what may be the prototype or best example of the class. In part two I follow wild children as they enter, as evidence or example, some of the major eighteenth-century philosophical and scientific debates about innate ideas, human nature, the state of nature, and the boundaries of the human. Part three examines the changes taking place in the early nineteenth century in both understandings of and responses to the wild child: how something was done to (and through) the wild child to change his or her wild condition, and how this process was explicitly devised and received as a medico-pedagogical experiment providing insight into the appropriate treatment and care of larger groups of "normal" and "abnormal" children.

In part four I discuss the more recent incarnations and meanings of the wild child – animal-nurtured children in "exotic" colonial and postcolonial locations; confined, abused, and neglected children; and children in perfect harmony with nature – and different forms of emotional investment in and identification with the figure of the wild child. In each section I focus on specific stories: the earlier cases in part one; Peter of Hanover and the wild girl of Songi in part two; Victor of Aveyron in part three, and the Indian wolf children, John of Burundi, Genie, Kaspar Hauser, and the gazelle boy in part four.

My account of the stories of wild children is partial, of course. In trying to lay hold of, and emphasize, certain levels of discourse and experience, I have unavoidably neglected, blurred, or excluded others. Someone else may disagree with my choices and conclusions and retell these stories in a different form, from a different perspective. I will welcome that other voice and the opportunity to continue the dialogue.

A NOTE ON THE TEXT

Unless otherwise indicated in the bibliography, all translations are mine.

PART ONE Telling Stories of Wild Children

CHAPTER ONE **The Accounts**

One cannot speak of anything at any time; it is not easy to
say something new; it is not enough for us to open our eyes,
to pay attention, or to be aware, for new objects suddenly
to light up and emerge out of the ground.

M. Foucault, *The Archaeology of Knowledge*[1]

WHAT IS A "WILD CHILD"? This is the question that will occupy us in the first two chapters. It is not my aim to formulate an accurate or definitive understanding, definition, classification, or characterization of wild children but to stipulate the discursive – epistemological and narrative – processes and mechanisms through which something like "the wild child" was constituted, in diverse times and places, institutional and textual locations. In other words, the first two chapters are about different approaches to the question of what a wild child is, from the perspective of description, classification, definition, and narration.

Let me say that, as a starting point, I take the wild child as a given. But what kind of a given? I take the wild children as they are given to me, at face value as it were, but not in unmediated reality. I do not accept the idea that some children are given to us as "wild" in reality (or in documentary evidence of past reality), that there may be something in such children that warrants the label in the same way that lack of hearing warrants the label "deaf" or being born in Argentina makes someone "Argentinian." This is not a blanket rejection of a correspondence theory of meaning or classification but a very specific claim about the way the class "wild child" functions. As my discussion will show, the wild child is given to us in the literature. This means both that there is something like a literature (or "discourse") on wild children and that "wild child" is to a great extent a literary or discursive class or kind. I argue that wild child is a discursive class and analyze it as such, because it is the discourse, in its many forms, repetitions, and transformations during the past four centuries, that both gives rise to the class and brings the cases together. But in what ways is the wild child given to us in and moulded by the discourse? What real affinities may be found between the cases?

The wild child is always a *strange* child, perceived as strange, but not any and every strange child is understood to be a wild child. There is no single reason why a child is labelled wild, but a series of contingent and often extrinsic reasons having to do with the (social, historical, intellectual) context in which these children appear and the motives and expectations of those who, directly or retrospectively, observe and label them. For instance, the fact that Genie was called wild child in 1970 is tangled with the release in Los Angeles of Truffaut's film *The Wild Child* about Victor of Aveyron and the desire, on the part of the doctors and scientists in charge of her case, to repeat the achievements of Jean-Marc-Gaspard Itard (1774–1838), Victor's doctor-teacher. More than one hundred and fifty years earlier, the "savage of Drôme" was *not* labelled "wild child" at the same time that Victor was being "expelled" from the Institute for Deaf-Mutes in Paris.[2] A wild child may be designated as such by journalists, government bureaucrats, or even ordinary people, but ultimately the label only sticks (that is, it is only legitimized) when the wild child is named, or when the name is accepted, by scientists, the legitimate speakers of the discourse or producers of knowledge. Thus Genie, named wild child by doctors and scientists, remained a wild child – as attested by Linda Garmon's 1994 television documentary *Secret of the Wild Child* – even though her mother strongly opposed the label: "When I saw the title of the book [Susan Curtiss's 1977 *Genie: A Psycholinguistic Study of a Modern-Day "Wild Child"*], I felt hurt ... My daughter ... classified as a 'wild child.'"[3] Yet it was not enough for the French minister of the Interior to suggest that the boy found in the Drôme in 1811 might be a wild boy like Victor of Aveyron; the experts who administered the Institute for Deaf-Mutes, including its director, the celebrated abbé Sicard, dismissed the suggestion and the boy was soon forgotten. Furthermore, not all children who are labelled "wild" can be said to share clearly identifiable traits or characteristics. There are many ways to be named and to be a wild child, to be described and to behave as a wild child. A significant consequence of this is that the label itself is fragile. It is always contested, qualified, or on the verge of being replaced by alternative labels or interpretations.

While I prefer "wild children" as the general name encompassing all the children and stories included in this study, it may be useful to consider alternatives and variations. In English there are two ways to translate the Latin "*ferus*" or the French "*sauvage*": "wild" or "savage." Not only does each word have slightly different connotations but "savage," like "*sauvage*," is also a noun. Using savage instead of wild underlines the relation between wild children and the *exotic* "savages" (non-European "primitive" cultures or nations); using it as a noun ("*Sauvage de l'Aveyron*") downplays the question whether the people concerned are children or adults. In Spanish, the labels attached to wild children exploit the etymological relation between "*salvaje*" (savage) and "*selva*" (forest or jungle): "*salvaje*" carries the meanings both of "forest-dweller" and of "uncivilized" or "ferocious." Other terms used in English and other languages emphasize the connection between wild children and animals, either in general ("beast-children") or in the distinct names coined for animal-nursed children: "wolf boy," "bear child," "swine girl," "gazelle boy." As a way to capture the phenomenon and experience of wild children in a word, Franck Tinland relies on the felicitous term "*ensauvagement*," which suggests that wild children are indeed children *turned wild* ("*ensauvagés*"), their wildness or savagery not an inherent quality or condition but the result of a process and a set of circumstances.[4]

Wild children are often referred to as "feral children." The term has a history: it derives from Linnaeus's "*Homo ferus*," popularized by anthropologist Robert Zingg in English as "feral man," and later associated exclusively or especially with children.[5] (In some of the recent literature, the purportedly more neutral and inclusive "isolated children" appears as a substitute for "feral.") I prefer "wild children": the notion of "feral child" conveys an aspiration to a certain type of objectivity and scientificity, and the acceptance of a set of assumptions about the proper way to produce knowledge about people, from which I want to distance myself, because this aspiration and these assumptions are part of what I set out to investigate. Rather than taking "wild child" as an unproblematic label that may be attached to a well-delimited group of objects or people in the world or as a class within a scientific system of classification – Linnaeus's *Homo ferus* is related and opposed to *Homo Americanus, Homo Asiaticus, Homo Europaeus, Homo Afer,* and *Homo monstrosus*; "feral child" is related and opposed to "normal (or civilized, or socialized) child" – I understand wild children as human beings whose names and stories were somehow linked to one another, in the course of recent history, in an active sense and by particular historical agents. The links between wild children were forged by knowledge producers – not the wild children themselves but other people who labelled the children, compared and contrasted their condition, characteristics, and changes, and put together a list of cases. The wild children are in effect related – Genie to Victor, Victor to the wild girl of Songi, the wild girl of Songi to the wolf boy of Hesse, all of them to Kamala, and so on – because those responsible for producing accounts and explanations fabricated those relations. And as Ian Hacking reminds us, what has been fabricated or "constructed" is by no means less real.[6]

In this chapter I present the accounts of what for lack of a better word I call "historical," or "real," wild children. The historical wild child is an individual with an often contested story. Usually what is contested is the very claim to the reality of the phenomenon and appropriateness of the name or class. The accounts monotonously include or bring about disputes as to whether the child indeed existed, whether the reports are authentic or credible, and whether the right label for that child is "wild" (rather than imbecile, deaf-mute, impostor, etc.). We must however take into consideration the significant difference between these wild children and the *figure* of the wild child, also given to us in discourse, mainly in two kinds of setting: as example, illustration, or evidence, used to support, prove, or disprove philosophical or scientific arguments and hypotheses, and as an image or theme that triggers the imagination, found in myth, fiction, poetry, film, and the visual arts. My goal is never to lose sight of the "real" wild children, especially insofar as they were involved in relations with no less real adults and were the occasion for the production of a kind of knowledge that directly or indirectly touched the lives of many other (non-wild) children. But I pay close attention to the interrelation and feedback between real wild children and the figure of the wild child. On the one hand, the wild child's changing value as example or evidence fuels the search for and curiosity about real wild children. In many cases, wild children were explicitly looked up, pursued, or visited because they were believed to possess high epistemic value. The Enlightenment controversies featuring wild children motivated the visits to Wild Peter and Mlle Leblanc, formerly the wild girl of Songi, by the eccentric Scottish philosopher and judge James Burnett, Lord Monboddo (1714–1799), a great collector of stories of wild children. Two hundred years later a similar desire for knowledge took psycholinguist Harlan Lane and psychiatrist Richard Pillard from Boston to Burundi in their quest for John, the monkey boy. Just a few years ago, the writer Michael Newton went to see John Ssabunnya during the Pearl of Africa Choir's tour of Britain "because of what might be true about him."[7] On the other hand, the mythic, literary and artistic renditions of the figure of the wild child serve as a background against which the stories of real wild children are played out, and from which tropes, themes, and explanatory models are often borrowed.[8]

The sources on wild children are diverse, varying in type of text, length, quality, publication history, and reception. We find some unchallenged "classics," frequently reprinted and widely circulated, like Itard's early-nineteenth-century reports on the wild boy of Aveyron and Anselm von Feuerbach's 1833 book on Kaspar Hauser. But most accounts and discussions of wild children appear in rare texts of uncertain status, some of them undeservedly forgotten (e.g., Daniel Defoe's *Mere Nature Delineated* [1726] and Monboddo's *Antient Metaphysics* [1779–99]), some wholly forgettable or ephemeral by their very nature (e.g., scores of newspaper and magazine clippings). The earliest "original" accounts have been cited or paraphrased so many times that, in Tinland's view, the literature on wild children risks being regarded as little more than a "monotonous repetition."[9] In fact, as we shall see, it is not only the accounts that are endlessly and monotonously repeated but also the arguments and disputes; and, I suggest, both the repetitions and the variations are significant.

Who writes about wild children, in what genres, and for whom? The writings on wild children belong to three types of discourse. The first type is journalism, current events reporting, and works by travellers and explorers describing their adventures in faraway places. The stories of wild children constitute or add to the sensational, spectacular, extraordinary, or exotic appeal of these texts. In works bearing no palpable relation to the topic, such as Bernard Connor's *History of Poland* (1698), J.-J.-S. Leroy's *Mémoire* (1776) on wood exploitation in the Pyrenees, and Sir William Henry Sleeman's *Journey through the Kingdom of Oude* (1858), accounts of wild children were inserted as asides or digressions merely because of their value as stories or curiosities. The second type of discourse is the human and social sciences broadly understood, including human and comparative anatomy and medicine. Most of the book-length biographical or historical studies of individual wild children were written within the context of debates in one or more of these sciences. The third type is the arts and other forms of cultural production. The range of imaginary representations of both real and invented wild children is wide indeed, from anonymous poems and pamphlets on Peter of Hanover published in 1720s London to contemporary works about historical and fictional wild children like David Malouf's *An Imaginary Life* (1978), Jill Paton Walsh's *Knowledge of Angels* (1994), Mordicai Gerstein's *Victor* (1998) and *The Wild Boy* (1998), and Michael Apted's 1994 film *Nell*, starring Jodie Foster.

The factual information on each wild child is made up of witness reports – reports by participants in the discovery or capture of the child, of which there are not many; reports by witnesses of the child's life "in the wild" or among animals, which are even rarer; hearsay, second- or third-hand reports of the capture and subsequent incidents; and official inquiries, scientific field investigations, and interviews conducted in some cases decades after the main events[10] – and observational and experimental data – gathered by people (scientists and intellectuals) who had access to the children a short time after their return to human society or many years later. In very few instances we have first-person accounts by the (ex-)wild children themselves. The commentary and controversy following publication of the original accounts and reports, and the ensuing waves of debate, layer upon layer of interpretation and reinterpretation, generally involve people who never had personal contact with the children. In most cases, the human sciences have no choice but to feed on non-scientific accounts, reports, and testimonies, while regularly distrusting the actual value or authenticity of the evidence.

The authors of the accounts may become interested in wild children by fortuitously coming into contact with one such child or story. They learn more about similar cases or already know about other wild children and go looking for a new case to observe and write about. The traveller Jean-Claude Armen knew nothing about wild children before his "astounding discovery" of the gazelle boy in 1960 but studied the literature after his return to Europe,[11] whereas in 1800 the naturalist Pierre-Joseph Bonnaterre (1751–1804) requested permission to observe the wild boy of Aveyron because he was familiar with Linnaeus's *Homo ferus*. There seems to be an intrinsic fascination in the topic that drives the search or research. The interest and fascination extend to the various audiences: the nameless crowds reported to have thronged to see many of the cases, demanding that the strange phenomenon be exhibited and sometimes paying a price for the show;[12] the readers of newspapers and magazines who never seem to tire of new reports on wild children, whatever their provenance and despite the fact that they have seldom (if ever) been authenticated to everyone's satisfaction; the scientific community, including the tempted, the convinced, the sceptics (and the tempted-turned-sceptics), and the cultural critics of the scientists' and philosophers' follies.[13] More recently, a different type of adult audience is growing: not the curious mob looking for thrills in a "freak" or "monster" but the psychologically deep individual who senses in the wild child an intensified representation of "the child" in general as the embodiment of innocence, nature, and the adult's past. In addition, wild children are being presented to children themselves in texts and cultural objects produced for them, like Jane Yolen's *Children of the Wolf* (1984) and Gerstein's *Victor* and *The Wild Boy* (the first two are novels for young readers and the third is a picture book).

The accounts of "real" wild children fall into four groups: the earlier and minor European cases; the major European wild children (Peter, the wild girl of Songi, Victor, and Kaspar Hauser); the "exotic" (non-European) animal-nurtured children, and the more recent cases (the gazelle boy, Genie, John of Burundi, Marcos, John Ssabunnya, and many others who never made it past a single or a few newspaper and magazine articles or were promptly dismissed as hoaxes or reinterpreted as instances of pathology). I introduce most of them in the rest of this chapter. While I focus on the earlier and "minor" accounts, my intention is to show the gamut of stories, texts, motifs, concerns, and authors. The accumulated evidence may be conceived of as a source of interesting parallels – or predictable repetition; as a display of the richness of the human powers of invention – or their undeniable limitations. Thus brought together, the many accounts, in their interminable repetition and variation, provide the necessary background for the discussion of classification and definition in chapter 2 and the more detailed examination of some of the stories in parts two, three, and four.

CLASSICAL ANTIQUITY bequeathed us many myths and legends of animal-raised heroes. The Byzantine story of Aegisthus, a baby nursed and protected by a goat after being abandoned in the course of Belisarius's recovery of Italy from the Gothic invasion, has been construed by modern writers as a precursor of the historical wild children. The story was told by Belisarius's secretary, the historian Procopius of Cesarea (d. 562?), in *The Gothic War* (550). Procopius's child was first mentioned in relation to other wild children in 1863 by anthropologist Edward Burnet Tylor (1832–1917), for whom the case "belongs to the category before us" and "is very likely true as matter of fact." In 1925 Eugene McCartney, a member of the Michigan Academy, gave more elaborate reasons why he distinguished Procopius's story from the other classical legends: one "very reassuring piece of evidence" was "the addiction of the infant to goat's milk" (because "real" animal-nursed children were by then known to "retain their wild dietary habits"); a second was that, unlike the protagonists in other myths, Aegisthus "was not destined to become a national hero." McCartney saw "no object in the fabrication of such a story" and viewed Procopius as "a matter-of-fact historian."[14]

In the story of Aegisthus, the turmoil and disruption of war cause the involuntary abandonment of a baby and furnish the occasion for "adoption" by an animal. Left "in its swaddling clothes lying upon the ground" as the inhabitants of Urbisalia fled or were taken captive, the baby began to cry, until "a lone she-goat, seeing it, felt pity and came near, and gave the infant her udder (for she too, as it happened, had recently brought forth young) and guarded it carefully, lest a dog or wild beast should injure it." Upon their return, the people "were utterly unable to comprehend what had happened and considered it very wonderful that the infant was living." The women attempted to nurse the baby but he would not accept human milk, "nor was the goat at all willing to let it go," insisting "upon claiming the babe as her own." The people left baby and goat alone and, when Procopius was staying in that place, they took him near the baby (whom they had called Aegisthus, from the Greek word for "goat") "and purposely hurt it so that it might cry out ... whereupon the goat, which was standing about a stone's throw away from it, hearing the cry, came running and bleating loudly to its side, and took her stand over it, so that no one might be able to hurt it again." Procopius stated that the goat cared for Aegisthus "for a very long time," yet he did not say exactly how much time passed between the mother's flight and the people's discovery of the baby's miraculous survival, or how much later Procopius himself saw Aegisthus. It cannot have been too long, since the child seems to have remained very young throughout the ordeal. Did he suffer any lasting or permanent consequences? At least for a while, he refused human milk, but Procopius did not register any other characteristic that might have separated baby Aegisthus from other children. Procopius tells the story as a wonder, placing the emphasis not on the effects of the experience on the child but on the marvellous phenomenon of an animal protecting and nursing a human baby.[15]

The earliest modern accounts of wild children present several obstacles to interpretation. In most cases the original account is a brief passage in an obscure work for some reason taken up, cited, or transcribed by a famous author (La Mettrie, Rousseau, Linnaeus, and so on) and from then on repeatedly quoted or paraphrased and commented on by writers who rarely, if ever, check the primary source or know much about its context. Moreover, the first accounts we have of some pre-eighteenth-century wild children may be one or more times removed from whatever may have been the original, unidentified source. Changing borders and place names have created misunderstandings with regard to the locations where some of the children were allegedly found. There is a further problem. The authors of the early accounts claimed (and believed) that their reports were reliable because they were based on what at the time were deemed to be rigorous observational methods. But as time went by, as the texts became increasingly remote, and as standards of scientific observation and authenticity became stricter, these early accounts were read by philosophers and scientists as unreliable descriptions, no more valuable than the legend of Romulus and Remus. Because the value of the evidence and the criteria for authenticity have changed since the time when the original accounts were produced, any attempt to decide on the reality of the early stories is doomed to failure from the start.

The first surviving account of the earliest wild child found in northern Europe, the boy of Hesse, is the one with which I opened this book: a dated entry in the additions, by an unknown monk of Erfurt, to Lambert of Hersfeld's medieval chronicle, printed in the late sixteenth century by Hessian historian and theologian Johann Pistorius (1546–1608).[16] Another, less detailed and slightly different version was inserted by geographer, historian, and architect Wilhelm Dilich (1571 or 1572–1655) in his chronicle of Hesse: "In the year 1341 a savage of about seven, or as others write, about twelve years of age, was found among wolves, captured by hunters and brought to the Landgrave. It ran sometimes on all fours and was able to jump wondrously. When they tried to tame it in the castle, it would dash away from men and hide itself under benches, and after a short time it died because it could not stand human food."[17] According to Dilich, the boy was found in 1341 (not 1344 as in the account printed by Pistorius) and died soon after being captured. Dilich did not identify his sources but hinted that there were more than one ("or as others write"). The unknown monk's account contains some of the central elements that crop up again in later stories of wild children: a boy, said to have been captured by animals (in this case, wolves) in early childhood, is found many years later; life with wolves leaves visible and persistent marks on the child (unusual locomotion and food habits, lack of speech, etc.); after being forcibly returned to human society, the boy manifests a strong desire to escape; he is presented to the country's ruling authority, becomes an object of curiosity and concern, and the target of attempts to "tame" or "humanize" him. What is less usual is that the boy of Hesse remembered, and was able to communicate, at least something about his time with the wolves.

The unknown monk and Dilich presumably included the story in their chronicles as a remarkable phenomenon, but they did not comment on its implications. In contrast, Nuremberg lawyer Philipp Camerarius (1537–1624) and Angevin lawyer and demonologist Pierre Le Loyer (1550–1634) cited it with a further purpose. The story made Camerarius wonder "at such conversing betwixt creatures so differing," which "custome" made "so agreeable and pleasing, that this boy had rather be a companion to wolves than to men whom humanitie and instinct of nature should assemble in troupes and companies." From this wonder he could thus derive a conclusion: the boy's fate verified the common saying, "*That Custome is a second Nature, and sometimes goeth beyond it.*" Le Loyer summoned the "wolf boy" as evidence to support his argument that in their ecstasies sorcerers were not really transmuted into animals. If natural causes alone made the boy behave like, and prefer the company of, wolves, "the Devil occupying the spirit of men" could easily persuade them that they were wolves or other wild beasts and make them behave accordingly. Although Camerarius noted that he found the story in the additions to Lambert's history and reproduced it almost verbatim, he (or his printer) changed the date from 1344 to 1544. Many future students of wild children would repeat the mistake and solidify the confusion in their lists and discussions.[18]

The unknown monk, and after him Camerarius, claimed that *another* boy was captured by nobles hunting wolves in the Wetterau in the same year (that is, in 1344 or 1544). The monk said that the boy lived with wolves for twelve years, and Camerarius (once more changing the meaning) that the boy was twelve years old. Camerarius mentioned a third case, "a certain peisant of Germanie, nourished and brought up (as himselfe avouched) in the mountaines thereby among beasts." Since Camerarius himself saw this boy at the court of the prince of Bamberg, heard his story and observed his strange behaviour, John Webster (1610–1682) saw in him (and in the boy of

Hesse) reliable empirical evidence proving that a human being could look and behave like an animal due to natural causes rather than "supposed witchcraft" (or the devil's persuasion, as Le Loyer had maintained). Linnaeus included the Bamberg youth as an example of his class *Homo ferus*, but some later authors, such as Johann Schreber in the eighteenth century, August Rauber in the nineteenth, and Zingg in the twentieth, did not accept this case as an instance of "real wildness."[19] But there is more: to undo Sir Thomas Browne's refutation of the legend of Romulus and Remus, Alexander Ross (1590 or 1591–1654) referred to several children nursed by wolves in recent times. To the boy of Hesse and Camerarius's boys he added the "strange story" recounted by Louis Guyon, sieur de La Nauche, "of a childe that was carried away in the Forest of *Ardenne* by Wolves, and nourished by them." After a few years, the child was "at last apprehended, but could neither speak nor walk upright, nor eat any thing except raw flesh, till by a new education among other children, his bestial nature was quite abolished."[20] The writings on the boys of Hesse, Wetterau, Bamberg, and Ardenne constitute the first identifiable cluster of texts on wild children. No matter how isolated they may have been in reality, in discourse wild children do not appear alone but in the company of others of the same kind. From the very beginning, the stories called for, or recalled, other stories; one account led to more accounts. But no single reason seems to have caused this, the first upsurge of interest in wild children.

The story of Jean of Liège appeared in the natural philosopher Sir Kenelm Digby's *Two Treatises* (1644). It begins like Procopius's account – there was a war going on and people escaped to the woods. The boy was not accidentally left behind like Aegisthus but stayed hidden in the forest because "being of a very timorous nature" he was afraid: "he ranne further into the wood then any of the rest; and afterwardes apprehended that euery body he saw through the thickets, and euery voyce he heard was the souldiers: and so hidd himselfe from his parents, that were in much distresse seeking him all about, and calling his name as loud as they could." He lived in isolation, ate "rootes, and wild fruites, and maste," and acquired strange habits, losing some skills (language) and gaining others (an acute sense of smell: "He said that after he had beene some time in this wild habitation, he could by the smell iudge of the tast of any thing that was to be eaten: and that he could att a great distance wind by his nose, where wholesome fruites or rootes did grow"). No animals are mentioned, but wild Jean is described as "a man so neere like a beast." When he was found again, "naked and all ouer growne with haire," people first mistook him for "a satyre, or some such prodigious creature as the recounters of rare accidents tell vs of"; when he was recognized, he was treated with kindness: "a woman that had compassion of him ... tooke particular care of him; and was alwayes very sollicitous to see him furnished with what he wanted." Back in human society, Jean underwent another transformation. He became dependent on his caregiver, learned to speak again but lost his notable sense of smell, and remained in good health.[21]

The story of Jean of Liège was part of Digby's discussion of the senses. The sense of smell is more perfect in animals than in human beings because the former use it to ascertain "what meates are good for them, and what are not." Men's smell would doubtlessly be as acute if they had no other means of knowing the quality of their food, as Jean's story demonstrates. The story is inserted as an example to support the argument, but once Digby starts telling it, he does not, or cannot, stop. In fact, the remarkable beautiful story breaks the argument, interrupts the discussion, and claims the reader's full attention. Digby did not himself witness the encounter with the wild boy but heard the story from people he trusted who "haue had it from his owne mouth; and haue questioned him with great curiosity, particularly about it." No ages or dates are given, but at the time of writing Digby believed Jean was alive and could "tell a better story of himselfe then I haue done." Enough mystery remains – what happened to the boy's parents? How did he survive in the woods? How old was he? – to keep interest in the story going, yet the story is also probable enough that it cannot be refuted once and for all. Years after Digby's death, Hermann Boerhaave (1668–1738), the renowned Dutch physician, chemist, and professor at the University of Leyden, used to mention Jean in his lectures. On Boerhaave's authority, French natural historian Julien-Joseph Virey (1775–1846) said that Jean was lost when he was five years old and found again sixteen years later; like Digby, Virey stressed his sharp sense of smell: "He distinguished from far away, by smelling, the woman who guarded him from all other women, as a dog discerns his master in the midst of a multitude of men."[22]

Nicolaas Tulp (1593–1674), famously portrayed in Rembrandt's *The Anatomy Lesson* (1632) dissecting the corpse of an executed criminal, included in his *Observationes medicae* (1672) the case of a boy "brought up from his cradle amongst the wild sheep in Ireland." Tulp saw the boy in Amsterdam and gave a first-hand description of him based on his observations. Because the boy, then sixteen years old, bleated and "had acquired a sort of

ovine nature," Tulp called him *Juvenis balans*. He attended to the boy's anatomical and physiological peculiarities, strange appearance and habits, and
good health: "His appearance was more that of a wild beast than a man; and
though kept in restraint, and compelled to live among men, most unwill-
ingly, and only after a long time did he put off his wild character." Before
he "fell into the power of the huntsman" he had lived "on rough mountains and in desert places, himself equally fierce and untamed, delighting in
caves and pathless and inaccessible dens," spending "all his time in the open
air," in winter as in summer. He disliked human food and "chewed grass
only and hay, and that with the same choice as the most particular sheep."[23]
Many points remain obscure: why was the boy "exposed to the eyes of all"
in Amsterdam, when he had been captured in Ireland? How long after the
capture did Tulp see him, and how "tamed" was he by then? Had he learned
to speak? If not, how did Tulp find out so many details about the boy's wild
life? Tulp's report was widely quoted and generally respected, and for Rauber this was "the most important case." But not everyone was convinced,
and Blumenbach argued that "there are many things which make the story
very doubtful, and of but indifferent credit."[24]

The case of the boys found among bears in Lithuania (at the time part of
Poland) is important because it was cited in major Enlightenment works.
The surviving accounts refer to two, perhaps even three boys, discovered
between 1657 and 1694. Gabriel Rzaczynski, a Jesuit, relying on the testimony of an eyewitness (another Jesuit), Wojciech Tylkowski (1629–1695),
and other printed sources, described a boy captured with bears in 1657 and
brought to Warsaw to the court of King John Casimir (according to one of
the sources cited by Rzaczynski, *two* boys were found among the bears, but
one managed to escape). The account contains elements that are by now
familiar: strangeness, animal habits, unusual food preferences, desire to
escape, and taming ("With much care he was taught to go erect, but his
movements were more bearlike than walking"). The new elements are the
many scars on his body ("His face was animal-like and would not have been
ugly had it not been disfigured by many scars, with which his breast was
also covered") and his initial aversion to clothes ("He was forced to dress
by means of blows"). The boy, who appeared to be twelve years old, had
been baptized and named Joseph.[25] The Jesuit polymath Athanasius Kircher
(1602–1680) discussed "wild men" ("*Homines Sylvestres*") in the chapter on
exotic animals in *China illustrata* (1667): "If anyone wishes to think that
they [hairy animals that look like men] are really wild men, he should know

that sometimes boys are left out in the woods and by Divine Providence, they are brought up by wild animals or in some other way. They do not develop properly due to their long solitude, they lead a life like animals, and they become hairy all over their bodies. When they are captured by hunters, they are thought to be wild men. In fact, they are true humans, but they lack human culture and lead a completely wild life. Such a boy, about 8 years old, was found about 1663 A D in Lithuania in the forest among the bears." Wild men (or wild boys) are now a class, and the Lithuanian boy an example of it. The date of discovery is 1663, and the boy is said to have displayed an assortment of strange traits, "the voice and the appearance of the bears," and a taste for raw meat. He was taught "with great effort" to be human again, to speak, and to eat ordinary human food.[26]

A travel account by Antoine de Gramont (1641–1720) points to 1663 as well. Gramont arrived in Warsaw with his brother, the duke of Guiche – banished from Louis X I V's court for his affair with Madame, the Sun King's sister-in-law – on 4 November 1663. The French visitors were effusively welcomed by Queen Maria Ludwika de Gonzaga, John Casimir's wife, and fêted by the local nobility during their two-week stay in the city. Part of the entertainment was the exhibition, in the garden of the palace, of the boy encountered six months earlier by villagers near Vilna among "five or six bear cubs" suckling a "mother bear." The queen, informed of the prodigy by the provincial governor in Vilna, had ordered the boy's immediate transfer to the capital and placed him in a nunnery near the palace to be educated. Six months later he was still unable to articulate a word but uttered a bear growl "to perfection." The child Gramont saw in the garden looked seven or eight years old and stood up with difficulty but moved easily with the animal gait "to which he had become used from birth." Noticing that a captive bear had been brought to the garden as well (to enhance the spectacle), the boy galloped towards it and caressed it "with indescribable tenderness." Then boy and bear devoured a piece of raw beef ("the boy's avidity even surpassed the bear's"). After carefully examining the boy, Gramont concluded that "his habits, his taste, his language and his knowledge" so resembled those of the animal with which he grew up that only his figure and lack of claws betrayed his human nature: "a man raised with an animal education, remains animal for the rest of his life." To his mind, "nothing in nature was more astonishing" than this boy.[27] The news reached the Royal Society of London through a communication from the Dutch scholar Isaac Vossius (1618–1689), attested by "a French gentleman" who had accompanied "the two sons of the marshal De Grammond." The phenomenon elicited the fellows' curiosity ("Sir Robert Moray was desired to make farther inquiry into the fact by a letter to Dr. Davison, living in those parts"),[28] but we do not know precisely what they wanted to find out: whether they sought confirmation of a strange event in nature or expected to learn something more substantial from it.

The accounts of Lithuanian boys most often cited by eighteenth-century authors were those in Louis Moreri's *Le grand dictionnaire historique* (1694) and in two works by Irish-born physician Bernard Connor (1666–1698). Moreri's entry "Ursin (*Joseph*)" was based on a poem by Johann Redwitz. A "monstrous Child" was captured among bears in the forests of Lithuania in 1661 by hunters, "though it defended it self with its Nails and Teeth"; he excited the curiosity of both nobility and ordinary townspeople; he was somewhat humanized and with great effort converted to Christianity ("at the Name of God he learn'd to lift his Hands and Eyes to Heaven"); he was given by the king to a Polish nobleman as a servant, and did not recover completely (he "could never be brought to speak, though there appeared no fault in the shape of his Tongue," nor could he "be brought to leave the natural fierceness that he had learn'd amongst the Beasts"). Two details, which echoed Gramont's report, would reappear in many later stories of wild children. First, the boy's general characterization: "his Senses were so abrutis'd, that it seem'd to have no more of Man than the Body." Second, his special relation to the "adoptive" animals: "It was observed, that he being in the Wood one day when a Bear had killed two Men, that Beast came to him, and instead of doing him any harm, play'd, and lick'd his Face and Body."[29]

After studying medicine in France, Bernard Connor arrived in Poland in 1694 in the company of the two sons of the Polish high chancellor. In Warsaw he was introduced to the court and asked to become King John III Sobieski's personal physician. He spent the last years of his short life in England as a lecturer at Oxford and Cambridge and an active member of the Royal Society and Royal College of Physicians. Connor first mentioned the Lithuanian boys in *Evangelium medici* (1697), a controversial work in which he suggested a natural explanation for some of the biblical miracles. But his full discussion of the cases is in *The History of Poland*, published in 1698 just before his death. The account has several layers: first Connor recounted the story of a boy captured among bears whom he saw during his own stay in Poland; then he remarked that there had been other instances of the same phenomenon, and as proof he reproduced a letter from Jan Pieter van den

Brand de Cleverskerk, Dutch ambassador to King William III, and cited a work by the Prussian historian Christoph Hartknoch (1644–1687).[30]

Cleverskerk's letter was written in January 1698 in response to Connor's inquiries regarding the boy Cleverskerk had visited in a nunnery in Warsaw in 1669.[31] Cleverskerk warned Connor that thirty years later his memory of the event was not entirely to be trusted: "having not with me the Book wherein I wrot my Observations in my Travels, I cannot possibly give you an exact Account of it." In Warsaw to attend the election of John Casimir's successor, Cleverskerk was directed to the nunnery upon inquiring "what was worth seeing in or about this Place." He found the boy, who looked twelve or thirteen years old, "playing under the Pent-house before the Nunnery Gate":

As soon as I came near him he leap'd towards me as if surpriz'd and pleas'd with my Habit. First, he caught one of my Silver Buttons in his hand with a great deal of eagerness, which he held up to his Nose to smell; Afterwards he leap'd all of a sudden into a Corner, where he made a strange sort of Noise not unlike to Howling. I went into the House, where a Maidservant inform'd me more particularly of the Manner of his being taken ... This Maid call'd the Boy in, and show'd him a good large piece of Bread; which when he saw, he immediately leap'd upon a Bench that was joyn'd to the Wall of the Room, where he walk'd about upon all-four: After which, he rais'd himself upright with a great Spring, and took the Bread in his two Hands, put it up to his Nose, and afterwards leap'd off from the Bench upon the Ground, making the same odd sort of Noise as before.

He could not speak, but "they hop'd in a short time he would, having his Hearing good." The scars on his face were thought to be "Scratches of the Bears." Once again, wild children are related to war – in the turmoil following the frequent Tartar attacks, children were sometimes left behind and lost: "This Boy might have been left behind after the like manner, and found and born away by the Bears; Of which there are a great Number both in *Lithuania* and *Poland*." In Hartknoch's work Connor found information on Joseph's later life: John Casimir had given him as a gift to Peter Adam Opalinski, vice-chamberlain of Posnan, "by whom he was employ'd in the Offices of his Kitchin, as to carry Wood, Water, &c." Joseph retained "his native Wildness" until his death and often went into the woods to be among the bears.[32]

Did Tylkowski, Gramont, Cleverskerk, and Hartknoch meet the same boy? How many children were found with bears in Lithuania between 1657 and 1669? There is no doubt that the boy kept in a convent in 1694, during Connor's visit, who looked about ten years old, was not Joseph. Still, Connor's description rings familiar: he had "a hideous Countenance, ... went upon all four, and had nothing in him like a Man, except his Human Structure"; he was "restless and uneasy, and often inclin'd to flight," yet was baptized and eventually "taught to stand upright, by clapping up his body against a Wall, and holding him after the manner that Dogs are taught to beg," and having become "indifferently tame" he "began to express his Mind with a hoarse and unhuman Tone." Unlike some of his predecessors, when this boy recovered speech he did not remember anything of his former life: "he could not give much better account of it, than we can do of our Actions in the Cradle." Connor insisted that these cases were not rare in Lithuania and speculated on how they came to happen. Like Cleverskerk, he gathered information on bears' habits and the likelihood of their adopting human babies. From the king and local nobles he learned that "if a hungry He-Bear finds a Child that has been carelesly left any where, he will immediately tear it to pieces," but "had it been a She-Bear then giving Suck, she would undoubtedly have carried it safe to her Den, and nourish'd it among her Cubs." From his experience and inquiries Connor inferred that the legend of Romulus and Remus "is not so fabulous as it is generally conjectured to be."[33]

The accounts of Lithuanian boys, then, make up the second cluster of texts on wild children. In them we find many elements already present in earlier cases (the children's strangeness, the people's curiosity, the involvement of authorities, the efforts to rehabilitate the children), as well as some attempts to check the stories, to ascertain their authenticity or ground belief in them, and to offer tentative explanations for the phenomenon – or, indeed, for that part of the phenomenon that could never be *directly observed*: the child's wild life.

Two other stories of wild children from the seventeenth century depart in important ways from the standard that has been gradually established so far. A short anecdote about a girl kidnapped by a bear in the mountains of Savoy, given by Nicholas Cox (1650?–1731) in *The Gentleman's Recreation* (1677), was first related to the stories of wild children in 1927, in a letter to the editor of *The Times*, and then taken up by J.H. Hutton, who in 1940 added it to his list of cases. No other writer on wild children mentions this

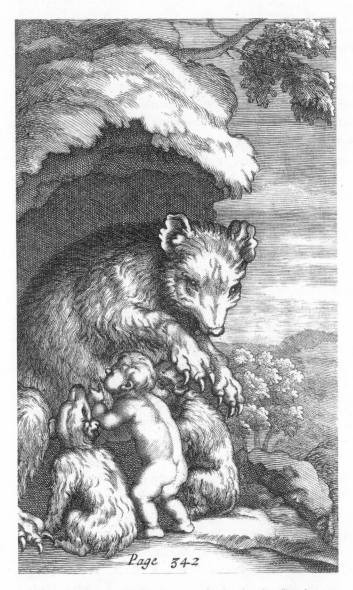

Page 342

From Bernard Connor, *The History of Poland*, vol. 1: "Had it
been a She-Bear then giving Suck, she would undoubtedly
have carried it safe to her Den, and nourish'd it among her
Cubs." Courtesy of the William Ready Division of Archives
and Research Collections, McMaster University Libraries.

story. This is the first wild *girl*, and in this case the sex reversal is meaning-ful: the animal is not a female mother-substitute but a male rapist who fed the child only to keep her in "bestial Captivity." As Cox tells it: "There is a strange report in History, (if it be true) That in the Mountains of *Savoy*, a *Bear* carried a young Maid into his Den by violence, where in a venereal manner he had the carnal use of her Body; and while he kept her in his Den, he daily went forth and brought her the best Fruits he could get, presenting them to her as Food, as courtly as he could do it; but always when he went to Forrage, he rowled a very great Stone to the mouth of his Den, that the Virgin should not make her escape from him: at length her Parents, with long search, found their Daughter in the *Bear's* Den, who delivered her from that bestial Captivity." Cox told the story of the girl of Savoy within a dis-cussion of bear hunting. Following a paragraph on the sex life of bears, it was but a titillating illustration of the bear's intense lust.[34]

The story of Francisco de la Vega, the amphibious man of Lierganes, in-vestigated and analyzed by the Spanish philosopher Benito Jerónimo Feijoo (1676–1764) in *Teatro crítico universal* (1734), was included by Lord Mon-boddo in *Antient Metaphysics* (Monboddo found it in Don Melchor Rafael de Macanaz's "Notas" to Feijoo's work). Francisco, an apprentice joiner, disappeared in Bilbao in 1674, at the age of fifteen, when he went swim-ming with other boys. He was "caught like a fish in the sea near Cadiz" five years later, seemingly "incapable of reasoning by himself; but capable of understanding what he was commanded to do," and having lost "the habit of speech" ("*Liexganes, pan, vino, tobacco*, were all the words that he spoke, and these not to the purpose"). He was returned to Lierganes, his native village, and recognized by his family, but after living with them for nine years he disappeared again "and was never seen, that we know, any more."[35] Although the story of Francisco de la Vega is replete with names and dates, what happened to him, why he "turned wild" and lost the use of speech, is a mystery. Like most of Monboddo's stories of wild children, this one was overlooked by later list makers.

The eighteenth century had its own crop of stories of wild children. For some there is still a single (and short) source, but for others we have entire dossiers (a number of texts written by different people on the same child). Here is an overview of what stands out about each of them. The story of the girl of Cranenburg, also known as the girl of Zwolle or Over-Yssel (now Netherlands), was told in two articles in the *Breslauer Sammlungen* (Jan-uary 1718 and October 1722). She was chased and captured in August 1717 by peasants, who "had known of her for some time," on a mountain near Cranenburg and subsequently identified as the child kidnapped on 5 May 1700 at sixteen months of age. The girl's origin is thus known (she was kidnapped rather than abandoned or taken by animals) but not when her wild life began. It was thought that her kidnappers "might have died before she had grown up and reached the age of reason." After many years of solitary life subsisting "on herbs and tree leaves" (no animals are mentioned) the girl "could rightly be considered a wild girl," was "monstrous in looks," and exhibited many signs of "savagery." When she was captured she had "thick hair ... like a bundle of straw"; her "hard, brown skin" later fell off "and she grew a new one." The 1722 report movingly depicted the girl's reunion with her mother and her striking transformation from monstrous to feminine (but still silent): "It is very interesting to notice that the wild girl is very kind and good-natured and likes to laugh. Since her arrival in Antwerp she has changed so greatly, that, when placed in the company of several women, it is not possible to see any difference except that she does not talk." The author of the report hoped she would learn to speak "so that the whole story of her strange adventure might be known." This wild girl's fate and condition were much more similar to those of the wild boys than the girl of Savoy's; however, gender-coded details set it apart: not only did she learn some feminine accomplishments (spinning) and evince "no desire anymore to live in the wilderness" but even when first found she was "almost naked, having on only a little apron made from a little straw."[36] (Virey found this sign of modesty in a nubile wild girl "remarkable.")[37] Though included in most lists of wild children, this case has been passed over by scientists and philosophers.

The case of the Pyrenees savages is elusive. They were mentioned in passing by Jean-Jacques Rousseau (1712–1778) in the *Discours sur l'origine et les fondemens de l'inégalité parmi les hommes* (1755): "In 1719, two other savages, who were found in the Pyrenees, ran about the mountains in the manner of quadrupeds."[38] Rousseau furnished no source or further details, but the case was taken up as authentic by Linnaeus and others. Two more stories of Pyrenees savages (a girl and a man) were introduced by J.-J.-S. Leroy (1747–1825), a French engineer employed to cut wood for the French navy, in the technical work reporting on his activities. Some later writers believed that Rousseau and Leroy referred to the same savages. Thus for Virey the two wild boys who "run about the mountains on all fours, like quadrupeds" were the ones "met by the men in charge of marking the woods destined for naval constructions." In contrast, Monboddo discussed the two mute savages found in the Pyrenean mountains in 1719 and Leroy's "solitary Savage," discovered in the same mountains several decades later, as separate cases.[39]

The story of Leroy's girl was poignant for it left no doubt about the disastrous consequences of an isolated existence. An ordinary girl lost in known circumstances was found, after a long period of isolation, wild, speechless, and forever inconsolable:

The forest of Issaux was so extensive & so dense before its exploitation, that more than thirty years ago a wild girl, aged about sixteen or seventeen, was caught there; she had lived in this forest for seven or eight years; she had been left behind by a group of other girls who were surprised by snow, & obliged to spend the night there; the following day they looked for their friend, but could not find her, & abandoned her. This girl, after she was captured by Shepherds, did not remember anything, having lost the use of speech, & did not want to eat anything but herbs; she was taken to the Hospice of the town of Moleon, where she lived a long time consumed by grief, always regretting her lost freedom, never speaking, & remaining almost motionless all day long, her head on her two hands; she was of regular size & there was something hard in her physiognomy.

In contrast, Leroy's wild man was cheerful and harmless. Discovered by shepherds in the forest of Yraty in the mid-1770s, he seemed to be about thirty years old, lived in the rocks near the forest, was tall, brisk, and "hairy like a bear." He approached the men's cabins but did not take anything and amused himself running after the sheep. Even though he had "a mild character" and "did no harm," the shepherds often sent their dogs after him and tried to capture him when he came to the door of a hut. He always managed to escape, fleeing "with the swiftness of an arrow shot from a bow" and laughing heartily. The common view was that "this solitary, but chearful creature, had been lost in his infancy, and had subsisted on herbs."[40] Monboddo cited yet another story from Macanaz's "Notas" about a wild man caught around 1723 by an inhabitant of Navarrens, a town of Bearnés in the South of France, who was hunting in the Pyrenean mountains. Was this wild man one of Rousseau's Pyrenean savages? Are the stories related or derived from some common source, however distorted? Monboddo did not make the connection, and no other writer mentions this account.[41]

Although the discovery of Peter of Hanover (in 1724) and the wild girl of Songi (or Champagne, in 1731) generated an explosion of writings, other wild children continued to inspire a single report. The girl of Fraumark (or Frauenmark), also known as the bear-girl of Karpfen, was found in 1767 in the course of a bear hunt, in a cave in a remote mountainous region in lower Hungary. Joseph Aigan Sigaud-Lafond (1730–1810), who related the story in *Dictionnaire des merveilles de la nature* (1781), did not explicitly associate her with any animal: "It is not known how she was left in those inaccessible forests, and how she was able to protect herself from the animals living in them." She was about eighteen years old, "naked, large and robust, with brown skin." At the hospice in Calpen (or Karpfen) where she was placed, she refused cooked foods but "ravenously ate raw meat, the bark of trees and different roots." We do not know what happened to her later or whether she changed at all.[42]

The long account of a wild boy found in the early 1780s in the Siebenbürgen-Wallachia border (now Romania) and brought to Kronstadt, written by an unidentified person who saw the boy on several occasions but was not his caretaker, is detailed and lively. It is also very different in style and content from all the earlier accounts. It lacks a narrative of discovery or capture, but the author imagines what the boy's origin must have been: "How the poor boy was saved from the forests, whether he left his parents in his childhood, or had been born of an unfortunate mother in these same woods, about these things I cannot tell. However one must preserve the facts, as they are, in the sad gallery of pictures of this kind." The account was thus written in relation to, and in awareness of, other equivalent cases. The carefully itemized physical and psychological description of the boy anticipates the reports on Victor of Aveyron, betraying a new way of observing behaviour. The boy's "wildness" now comprises not just a strong desire to escape but a deep longing for mountains and trees ("to control this wild urge, as soon as he came near to the gates of the city, and approached the gardens and woods, they used to tie him up"); not just strange appearance and habits but apathy, indifference, inattention, and noticeable absence of reason: "On the first glance at his face, from which a wildness and a sort of animal-being shone forth, one felt that it belonged to no rational creature, which presents new evidence for the observation that the special stamp which reason imprints on the human form is more or less missed by those who are not able to use reason in a higher or lower degree. This is also in evidence in insane asylums ... Aside from the original human body which usually causes a pitiful impression in this state of wildness, and aside from walking erect, one missed in him all the characteristic traits through which human beings are distinguished from the animals." The author registered a transformation in the boy's condition after some years in human society, but nothing like a full recovery. Tamer and softer but still speechless, while at first he had shown "not the slightest emotion at the sight of women" he now manifested sexual interest, and when in the presence of a woman he "broke into violent cries of joy." The wild boy's senses and skills were informally tested. If he was shown a mirror, he "would look behind it for the image before him"; if the author played the piano for him, he listened to the music with apparent pleasure but was afraid to touch the keys himself. Interestingly, this "wild boy," believed to be in his early twenties, was compared to a child: "Chiefly he was in every respect like a child whose capacities had begun to develop, only with this difference: that he was unable to speak and could not make any progress in that regard."[43]

Tomko, a "half-wild man," was described by the person who found him in the baths of Reischenbach, in the Hungarian county of Zipser. "Since this time he has always been at my house," the author indicated, "where he has earned the affections of everyone through his good-natured behaviour. It was very interesting to me to watch step by step the entire course of his education." Long and detailed like the account of the boy of Kronstadt, this one is less clinical and more personal, indeed quite endearing. Before meeting his new guardian, Tomko had lived in the forests in summer and in winter came to the villages "where, mostly, a stall, a shed, or sometimes the hut of a compassionate peasant served him for quarters." Tomko's strangeness and difference were acknowledged ("His condition was not so much one of stupidity or insanity, as one of wildness caused by neglect") but he was accepted within his community and given care and affection. The author stressed the wild man's growing communicative ability, his intellectual idiosyncrasies, loyalty, good heart, and love of freedom:

First he began to understand gestures of others, and then speech; and finally he learned to speak Slovak. But much more he formed a speech of his own, which he has retained until now. Thus he would call burning the rustle of the wind. Anyone who wore a wig, he called a soldier; and snow, he called Simon and Judas, since it usually starts to snow about on the day of these saints. He could never learn to count; and he never had any idea at all of a number, although he does know when one of the calves he herded gets away ... His chores are to bring letters and papers from the post office, to carry wood, and to herd the cows. He is very zealous and punctual in these little tasks and shows great loyalty and constancy to his benefactors. He calls me his consolation ... He loves his freedom extraordinarily well; and chains are for him the most feared punishment.

Like most wild children, Tomko was sexually confused: after a girl "tried to seduce him" while he was herding sheep, he told the story "with much disgust and repugnance." But in general he was a happy fellow, whom his guardian saw as an exemplar of Rousseau's "natural man."[44] The reports do not say what happened in the end to the boy of Kronstadt or to Tomko.

The remaining eighteenth-century accounts of wild children are stories Monboddo heard from various people or found in newspapers and then retold in *Antient Metaphysics*. From the Reverend Mr Maddison, a professor of mathematics at the University of Williamsburg, he learned about two young savages found in a swamp in Virginia who did not speak but used signs and strange gaggling sounds to communicate with one another, and who at first ran away from people but then "were become domestic" and learned some English. The common belief was that their parents had died after fleeing to the swamp to escape creditors, so that from a very young age the savages "made a shift to live upon wild roots and fish." From a French gentleman, then a prisoner in Scotland, Monboddo heard about another dumb savage, believed to be "a native of the Maldiva Islands," found four or five years earlier on the small desert island of Diego Garcia in the Eastern Ocean. When found he ran away from men and had lost the use of speech. Finally, Monboddo reproduced a report from a Devonshire newspaper about a boy and a girl, ten and twelve years old, who "have been suffered, by their mother, to run wild from their infancy rather than accept of the parish assistance." Both children were "in a state of nature, feeding only on wild berries, and running on *all fours* with amazing celerity." They did not speak but kept "a distant and fearful communication" with their mother; if pursued, they uttered "a terrific scream." Monboddo ordered an inquiry to be made into the case.[45]

The nineteenth century opened with the capture of the boy who would become Victor of Aveyron. Only Kaspar Hauser, who arrived in Nuremberg in 1828, rivals him in popularity. The rest of the nineteenth-century wild children pale in comparison to Victor and Kaspar but deserve to be remembered here nonetheless. In 1863 Tylor mentioned two wild boys, taken in at Count Adelbert von der Recke's asylum at Overdyke after Napoleon's German wars, whose initial condition showed "in what a state of degradation human beings might be found living in civilized Europe, not half a century ago." The boy named Clemens, forced to spend his early life with pigs, had adopted some of their behaviour patterns and never lost his affection for them: "His pleasantest recollections and his favourite stories were about his life with them in his childhood." Tylor's portrayal is ambivalent: Clemens was "not actually an idiot" but "probably of imperfect powers of mind from his birth"; he could speak but at first most of what he said was unintelligible; he was "of a joyous disposition" but sometimes "subject to uncontrollable fits of passion" (once he tried to murder his benefactor). The second boy, the orphan Wilhelm Ritter, had lived alone in the forest and there "learnt to live almost wild ... only approaching villages for the purpose of stealing food." He climbed trees with extraordinary agility and knew all about birds. Whereas Clemens adjusted to the institution, gained "the affections of his companions," became "a favourite with his teachers," and "cheerfully" repaid his benefactors by "employing his strength in the lowest services," Wilhelm refused to stay "where he could not get plenty of eggs to eat" and fled back to the woods.[46]

Zingg listed the cases of a strange man met by John Macdonald Kinneir (1782–1830) in June 1814 on entering the harbour of Trebizond (in Turkey), who had supposedly been "found wild in the woods" and was treated with respect because "Turks regard fools as the favourites of heaven," and of a girl noticed by Dr Horn in the infirmary of Salzburg and described by Feuerbach in his book on Kaspar. In her early twenties "and by no means ugly," she had been "brought up in a hog-sty among the hogs," sitting there for many years with her legs crossed: "One of her legs was quite crooked, she grunted like a hog, and her gestures were brutishly unseemly in a human dress." Feuerbach related the girl of Salzburg and Kaspar as victims of horrible crimes: "In comparison with such abominations, the crimes committed against Caspar Hauser may even be considered as acts in which the forbearance of humanity is still visible." But once the link between the two was thus established, Zingg could lift the account of the girl of Salzburg as another example to be added to his collection of "feral" cases, and from then on she was routinely listed among the wild children. In this story, as in that of Clemens of Overdyke, the association with animals did not take place in the wild, nor did it fit the "adoption" model.[47]

From the 1840s, a new type of wild-child story began to circulate: accounts of children found with wolves in India. There are many such cases, forming both a significant cluster (and several subclusters) of texts and a whole subclass of wild children. The main groups of cases are the wolf boys reported by Sleeman in 1852 and the wolf children who lived in the orphanage of Sekandra (or Secundra) in the second half of the nineteenth century. There are also many minor reports of Indian wolf children produced in the late nineteenth century and throughout the twentieth century, and in trying to sort them out we face some of the same difficulties surrounding the earlier European accounts: repetition and imprecision, uncertainty as to whether some reports refer to different or the same children, etc. In the twentieth century, some of the Indian wolf children became very famous, or infamous, among them Amala and Kamala of Midnapore, the boy of Miawana, Ramu of New Delhi, Parasram of Agra, and the boy known as Shamdev, Shamdeo, or Pascal.[48]

Other nineteenth- and twentieth-century accounts tell stories of children nursed or raised by various wild animals usually in "exotic" places, like the young girl "discovered by some coolies belonging to a tea garden in the den of a bear" near Jalpaiguri, India; the "leopard-boy" found in the North Cachar Hills of India and described by E.C. Stuart Baker; the European girl found living with jackals, who was "kept for a time by the Maharani of Cooch about 1923, but [who] 'proved far less responsive than the children brought up by wolves'" and died within a few months of her capture; the "Mowgli Girl" found by hunters near Mount Olympus, Turkey, "where she lived for eight years as the adopted child of a huge she-bear," and then taken to the hospital for mental illness at Bakirkey; Lucas, the South African baboon boy; the boy who lived with ostriches for ten years in the Sahara and tells his own story; the boy who lived with gazelles also in the Sahara; another boy who lived with gazelles, this time in the Syrian desert in the 1940s; John, allegedly found with monkeys in Burundi in the early 1970s; two-year-old Joel Zacarias, a starving slum child of Manila, Philippines, nursed back to life by "a mongrel dog that allowed him to suckle her milk for more than a year"; Robert, found living with a tribe of monkeys in a Ugandan jungle in the mid-1980s and "believed to have been nurtured by wild animals for as long as four to nine years"; Ivan Mishukov, who lived in the streets of Moscow with a pack of stray dogs in the late 1990s, and John Ssabunnya, who spent some time living with monkeys in Uganda in the late 1980s and was hailed, during his visit to the United Kingdom to sing with the Pearl of Africa Choir (directed by his foster father Paul Wasswa), as "the last wild child of the twentieth century."[49] Still other stories are about wild children not presumed to have been raised by or associated with animals, like the "half-human, half-animal creature" discovered on the Pindus in

Greece and brought to the village of Trikkala; Tarzancito, Ruben, or Tama-sha of El Salvador, and Marcos of the Sierra Morena in Spain, seized in 1965 and later studied and interviewed by Gabriel Janer Manila.[50] Also in the twentieth century, children who suffered extreme isolation through con-finement, abuse, or neglect were discussed together with "feral children," like Anna of Pennsylvania and Isabelle of Ohio; Anne and Albert; Yves Cheneau of Saint-Brevin, and Genie of Los Angeles. Their stories appear in press reports and in doctors' or other practitioners' case histories.[51]

Most of the recent stories of wild children uncannily resemble the accounts of Aegisthus, the boy of Hesse, or Jean of Liège. Consider the four cases reported by Paul Sieveking in 1991: Djuma, whose story I quoted in the introduction; Kunu Masela, an abandoned boy who lived for years with a dog, scavenging for food, in the Kenyan town of Machakos ("Poppy my mother," he told a reporter. "Poppy give me milk"); Wang Xianfeng, a peas-ant girl from Liaoning Province, China, who was raised by the family pigs "because her deaf-mute father and mentally retarded mother were unable to care for her and no one else lived near them," then rescued and re-educated by experts from the China Medical Science University and Anshan Institute of Psychometry; and Imiyati, discovered by hunters in a swamp in southern Sumatra in 1983: "At first they thought she was an orang-utang, because she was covered in moss and couldn't talk. It turned out that her name was Imi-yati and she had not been seen since 1977, when she went on a fishing trip with her sister and three other children. Their boat had capsized in a strong current, and the four other children were drowned. Imiyati was presumed dead, but somehow she survived and was only 12 miles from her home when she was found."[52] The latest wild children invariably come from non-Western, exotic, or developing places, ravaged by war, poverty, famine or natural disaster. They are still strange, but now they all have names.

CHAPTER TWO

The List, the
Class, the Story-Form

Perhaps the problem which really deserves attention is an attempt
to ascertain why this tale has been so uniformly attractive to men of
various times and places. We are not greatly surprised when ancient
or aboriginal peoples accept myth motif as historical occurrence.
When men of science accept evidence as tenuous as this, we may
well wonder about the pervasive appeal of the ancient motif.

D.G. Mandelbaum, "Wolf-Child Histories from India"[1]

ALTHOUGH WILD CHILDREN are children who, for one reason or another,
have spent a long time in isolation from other human beings, their accounts
are never isolated but always linked to other stories of the same kind. Since
the early seventeenth century, accounts of strange children encountered in
strange circumstances have been produced and positioned *as* stories of wild
children. The children, and the stories, have been related to one another.
This chapter examines the emergence of the wild child as a class. Following a discussion of historical attempts to compile a list of cases and of the
different ways in which the "wild child" is understood and defined in the
literature, I suggest that the prototype of the wild child must be sought not
in what the wild children themselves are or are deemed to be but in their
stories – both what happens to them and how what happens to them is given
narrative form. The attempts at classification are themselves part of the stories of wild children.

We owe the concept and classification of what would eventually become
"wild children" to that epoch-making taxonomist, Carolus Linnaeus (or
Carl von Linné, 1707–1778). In the tenth edition of his *Systema naturae*
(1758), Linnaeus introduced "*Homo ferus*" (wild man) as the first variety of
the species *Homo sapiens* within the genus *Homo* and the order *Primates*.
This is the full classification:

[*Homo Sapiens*] *Ferus.* tetrapus, mutus, hirsutus.

    Juvenis Ursinus lithuanus. 1661.

    Juvenis Lupinus hessensis. 1344.

    Juvenis Ovinus hibernus. Tulp. obs. IV: 9.

    Juvenis Hannoveranus.

    Pueri 2 Pyrenaici. 1719.

    Johannes Leodicensis.

Homo ferus differed from other classes in this, earlier, and future editions of the *Systema naturae* in that, besides the three specific differences that characterize the class (*tetrapus, mutus,* and *hirsutus,* i.e., quadruped, mute, and hairy), Linnaeus furnished not a more general description of features deemed to be common to all its members but a list of individual examples. The 1758 edition of the *Systema naturae* listed six examples, and the twelfth edition (1766) added three more: *Juvenis bovinus Bambergensis, Puella transisalana* 1717, and *Puella Campanica* 1731.[2]

We should have no difficulty identifying Linnaeus's examples. The first list of *homines feri* consisted of the bear boy of Lithuania, 1661; the wolf boy of Hesse, 1344; the sheep boy of Ireland, mentioned by Tulp; the boy of Hanover; the two boys of the Pyrenees, 1719; and Jean of Liège. The cases added in the twelfth edition were the cattle boy of Bamberg; the girl of Cranenburg, 1717; and the girl of Champagne (or Songi), 1731. Most of these cases were in all likelihood known to Linnaeus's readers, because they had already appeared in major works and discussions in the earlier half of the eighteenth century; but Linnaeus for the first time brought them all together, arranged the examples in a list, and gave them both a common label and individual "scientific" names. In the 1758 edition of the *Systema naturae* Linnaeus proposed a new classification of man. He divided the genus *Homo* into two species or major subgroups, *Homo sapiens* and *Homo troglodytes* (a confused admixture of apes and albinos), and subdivided the species *sapiens* into six varieties, *ferus, Americanus, Europaeus, Asiaticus, Afer,* and *monstrosus.* In this revised classification, Linnaeus created "*Homo ferus*" as a separate class to hold these rare individual cases and, even more strikingly, granted it the rank of a variety of the human species, seemingly on the same level of importance as "European" or "African."[3] The individual examples were identified or named following a pattern. Each name (e.g., "*Juvenis Ursinus lithuanus.* 1661") comprises identification as "child" or "youth" (*puer, puella,* or *juvenis*), an animal, a place, and a date. In light of

1. HOMO noſce Te ipſum. **(*)**

Sapiens.   1. H. diurnus; *varians cultura, loco.*
Ferus.   tetrapus, mutus, hirſutus.
           Juvenis Urſinus lithuanus. 1661.
           Juvenis Lupinus heſſenſis. 1344.
           Juvenis Ovinus hibernus. Tulp. obſ. IV: 9.
           Juvenis Hannoveranus.
           Pueri 2 Pyrenaici. 1719.
           Johannes Leodicenſis.

Homo ferus: Linnaeus's classification and list in *Systema naturae*, 10th ed. (1758).

1. HOMO. Noſce te ipſum. **(*)**

Sapiens.   1. H. diurnus; *varians cultura, loco.*
Ferus.   Tetrapus, mutus, hirſutus.
           Juvenis Urſinus lithuanus. 1661.
           Juvenis Lupinus heſſenſis. 1544.
           Juvenis Ovinus hibernus. Tulp. obſ. IV: 9.
           Juvenis Bovinus bambergenſis. Camerar.
           Juvenis Hannoveranus. 1724.
           Pueri 2 Pyrenaici. 1719.
           Puella Tranſiſalana. 1717.
           Puella Campanica. 1731.
           Johannes Leodicenſis. Boerhaav.

Linnaeus's classification and list in *Systema naturae*, 12th ed. (1766).

later incarnations of the list, these markers may be understood as an abbreviated story. Only one of the examples, *Johannes Leodicensis,* or Jean of Liège, was given a proper name.

Thus in the first comprehensive attempt to classify nature and to include human beings within the system of nature, wild children were granted a place and a class *and* they were distinguished as individuals. From the very beginning, the class was made up of individual examples brought together to form a list. Moreover, the list was something to be added to, as new examples of the class were discovered. But even though each case was individually referred to as "child" or "youth," at this point the classification was "wild *man*." The class *Homo ferus* and the list of cases originated at exactly the same time. And from Linnaeus on, the class and the list had a parallel history. The individual cases have an ambiguous status both as examples of the class and the only known instances of it. The examples of wild children exhaust the class "wild child." For this reason, if we want to understand something about the class we must follow the vicissitudes of the list: how it was put together and gradually expanded; how the particular accounts, turned into cases, were included in or excluded from it; how principles of classification were established to give coherence to the list and solidity to the class; and how the list makers never completely succeeded in transforming the list into a fully recognized class.

The tendency to bring stories of wild children together was already noticeable in early accounts such as those of the unknown monk of Erfurt, Camerarius, Ross, and Connor. Only a few years before the tenth edition of the *Systema naturae*, Rousseau, in a note to the *Discours sur l'origine de l'inégalité*, had listed the "savages" known to him when discussing whether, as some philosophers and naturalists thought, the quadruped form of locomotion was the most natural to man. Rousseau's "examples of quadruped men" were the child found in 1344 near Hesse, who had been raised by wolves; the child found in 1694 in the forests of Lithuania, who lived among bears; the little savage of Hanover; and the two savages found in the Pyrenees in 1719. Rousseau's enumeration was embedded in a philosophical discussion. The examples were classified together according to the principle that they were "quadruped savages," yet in all but one instance the individuals were expressly identified as children. Linnaeus himself returned to the *homines feri* in the dissertation *Anthropomorpha* (1760), this time offering a list of men who "passed their whole lives in woods among the Brutes," of whom "ingenious descriptions" exist:

I. The boy found among the BEARS in the Grand Duchy of *Lithuania*, in 1661.

II. The boy caught among the WOLVES in 1544 in *Hesse*.

III. The boy discovered among the CATTLE in *Bamberg*, and described by Camerarius.

IV. The boy captured by accident amongst the SHEEP in *Ireland*, described by Tulp. I shall pass over the boy found in *Hannover* in 1719, the boys found in the *Pyrenees* in 1719, and the girl of *Champagne*, and all the remaining ones, of whom there is quite a multitude.

The descriptive phrases echo those used by Rousseau. Four of the cases were numbered, a few more were mentioned, and even more ("quite a multitude") merely insinuated.[4]

Linnaeus's list of wild children inspired others in works of philosophy and natural history by Cornelius de Pauw (1739–1799), Delisle de Sales (Jean-Claude Izouard, 1741–1816), and Sigaud-Lafond.[5] Johann Christian Daniel Schreber (1739–1810), who studied in Uppsala with Linnaeus and later taught medicine and directed the botanical gardens and natural history collections at the University of Erlangen, took up Linnaeus's *Homo ferus* in his discussion of man's natural state in *Die Säugthiere in abbildungen nach der Natur mit Beschreibungen* (1775). Schreber's list included ten numbered entries, and its principle of classification was as it were intrinsic: Schreber's cases were those he found in his teacher's work. Despite his doubts about the authenticity of some of the reports (for instance, the story of the boy of Hesse was "evidently a legend of which we do not even know the author"), Schreber had no alternative but to discuss (and assess) the list of cases already brought together and classified by Linnaeus. This is what I mean by the "givenness" of wild children. Schreber's list was novel in a significant way: unlike Linnaeus's, it was not a list of names and labels but of *stories*. Each entry is a brief account relating the salient aspects of each case: gender of the child; circumstances of discovery (place, date, age of the child, people involved); what was known about the child's earlier life; description of the child, stressing unusual traits or habits (food, locomotion, language, dress); later changes or learning, if any (noting taming or treatment); presence or absence of memories of the time spent in the wild; and sources. The narrative elements implicit in the other lists were now fully spelled out, henceforth becoming an essential component of the list and the classification. In putting together his list of stories, however, Schreber selected from all the available data what would be appropriate for each entry. He gave each wild child about the same space (a paragraph) and omitted much of the information contained in the longer accounts. In this way, the accounts were homogenized and the stories made to parallel one another. Schreber brought together not only the cases but also the accounts, by presenting them in such a way that they could be compared and contrasted as ordered series of events and traits.[6]

In 1800 the naturalist Pierre-Joseph Bonnaterre published his detailed first-hand observations of the "savage of Aveyron." To shed light on the boy's condition, Bonnaterre included the list, handed down by "the celebrated Linné," of similar cases of "children isolated from a very young age and found in the wild, far from the society of men." First he listed the cases and then he reported in chronological order "the circumstances known of their stories." After the list came the work's main section: Bonnaterre's extended account of the savage of Aveyron, ending with a comparison between him and the "other savages." Bonnaterre's argument was that the boy of Aveyron must be added to the list because he resembled the other savages in external organization, tastes, and habits. What is noteworthy about this list is that it was motivated by the actual presence of a wild child (the boy was then living with Bonnaterre at the Central School of Rodez). Other than that, it was largely derivative: Bonnaterre reproduced Schreber's list and accounts, with minor changes in numbering and sources, and added the cases of the girl of Karpfen and the boy of Aveyron. Only a few months earlier Julien-Joseph Virey had put forward the example of those "wretched youths" abandoned by their parents in childhood who nevertheless survived in isolation as evidence that human beings have instincts, giving a list of the known cases and noting, in a footnote, that "a young savage has just been found in the department of Aveiron."[7]

Like other naturalists, Johann Friedrich Blumenbach (1752–1840) pondered the class *Homo ferus* and the examples of wild children in response to Linnaeus's work. A professor at the University of Göttingen, and generally considered the "father" of physical anthropology for his studies of the varieties of the human species, Blumenbach approached wild children in two different ways. On the one hand, he estimated their value as examples of the natural condition of man. From this angle he criticized the use many naturalists and philosophers had made of the stories but on the whole accepted the evidence. On the other hand, he rejected Linnaeus's class *Homo ferus* as a variety of man. In his attempt to dissolve the class, and because the class was coextensive with the examples, Blumenbach also rejected the accounts of the individual wild children. From this second perspective he maintained that the cases were not only irrelevant (wild children do not stand for what philosophers think they stand for – natural man) but also mislabelled (the so-called *homines feri* were in fact deformed individuals who would have been better classified under Linnaeus's *Homo monstrosus*) and unreliable (the evidence is inadequate, unsubstantiated, unscientific, etc.). Blumenbach thus produced an *anti-list*: an openly sceptical examination of the accounts of wild children with the purpose of debunking them altogether.

Blumenbach questioned the authenticity of much of the evidence. In the third edition of *De generis humani varietate nativa* (*On the Natural Variety of Mankind*, 1795) he listed the cases but introduced internal distinctions according to the reliability of the sources: "If we look a little more closely into these stories of wild children, it is more likely to turn out in the instances which are the most authentic, and placed beyond all doubt, as that of our famous Peter of Hameln (Peter the wild boy, *Juvenis Hannoveranus* Linn.), of the girl of Champagne, the Pyrenæan wild man, and of others, that these wretches used to walk upright; but in the stories of the others who are commonly said to go on all-fours, as the *Juvenis ovinus Hibernus* Linn., there are many things which make the story very doubtful, and of but indifferent credit." The more recent accounts seem more reliable, but with the passing of time they are disputed as well. Whereas in 1795 Blumenbach conceded that Peter's story was "placed beyond all doubt," less than twenty years later, in "Vom Homo sapiens *ferus* Linn. und namentlich vom Hamelschen *wilden Peter*" ("On the Homo Sapiens *Ferus* Linn.: and particularly of Wild Peter of Hameln," 1811), he asserted that Peter was just like "all the other instances of so-called wild children," whose stories, "almost without exception, are mixed up with so many beyond measure extraordinary and astonishing untruths or contradictions, that their credibility has become in consequence highly problematical altogether." In this work Blumenbach proffered a sustained critique of the evidence on Peter and reviewed Linnaeus's cases. The Irish boy, mentioned by no other author besides Tulp, was obviously "an imbecile, dumb, and also outwardly deformed creature" who "could hardly have grown up from the cradle among wild sheep in Ireland, because they exist no more there than anywhere else." He in turn dispatched the stories of the savage of Bamberg, the boy of Hesse, the Lithuanian boys, the *Puella Transisilana*, the *Puella Campanica*, *Johannes Leodicensis*, and the Pyrenean boys, hoping that his analysis would "give the proper value to those wonderful and various stories about these pretended men of nature in a philosophic natural history of mankind." Oddly enough, Blumenbach did not refer to Victor of Aveyron. The possibility that he might not have heard anything about Victor from 1800 to 1811 does not square with his extensive acquaintance with the literature on wild children.[8]

The early-nineteenth-century lists of wild children betray Blumenbach's influence. Karl Asmund Rudolphi (1771–1832), one of Blumenbach's students, continued the debunking and unmaking of the class, claiming that all the known cases, including the wild boy of Aveyron, were idiots or inventions (only the wild girl of Songi "seemed to have more reason"). M. Bory de Saint-Vincent (1778–1846) criticized the "judicious Linnaeus" for inventing the class "*Homo ferus tetrapus*" to gather "certain individuals of the civilized European species, found in a state of imbecility resulting from their having been abandoned by no doubt poor parents." Like Blumenbach and Rudolphi, Bory declared that nothing of importance could be learned from these "so-called children of Nature"; nevertheless, immediately after dismissing the class Bory proceeded to list the cases. In contrast, Johann Friedrich Immanuel Tafel (1796–1863), professor of philosophy at the University of Tübingen and leading Swedenborgian, affirmed that *Homo ferus* was the natural condition of man. Because Tafel's position was directly opposed to Blumenbach's, to defend it he had to counter the latter's objections to the evidence and propose an alternative explanation of the children's condition. Tafel's argument, based on his reinterpretation of the accounts and on current expertise on idiocy, was that the condition of wild children did not indicate congenital idiocy but resulted from their isolation.[9]

Blumenbach's shadow extended much further. He was the first to articulate fully the three sets of interrelated questions within which *all* subsequent lists, classifications, and definitions of wild children would operate. First, the question of *evidence*: was the evidence good? Must we accept the accounts as fact or dismiss them as fiction, myth, or fraud? Second, the question of *explanation*: if we accept the accounts as fact, how should we explain the children's condition? Were they examples of natural man, anomalies, or monstrosities? Third, the question of *causation*: if wild children were indeed anomalies, was their strangeness (or defect) due to congenital causes or to the very effects of isolation (or an accident)?

The next consequential list of wild children, in Edward Burnet Tylor's "Wild Men and Beast-Children" (1863), was still very much indebted in tone and spirit to Blumenbach's work. The article may have been prompted by the publication of Sleeman's account of Indian wolf boys, which revived the idea of animal-nurtured children. Tylor's purpose was to assess "where the lowest limit of human existence lies," and thus he intended to separate fact from fable in "stories of man living as beast among beasts, or in a state of degradation not far removed from this." He incorporated many new cases, in some instances reproducing the accounts, partially or in full. The organizing principle of his list was not chronology (temporal markers are vague throughout the article) or reference to earlier lists but decreasing verisimilitude: "I have arranged and sifted, to the best of my ability, the stories of this kind which I have met with, beginning with some which are certainly true, and ending with others which are as certainly fabulous." Tylor did not elaborate on what exactly linked these disparate individuals and stories besides the two labels in his title ("wild men" and "beast-children") and the unspecified notions of "degradation" or "brutalization." This is how he summed up the evidence: "In different parts of the world children have been found in a state of brutalization, due to want of education or to congenital idiocy, or to both" and people have accounted for "their beast-like nature" by supposing that they were "caught living among wild beasts." Tylor discarded the accounts in two respects: as evidence that human children had indeed been nurtured by animals (he believed animal nurture was a myth to explain idiocy) and as supposedly valuable instances of man's natural state: "It is impossible to say in the case of any one of them how far their miserable condition was the result of want of civilization and how far of idiocy. Casper Hauser's case is of more value than all of them put together, as he, if the published accounts may be believed, seems at least to have been naturally of full powers of mind." Why did Tylor introduce Kaspar Hauser here? How did Kaspar's story of confinement and victimization fit Tylor's picture of wild men, beast-children, degradation and brutalization? Tylor stressed what he perceived as a crucial difference between Kaspar and wild children, but the very fact that he discursively connected them had unintended consequences. Later list makers would find Kaspar *there* and add him to their lists without hesitation.[10]

Lists of wild children continued to appear towards the end of the century. As its title indicates, *Homo sapiens ferus*, by August Antinous Rauber (1841–1917), was a book-length study of the class first named by Linnaeus. The work opens with a list of cases presented according to the old Schreber model (numbered list, German and Latin names, accounts), but rather than summarizing each child's story, Rauber reproduced the reports. He cited long passages from the primary sources and assessed the availability, adequacy, and reliability of the evidence for each case. Rauber's list did not include the cases added by Sleeman and Tylor, or the story of Kaspar Hauser. It remained one of "savage" (feral) children, who lived alone in the wild or with animals.[11] Dr William W. Ireland's list was appended to his textbook *The Mental Affections of Children, Idiocy, Imbecility and Insanity* (1898). He enumerated the cases and sifted the evidence (he was particularly concerned with the possibility of finding definitive confirmation for the contemporary Indian accounts), concluding "that idiots have occasionally been found straying in the woods, and that people accounted for their wildness and stupidity, their want of speech, and their abnormal sense of taste, by supposing that they had been brought up by or lived in the company of wild beasts." Ireland drew a distinction between children "straying in the woods" and children "brought up by or living in the company of wild beasts." He accepted the former (but as idiots, not savages) and reduced the latter to idiot wild children (without animals) plus myth.[12] Then in his article "On Some Psychical Relations of Society and Solitude" (1900) Maurice H. Small had a subsection on "Caspar Hauser" and another on "Feral Man," with a list of cases whose "present significance becomes greater when we compare them with The Imbecile Type."[13] Despite the proximity or contiguity Small established between Kaspar, "feral men," and "imbeciles" – his organizing criterion was isolation (or solitude) – he did not make them all part of the same class.

After several decades of silence, the list makers set to work again in connection with the huge rise of interest in wild children provoked by the reports of the girls of Midnapore. J.H. Hutton's presidential address to the Folk-Lore Society (21 February 1940) was the first list of *wolf children* (children reared by wolves or other animals) excluding any other type of wild child. The main issue was to ascertain whether the stories were credible, whether animal nurture had ever happened and whether it was at all possible, and, if not, what the origin of the stories was. After carefully weighing the reasons for and against the reports' authenticity, Hutton was unable to reach a definitive conclusion, especially since "the capture of a child from the company of carnivorous animals believed to have suckled it has seldom if ever been witnessed by a European, at any rate since the seventeenth century." However, he declared that "if a single case can be taken as satisfactorily proved many others become credible."[14] In contrast to Hutton's list, which was both restrictive (regarding the type of cases included) and cautious (regarding the value of the evidence), the two lists of wild children published by Robert Zingg shortly after were inclusive and overtly favourable. Zingg was just then editing J.A.L. Singh's diary of the Midnapore girls and firmly believed it purveyed the conclusive proof Hutton was looking for. Zingg was the most consistent collector of cases, evidence, and accounts, and his lists, the most comprehensive so far, brought together for the first time *all* the cases of wild and animal-reared children as well as the cases of "extreme isolation" (e.g., Kaspar). Still, in his pursuit of academic recognition for "feral man" Zingg was careful to exclude any case that was not sufficiently "authenticated" (e.g., the Miawana boy and Lucas of South Africa) and to downplay the mythical and fictional references. In its first version, which appeared in the article "Feral Man and Extreme Cases of Isolation"

(1940), Zingg's list consisted of thirty-one cases (plus the boy of Bamberg, not given a separate number). Zingg had a chance to correct and add to the list in his contribution to *Wolf-Children and Feral Man* (1942).[15]

Zingg's comprehensive list and unabated enthusiasm inevitably called forth some anti-lists, in which the cases were enumerated and the evidence reviewed only to conclude in the end that they were invalid or inauthentic. Wayne Dennis's "The Significance of Feral Man" (1941), a response to Zingg's article, was another attempt to evaluate the accounts and the conclusions that might be rightfully drawn from them. "Unless this is done now," Dennis warned, "these stories will be accepted without scepticism, and soon will take a place in our textbooks as 'established facts.'" For Dennis, the evidence, resting mostly on hearsay, was weak: "The burden of proof rests upon those who want to draw some conclusion from these accounts." David G. Mandelbaum's "Wolf-Child Histories from India" (1943), written in response to the publication of Gesell's book on Kamala, listed sixteen cases of "wolf children" and three "recent cases of adoption by a bear, leopard, and a jackal," leaving out a number of cases where "there is little more than the bare report." The style of presentation resembled Schreber's: the summary of each story was written in such a way that the accounts were homogenized and the cases could be more easily compared. Mandelbaum complained of the quality of the evidence ("Most accounts are bedecked with so much philosophical speculation and irrelevant comment that it is difficult to winnow out the descriptive essence, factual or pseudo-factual, of each report") and noted that "the actual capture or rescue of the children, like the famed Indian rope trick, is always seen by someone who is not the one who is writing or telling about it."[16]

In 1951 Dennis returned to the subject of wild children because what he had earlier feared had happened: the stories were being cited in textbooks as "established facts" from which conclusions could be drawn about the effects of early experience on children's development. While in his first article Dennis had challenged the belief that wild children were originally normal and were reared by animals, now his strategy was different: "I am accepting the data on wild children at their face value, for a while, to see what conclusions follow from the data." The "data" were yet another list of cases, selected from the second version of Zingg's but limited to those cases "in which some statement is made concerning the probable age of the child during his animal association." This list was thus arrived at by applying a more selective principle of organization, itself subordinated to the author's interpretive goal, to a previous list. Dennis abstracted the information he considered relevant from Zingg's list, kept Zingg's numbering, and added comments, as in the following example:

Case 11 – A Wolf-Boy of India
estimated age at isolation: 3 years
estimated age at discovery: 9 years
behavior at isolation: was led by his mother to the field from which he was stolen; no other data
behavior at discovery: ferocious, bit at captors, ate nothing but raw flesh, dipped face in water to drink, went on all fours, tore off his clothes
recovery: never learned to speak, very little improvement
comment: habits learned before 3 years of age disappeared; habits learned between 3 and 9 years persisted.

Then in 1954 Marian W. Smith claimed to carry Dennis's analysis "a step further," using the latter's list as the basis for her reinterpretation.[17] In these lists we see how, by the mid-twentieth century, the list of cases of "feral man" (increasingly "feral children") is already a given, something to be discussed, reviewed, accepted, modified, or rejected. Although the boundaries of the class are somewhat flexible, some examples are more or less unanimously challenged or outright excluded from the list due to insufficient evidence or lack of certain conditions. The class implies some kind of animal association but also isolation. The question of idiocy is central, as is the fact that many authors are using the stories to make generalizations about childhood and development.

The most famous recent list of wild children is the one social psychologist and jazz critic Lucien Malson attached to his edition of Itard's reports on Victor. Malson admitted that some of the stories might be hoaxes but believed that was no reason to reject them all: "The simplest way to proceed would be to present each account regardless of whether it is legendary, historical, authentic or obviously invented." He listed an impressive total of fifty-three cases. Like Zingg's, Malson's is an inclusive list of cases (this time arranged in chronological order), yet even though Malson presents it as a corrected and expanded version of Zingg's, it contains many surprising mistakes and unwarranted inferences. Malson fixed some ages that had been offered as guesses in the original accounts while omitting a few of the more certain age indications in the sources. His choice of "first important accounts" is idiosyncratic, and he threw in some wolves where the reports had featured none (e.g., in the stories of the second boy of Overdyke and the boy of Kronstadt). And because Malson's has become the standard list of wild children, his mistakes and misreadings repeatedly show up in other texts.[18] To add to the confusion, in 1977 the psychiatrist Armando R. Favazza put forward a "List of recorded cases" that, he says, was "adapted, corrected and expanded from that of L. Malson's *Wolf Children*." Malson's list certainly stands in need of correction, but one wonders why Favazza himself felt obliged to undertake the task, for he not only dismissed the entire topic of wild children as "a bizarre chapter of psychiatric history" but also introduced more mistakes in his revised list than he eliminated from Malson's. In any case, by adding and "correcting" Favazza managed to bring the grand total to sixty cases.[19] Most recent attempts to re-examine and reinterpret the evidence usually incorporate some version of the list, sometimes subdividing the class "feral children" into subgroups, e.g., "(a) children reared by animals, (b) children reared in isolation in the wilderness, (c) children reared in isolation in confinement, and (d) children reared in isolation with limited human contact."[20]

I have reviewed the history and multifarious appearances of the list of wild children – how it was put together, how it was transmitted and modified, how it grew, how new wild children were integrated into it or excluded from it, how internal distinctions and subcategories were introduced. I have shown how lists (and anti-lists) were compiled according to varying principles of classification and presented in different styles, more or less comprehensive or exhaustive. Some lists adhere to more restrictive principles (e.g., they only include the fully authenticated cases), some highlight representative examples of the class as a whole, and some list exclusively the cases fitting one of the subgroups within the class (e.g., wolf children). In general there is a desire or compulsion to *complete* "the list" by identifying more and more cases and "correcting" the mistakes in previous versions. But what does the list, in its escalating inclusiveness and length, signify? Of the many scientific and non-scientific writers interested in wild children in the last four centuries, only a handful were directly concerned with questions of enumeration and classification. However, the list is significant in general because it grounds all treatments, definitions, and characterizations of wild children, and because, I argue, it is what brings the cases (individuals, accounts, stories) together. Other discussions of wild children draw from the list, that is, they relate the wild children on the basis of previously established links between them. In recent "discoveries" of wild children, the adults who find the children and write the accounts (Armen, Janer Manila, Lane and Pillard) present or refer to some version of the list, into which they integrate, and in relation to which they discuss, their own child (the gazelle boy, Marcos, John of Burundi). And wild children are brought together in literature on the basis of the list as well: in his book of poems *Wild Children*, John Fairfax mentions fifty-three cases – Malson's number.[21]

NOW THAT WE have seen how the accounts of wild children have been pre-served and collected and the list of cases compiled, it is possible to examine the class "wild child" – and whether there is such a thing. As we know, wild children are *strange*. The people who encountered, observed, and wrote reports about them were struck by their strangeness. They believed that there was something specific about it that made wild children stand out, that separated them from other human beings, that approached them to children even when they were already past childhood, and that put their very humanity in question. They called the strangeness "wildness" and wondered what had caused it. At first, *homines feri* were understood as chil-dren who, abandoned or lost, had survived in "the wild" (forests, moun-tains, jungles, or deserts) by their own means or with the help of animals. Wild children seemed to have been born of "civilized" (European) parents and yet displayed the characteristics and habits of savages. They were indis-putably human and yet behaved like, and resembled, animals. At this point the diacritical lines were those dividing *savagery* from *civilization* and *ani-mality* from *humanity*. Wild children's "wildness" pointed to i) a relation to "savages" and ii) an affinity with (other) animals but also iii) something recognizably, often disturbingly, human. The affinity with animals could be a real connection, in the cases of children believed to have been nurtured by or to have lived in close contact with animals, but also animal-like ("brut-ish") traits, habits, or behaviour, or a startling resemblance to animals. All the accounts of wild children are pervaded with animal references, and most of the children were given names that stressed the same connection.[22]

Until roughly the end of the eighteenth century, then, wild children's strangeness was attributed to their early isolation from other human beings and from the civilizing influence of (European) society. This way of under-standing wild children continues to this day. I like the definition given in 1833 in an article in the *Penny Magazine* of the Society for the Diffusion of Useful Knowledge because it is both representative and matter-of-fact: "There are several well-authenticated cases on record of children having been found in solitary places, leading a brutish life, incapable of communicating ideas by language, and apparently completely ignorant of the social uses of mankind."[23] But since the early nineteenth century, marked by the debates on Victor of Aveyron and Blumenbach's discussion of Peter, there has been a competing set of terms of reference: the wild children's strangeness was construed as a sign of abnormality within an emerging model of human development that charts the "normal" stages of becoming human and diagnoses any deviation from them as pathological.[24] Wild children were idiots or imbeciles, lacking reason and perfectibility. Later on they were mentally retarded or defective. The question of causality remained open: was the wild child's retardation due to congenital defect or early isolation? Wild children's "wildness" increasingly came to signify strangeness or extreme isolation in general, and the class "wild child" absorbed the cases of confinement and abuse. Zingg's definition of "feral man" is thus all-inclusive: "Feral (L wild) man is the term for extreme cases of human isolation either ... of abandoned infants adopted and suckled by animals; or of older children who have wandered away into the forests to survive by their own efforts unaided by human contact. Similar cases of children shut away from human association by cruel or insane parents furnish a commoner case, reported in the press from time to time."[25] Zingg's definition distinguishes between the three separate "types" of wild child: alone in the forest, raised by animals, and confined. New interpretations and diagnoses have been proposed closer to our time: child psychosis, autism or some kind of emotional disturbance, child abuse and neglect. As the "bestial" associations of the earlier wild children touched the modern victims of confinement and parental cruelty, the meaning of "wildness" in the wild child itself changed.[26]

Let us look more closely at how the class wild child functions. Whereas the "classical" theory of categorization held that membership in a category is based on properties shared by all its members, the philosopher Ludwig Wittgenstein noticed that members may instead be related by a kind of "family resemblance." The members of a family resemble one another in various ways, but there need be no single collection of properties shared by every member; in the same way, the members of other categories may resemble one another in different ways without all of them having any common properties that define the category. Wittgenstein showed that, within a particular category, some members are more central than others. More specifically, Eleanor Rosch claimed that categories have *best examples* or *prototypes*, which people take to be more representative of the category than other members. "Prototype effects" are superficial and may result from many factors, like the degree of category membership in "fuzzy" categories without rigid boundaries (e.g., tall men) or some other aspect of internal category structure in those with rigid boundaries.[27] Since it should be clear by now that the members of the category or class wild child do not all share a single set of characteristics or properties, prototype theory offers a useful model for thinking about wild children.

But what (or who) may be said to be the prototype of the wild child? I suggest that, for different authors, in different contexts, and for different purposes, different individual wild children function as the prototype. Depending on the occasion and on questions of credibility and authenticity, as well as of distance and closeness – from other children, from civilized or socialized human beings, from the state of nature, from the normal, and so forth – different wild children, or *kinds* of wild children, may be seen as the core of the class. For Zingg, the children "shut away from human association by cruel, criminal, or insane parents" are not *strictly* feral: "They show the same effects from isolation; but they more commonly recover normal minds and personalities not only due to the shorter period of isolation involved before they attract the attention of neighbors or child protective societies, but also due to the fact that they do not have animal or other wild conditioning to unlearn." Likewise, McNeil, Polloway, and Smith assert that, of the four groups into which they subdivide the class "feral child" (reared by animals, reared in isolation in the wilderness, reared in isolation in confinement, and reared in isolation with limited human contact), "the term feral is most appropriate when used to refer only to the first and, to a lesser extent, the second."[28] Malson holds that Victor, Kaspar, and Kamala deserve the special chapter he devotes to them in his book because they are indisputable and exemplary (they illustrate the capacity to profit from education and develop cognitively and emotionally) and also because "they offer, in their diversity, the triple aspect of 'wildness': the child in confinement, the 'animalized' child, and the solitary child." Many decades earlier, Rauber had faulted Blumenbach for making Peter the focus of his discussion of wild children: "The very fulness of the data might induce one to regard a case as typical, when it lacks this quality entirely."[29] Some wild children are always more representative of *the* wild child than others, but not always the same ones, nor for the same reasons.

Contemporary supporters of prototype theory may readily accept a class without identifiable properties shared by all its members, but for a long time the writers of accounts and lists of wild children endeavoured to pinpoint the characteristics of "the wild child" by looking for similarities among the cases. The shared features of wild children would moreover signal the difference, or boundary, between them and *us*. For Linnaeus, as we have seen, *Homo ferus* was *mutus*, *tetrapus*, and *hirsutus* (mute, quadruped, and hairy). In the *Anthropomorpha* he noticed that all the cases agree in these points:

1 That they could not *speak* at all.
2 That they were all *hairy*.
3 That they ran about on their *hands* and *feet*, climbed up trees in a moment, were astonished at the approach of a man, resembled beasts and apes.[30]

Two centuries later, Zingg discerned other common traits or similarities: a) highly unusual food tastes and habits (voracious appetite, preference for raw food and often raw meat, smelling food before eating, etc.); b) illnesses caused by the return to social or civilized life and change in diet;[31] c) apathy and indifference – besides hunger, "we apparently have no evidence of other motivations in feral man strong enough for the invention of tools, houses, or the use of fire"; Zingg seems to regret that, unlike Robinson Crusoe, Condillac's statue, Émile, and the other subjects of imaginary experiments in isolation or natural education, "feral man" did not prove capable of reconstructing or reinventing culture and language on his (or her) own; d) refusal to wear clothes and shoes; e) a lack of shame – "Such data as we have from feral man regarding a sense of shame suggests an infantile naïveté, which develops into the human attitude through social conditioning"; f) peculiar or inhibited sexuality – "Feral cases yield unexpected evidence of inhibition of the sexual impulse apparently due to unfamiliarity in the new situation and impossibility in the old"; Zingg was baffled by the odd mixture of voracious appetite and absence of lust in wild children; g) sensory and perceptual modifications (ability to see at night, sharp sense of smell, defective hearing, insensitivity to heat and cold, etc.); h) emotional disturbances – the data "show the expression of violent emotions of anger and impatience … So human an expression of emotion as laughing, or even smiling, is not recorded for feral cases" (this is not true – the inability to laugh frequently imputed to wild children as a way to underscore their "inhumanity" is belied by observations reported in many of the accounts); i) selfishness and absence of sociality – "The material of feral man deals a hard blow ... to the 'social instincts' of gregariousness"; j) a special bond of sympathy between feral children and wild or other animals and between pairs of wild children found together (such as Amala and Kamala).[32]

Malson and Tinland also indexed the common characteristics of wild children, in general agreeing with Zingg. For Malson, their alleged hairiness may be discounted as "probably a literary survival" but all-fours locomotion and inability to speak may be "accepted as typical characteristics." Tinland ascribes wild children's hairiness to inadequate care and perhaps to the "blackness" caused by exposure to sun and air, "this 'blackness' which seems to have strongly impressed the observers." He insists that, even if each wild child showed singularities explained by the duration of savage existence, age at abandonment, and presence of a companion or animals, it is possible to draw a general picture of typical or constant effects of isolation. To Zingg's catalogue Tinland adds the children's vivid desire to return to their old way of life: "'Reeducation' appears like a true 'domestication,' and at the beginning it entails a state of prostration comparable to that in which certain wild animals fall following capture." The similarities between members of a subgroup of wild children have been highlighted too. Tylor remarked that Sleeman's accounts of wolf boys were "so curiously consistent with one another that it is possible to make a definition of the typical wolf-child, or rather wolf-boy, as we hear nothing of wolf-girls. He should be about ten years old, more or less, brutal and hideous in appearance, idiotic in mind, given to eating raw meat and garbage in preference to anything else, generally averse to wearing clothes, incapable, or almost incapable, of learning to speak, but able to understand and express himself by signs to some slight extent."[33] The perceived and reported similarities between wild children, or between some particular aspect of their stories, afford the grounds on which the cases are linked – sometimes in convoluted ways. Zingg declared that Kaspar, "a case of *isolation amentia*," was "comparable to feral ones because his only remembered associations were with toy hobby-horses. These conditioned him to horses as feral cases are conditioned to the species of their animal associates."[34]

The similarities between the accounts of wild children, and the singular portrait of "the wild child" that emerges from them, are sometimes proffered as proof that the stories cannot be mere inventions. In defence of the reliability of Itard, Feuerbach, and Singh, Malson writes that "any final hesitations must surely be overcome by considering the resemblance between these accounts, written as they were by careful and scrupulous men who could not possibly have communicated their results to each other." Not everyone draws the same conclusion from the stories' commonalities. Whereas the convinced see in them a guarantee of truth (how could all the accounts agree otherwise?), for the sceptics the very fact that the stories of wild children so resemble each other reveals that they are myths derived from the same mythic source or complex (how could all the accounts agree otherwise?). Other sceptics prefer to stress the *differences* between the cases. Blumenbach highlighted these differences ("Taken altogether, they were very unmanlike, but each in his own way, according to the standard of his own individual wants, imperfections, and unnatural properties") and used them to demonstrate that wild children can tell us nothing about human beings in general. But for Tinland these same differences made wild children important. Their singularities and the extreme variation in some of their reported traits and behaviours (e.g., posture and eating habits) show that there is no such thing as an original human nature or instincts. The differences confirm "the weakness, and almost non-existence, of preformed behavioural schemes in human beings ... and the importance of processes of imitation and identification in the structuration of human behaviour."[35] Regardless of whether they choose to stress the similarities or differences between the cases, critics and defenders concur on a crucial point: isolated existence cannot be *human*. In Tinland's view, wild children disclose "the teratological character of human existence reduced to isolation for a more or less prolonged period of time." As Malson puts it, the central question is, "now that it is generally recognized that the human environment plays an indisputable, fundamental role – without precise limits – in the formation of a human being, should we continue to be surprised if, when this environment is lacking, what we find facing us are only spectres?" And Zingg: "Feral man has the sensory and other biological equipment that man shares with the animals. The biological foundation is there; but the human superstructure is vastly lacking, when the children are found."[36] Wildness is not merely "savagery" or lack of civilization but *inhumanity*.

We will return to wild children's questioned humanity in later chapters. Here I want to consider whether wild children constitute what Hacking calls a "human kind." According to Hacking, all human kinds, or kinds of people, share a peculiar feature that separates them from "natural kinds," namely a "feedback" or "looping" effect between people and knowledge about people. Still, Hacking advises that there is no unified theory of human kinds; conversely, there are different types of human kind and different stories to be told about the origin and history of each one of them. From Hacking's "Looping Effects of Human Kinds" (1995) I have distilled seven elements of human kinds, and I present them alongside some aspects of the class "wild child" (and its predecessor, *Homo ferus*).[37] 1) Human kinds are the kinds discovered and described by the "marginal, insecure, but enormously powerful" human and social sciences. – The class *Homo ferus* surfaced in the first systematic effort to classify human beings within the system of nature. From then on, wild children haunt every attempt to study human beings and societies scientifically. 2) The term human kinds indicates "kinds of people, their behaviour, their condition, kinds of action, kinds of temperament or tendency, kinds of emotion, and kinds of experience." Hacking prefers to emphasize the *kind* as a system of classification rather than the people and their feelings. – Wild children are labelled and classified with reference to a set of circumstances and appearances. The stress is on something visible and exterior rather than the interiority or selfhood of the individuals involved. 3) Human kinds are, "at least at first sight, peculiar to people in a social setting." – Although it is meant to designate the "other" of society and culture, the class wild child is possible only within them. The wild child is recognized and labelled as such in a socio-cultural context. In fact, it is the social (and sociable) context that marks the wild child's difference (isolation, animal affinities, lack of civilization, and so on). 4) Human kinds are kinds "about which we would like to have systematic, general, and accurate knowledge" useful to reform other people and predict their behaviour. – The "wild child" is someone about whom philosophers and scientists wanted, and still want, to have accurate and systematic knowledge that may be generalized to other kinds of people, even if the content of the knowledge sought and its intended uses vary. 5) The systems of classification in which human kinds arise are inextricable from industrial bureaucracies. – Wild children became "an issue" for science in the early eighteenth century, and in their successive stories we see an increasing involvement of centralized governments and institutionalized science. But they stubbornly resist statistics.[38] 6) Human kinds are "relevant to some of us." – Students of wild children believe they are relevant, and fascinating. 7) The kind and the knowledge about the kind appear and grow together. In other words, the classification of people into kinds often produces the very people needed to fit those kinds. – I hope to have shown that the class wild child and the "knowledge" about wild children emerged at the same time, even if it may be argued that neither class nor knowledge has ever grown, or only did so by adding individual cases to the list and disappointments to the history of scientific knowledge.

For Hacking, the most distinctive property of human kinds is that the people who have been classified react to the classification in various ways, affecting what they are and how they act and in turn changing the knowledge to be had about the kind. This is the looping effect of human kinds. But he posits a special kind of human kind "in which the people classified cannot take in how they are classified" (e.g., infants or autistic children). In these "inaccessible" kinds, there cannot be "self-conscious" feedback but "there can be looping that involves a larger human unit, for example the family." Wild child is an inaccessible human kind because the majority of wild children do not understand or use the name themselves (there are some exceptions, like the wild girl of Songi or John Ssabunnya). Yet as Hacking noticed in relation to autistic children, "the lives of the named are arranged to fit the categories into which they are fitted."[39] The kind "wild child" is inaccessible in another sense as well: by its very nature, the type of isolation that determines the "wildness" in the wild child cannot be systematically observed. It is for this reason that wildness can never be definitively proved, and that the number of cases is inherently limited. In *Rewriting the Soul* (1995) Hacking described the transformation of multiple personality from an extremely rare disorder, a mere curiosity, a number of stories that could be arranged in a list, to a veritable epidemic, "so overwhelming that only statistics could give an impression of the field."[40] This could never happen to wild children. In their case, a comparable transformation – the instances multiplying to such an extent that the individual names would come to exceed any manageable list and be submerged into the anonymity of statistics – is ruled out from the start.

By making lists of cases, by enumerating and analyzing shared traits and formulating explanations for them based on the children's isolation, some human scientists strove to establish "wild child" as an independent, relevant, and real human kind. In parallel, other scientists engaged with the lists, accounts, and cases to debunk them or propose alternative explanations for the children's strangeness. Many scientists jettison wild children as the stuff of myth and legend. Others denounce the accounts or evidence as fraudulent or see the children themselves as frauds. While some critics challenge the factuality of the stories (or some aspect of them) and the authenticity of the reports (or some aspect of them), others attempt to dissolve or erase the class wild child (to dismiss wild children as an independent phenomenon) by reducing wild children to unrecognized or mislabelled instances of other, usually "biologized," classes, already existing or in process of formation.[41]

The most influential and lasting alternative explanation for the wild child phenomenon is congenital defect: idiocy, imbecility, and the other labels progressively coined to refer to the same "thing" in supposedly less offensive ways: mental defect, mental retardation, feeble-mindedness, mental handicap, learning or developmental disability, special needs, and so on. To the view that wild children's "savage" condition resulted from their early deprivation of human contact some scientists opposed the theory that the children were abandoned *because* they were (naturally) defective. The observational reports on the wild boy of Aveyron produced in 1800 by the naturalist Bonnaterre and the physician-alienist Philippe Pinel sharply illustrate the clash between the two positions. To identify, classify, and diagnose this boy, presumed to be a wild child, Bonnaterre and Pinel used the same method: they compared him with known instances of a class with which they were familiar, the former with the other "savages" in Linnaeus's list, the latter with a list of inmates of the Bicêtre and Salpêtrière hospices. After their respective comparisons, Bonnaterre concluded that the boy was really a savage and Pinel that he was no different from his child and adult patients with damaged intellectual or affective faculties.[42]

The congenital defect explanation sufficed to eliminate the concept and class of wild children from the sphere of legitimate scientific and intellectual inquiry in many a sceptic's view; however, the believers in the class wild child attacked it on several fronts. Firstly, they claimed that while idiocy might indeed account for some of the cases, it would be too much of a coincidence if *all* the wild children turned out to be idiots. Many common people (non-scientists) who encountered and observed the wild children obviously must have had contacts with children with mental defects and yet they did not confuse the two. There seemed to be something else or different about the wild children, something in their appearance and behaviour, perhaps some mystery about their origins, that clearly separated them from your usual "village idiot." And if wild children were just idiots, how could they have survived the harsh conditions of isolation or life with animals, which seem to hint at special skills and superior adaptability instead? They conceded that the clinical picture observable in many wild children on their return to society matched many symptoms of congenital idiocy but argued that wild children's initial retardation was of a special kind, acquired rather than inborn (some scientists propounded special names to designate this type of idiocy, e.g., A.F. Tredgold's "*isolation amentia*").[43] Retardation was made a consequence of isolation. The sceptics presented another objection. If wild children were not originally defective, why did so few of them ever recover (learn speech, develop intellectually, lose at least part of their strangeness)? Already in the eighteenth century reflection on the condition of wild children led Defoe and La Mettrie, and later Herder and most notably Itard, to the notion that the ability to learn may decrease or disappear after a certain age (what contemporary experts call a "critical period" for learning or acquiring certain skills).

To complete the discussion of questions of definition and explanation in the stories of wild children, here are some combinations and variations. i) Idiocy and isolation: the *Penny Magazine* author suggested that Peter and the Savage of Aveyron "were probably idiots from their birth; but their mental defects were greatly increased by their wild life;—for education did something for the mitigation of their calamity." ii) Acceptance of part of the wild child phenomenon only: some writers believe that some wild children did survive alone in the wild but the animal association was an imaginary addition. De Pauw doubted "that any of these human creatures ever received the least help, the least care from bears or any other animals"; rather, they must have been lost or exposed when they were old enough to survive on their own and luckily avoided the attacks of carnivorous animals until they learned to defend themselves. For Rauber, the boy of Hesse may have been "a wild and unruly child who was discovered by hunters in the woods ... In the same woods, wolves may not have been completely lacking." Mandelbaum admitted that the observers of so-called wolf children saw "some sort of odd children" but certainly not "wolf wildings." Children who were abandoned, lost in the forests, or carried off by animals and survived a period of isolation would become "local wonder children" when brought back to society: "Villagers need some explanation of their survival and the stereotyped motif of animal adoption is propounded." And Werner Stark: "There were no wolf children or bear children or tiger children, but disbelief in the alleged suckling of them by animal foster mothers need not be connected with skepticism concerning the other reported circumstances." iii) Idiocy and animal-nurture: Hutton refers to "the hypothesis that [wolf-children] are idiot children who have wandered into the jungle and have taken up their abode in the dens of wolves, the natural inmates of which have tolerated them." iv) Autism (or, in other versions, child psychosis or emotional disturbance), first proposed by Bruno Bettelheim. v) Child abuse and child sexual abuse (the explanation proffered in Money's *The Kaspar Hauser Syndrome of "Psychosocial Dwarfism"* and Masson's *Lost Prince*). vi) Some writers hold that the wild child is a popular myth intended to account for something else that the group or community concerned finds disturbing or uncomfortable, like idiocy (Tylor, Ireland), autism (Bettelheim), repressed Oedipal desires (Carroll), or child sexual abuse (Masson). vii) Boris Porchnev argues that hairy and speechless wild children (the first Lithuanian boy, Tulp's boy, the boy of Kronstadt) were neither raised by animals nor mentally defective but unrecognized instances of "living Neanderthals" (*"paléanthropes reliques"*).[43]

To this day, the question remains open. The attempts both to make a universally recognized kind out of the stories of wild children and to dissolve the kind altogether (into myth or other kinds) have been unsuccessful. It seems that wild children, *as wild children*, resist being turned into a human kind: the cases are too few and too individualized; they cannot be experimented with and do not allow for the use of statistical methods, etc. Moreover, any effort to prove or disprove that isolation explains wild children's strangeness is bound to fail. Since nobody can be a witness to another person's isolation, and since, the lasting consequences of isolation being disturbances in speech, memory, perception, cognition, and affectivity, wild children seldom tell their own stories, the period of isolation (wild children's "wild life") remains unfathomable, forever beyond the investigator's grasp. It can be neither definitively documented nor definitively refuted. Like those fairy-tale heroes who survive inordinate perils and achieve extraordinary feats only to be told that there is one more thing to be done before they can marry the princess, the defenders of the reality of wild children, in their quest to establish the stories' authenticity beyond any doubt, are always short of fulfilling one more condition, finding one more witness, securing one more testimony, making one more observation, the only one that would satisfy the sceptics – but never does. Yet the human sciences have been ceaselessly haunted by wild children, by their unbridgeable inaccessibility, their irreducibility to a spot on a bell curve, and the limitations to knowledge of the *other* inseparable from the notion (and experience) of "wildness" as prolonged isolation from other human beings. The relation between the human sciences and wild children conforms to a dialectic of temptation and disappointment. Every time a wild child is identified, exorbitant hopes are raised, and every time they are frustrated.

Because extant efforts to classify and define wild children are inconclusive and leave us unsatisfied, I would like to offer another way of understanding what brings wild children together. The prototype of the class wild child must be sought not in a sketch of a type of child or person, a set of traits or characteristics, something intrinsic or visible in the children themselves, but in a type of narrative, a *story-form*. For "wild child," the prototype is a narrative prototype. The narrative element, already present in embryonic form in the "names" Linnaeus invented for the examples in his list, is a constant in the stories, and history, of wild children. The story-form or narrative prototype provides the basic framework with which every story accords or from which it more or less deviates. As handed down in accounts, lists, and classifications, it establishes for the child a type of relation to the observing and concerned adults, a relation to knowledge-production, and a pattern of possible responses. It allows and invites a great range of "moves" but also imposes constraints by making some moves easier to think and do than others. The narrative prototype of wild children comprises distinct moments that appear, in some form or another, abbreviated or maximally expanded, in all the stories: 1) encounter/discovery, 2) capture/rescue, 3) curiosity/concern/diagnosis, 4) response/care/treatment, 5) knowledge-production/controversy, 6) disappointment/indifference.

1) The first moment is the encounter with, first sighting, or "discovery" of, the strange child. In most accounts it is explicitly present, but more rarely it is only implied. In some accounts this moment is barely noted or fused with the second (capture). But usually some time elapses between discovery and capture, filled by astonishment and confusion. The first sighting may involve a single individual, a small group of people, or an entire community. The child may be encountered in the wild or for some reason appear amid the human community. In some cases there is a succession of sightings before the definitive capture or rescue. Following discovery, special preparations may be made to track down, chase, or entice the wild child. In almost all cases, once "discovered" the child is not left alone. The encounter with the wild child parallels and re-enacts the historical encounter with "the savage." Both are encounters with radical otherness that challenge *us* – the civilized adults who discover the wild children, the Europeans who discover the American Indians and other "savage nations" – to redraw the boundaries of

the human and rethink our own identity as human beings. But the pervasive rhetoric of discovery needs to be probed. What does it mean to say that an individual or group is *discovered*? To complicate matters, in many cases the child is first seen by subordinate people, who rank low in the hierarchy of knowledge-production (peasants, lumberjacks, soldiers, natives) and are therefore not granted full status as "discoverers."[45] This leads to endless suspicions, inquiries, and efforts to restage the moment of discovery.

2) Discovery is followed by capture. In some cases discovery and capture coincide almost completely; much less often, capture does not follow at all (i.e., the gazelle boy). There may be a significant shift, a definite moment when a strange child known to a certain community is no longer permitted to carry on his or her "wild" existence but is captured, put under surveillance, and actively hindered from escaping. This, the moment when society, government, and science take in the child as an object of concern, is the precise moment when the strange child becomes a *wild child* (e.g., the morning of 9 January 1800 when the boy later known as the savage of Aveyron was found at tanner Vidal's in Saint-Sernin). We must try to understand, in each story, what causes this shift and brings about this moment. The capture of the wild child may be seen as *rescue*. But it is never entirely clear, even in the minds of the actors themselves, whether the wild child has been "rescued" or "captured," and whether this, the first crucial response on the adults' part to the child's plight and needs, was right or wrong (was it right to interfere, to take away the child's freedom, to pursue the child every time he or she escaped?).

3) The third moment refers to people's first and subsequent impressions of the wild child. How is the child described, and by whom? What exactly in the child's appearance or behaviour catches people's attention? What is noticed and registered as strange (or bestial, brutish, repulsive, frightening) in the wild child depends on the observers' own relation to, and place in, what Norbert Elias called the "civilizing process."[46] The wild child is often related and compared to other kinds of people (savages, children, idiots, deaf-mutes). There is generally a first, "popular" perception or image of the child, and then a more "objective" scientific diagnosis. These correspond to two types of curiosity: the curiosity excited by a freak or monster, a "devil" (Songi girl) or "ghost" (Amala and Kamala), and the curiosity of the scientist facing a problem, confronting a new object of knowledge, observation, and experiment. The scientific or philosophical observer raises questions about the child (who and what is this child? How did the child get to be

what she or he is? Is "wild child" the appropriate label?) but also asks questions *of* the child (what problems does this child hold the key to?). While certain characteristics of the wild child are immediately noticeable (nakedness, gait, food tastes, and habits), others, like muteness or deafness, require confirmation by means of specialized testing, expertise, and apparatus (systematic sensory tests, autopsies, the brain tests performed on Genie). In time, observation, testing, and re-education become one: only after the child has been socialized, reached his or her limit, or been taught to speak can we now really know what or who that child is.

4) The community responds to the newly discovered wild child, and this response is informed by specific concerns. Something is always done to and with the child. We must inspect what it is, who does it, and whether there are any debates as to what is to be done and who is to do it. The response to the wild child is connected to questions of power. All the stories feature powerful authorities (royalty and nobility, churches and missionary societies, the military, different levels of government and administration, scientific academies, universities, foundations and granting agencies), and most of them contain some type of dispute about jurisdiction. Wild children may become an amusement for the aristocracy, an affair of state, or a charge of the welfare state. They are commonly provided for, through patronage, pensions, charity, or government relief. They are placed in nunneries, hospices, asylums, orphanages, or foster homes. Most accounts tell of attempts to transform (civilize or humanize) the wild child. The approaches used vary widely, from direct and unashamedly violent "taming" or training to more "rational," non-violent, and medicalized forms of education, treatment, and rehabilitation. The changing response to the wild child intersects with the historical emergence and progressive refinement of medical and pedagogical technologies of intervention in all children's lives.

5) Wild children give rise to knowledge and controversies. Philosophers and scientists who become aware of their existence (directly or through others' reports; during the child's life or at a distance of decades or centuries) may "receive" them as privileged objects of knowledge, the holders of answers to fundamental questions. In some cases no first-hand knowledge is produced because no scientist comes in direct contact with the child. The wild child may be studied by a single scientist or by a whole scientific community whose members hold radically diverging views on him or her. The scientific communities that investigate wild children differ in their structure and characteristics, in the way they construct the "wild child" as an object

of knowledge, in the amount of funding and support they obtain from the state or other authorities. But in every case the involvement of the scientific establishment in the lives of wild children comes at the expense of other, non-expert forms of knowledge and forms of caring for the child. Scientific intervention and knowledge-production disqualify other interventions and types of knowledge. Many wild children have significant "afterlives": their stories appear in later controversies and are subject to competing retrospective diagnoses and interpretations. The accounts are eventually challenged and fears voiced that something about them is "not true" or "not real."

6) There are several reasons for the ultimate indifference towards and disappointment in the wild child. If the child is "far away," inaccessible, or dead, then the growing suspicions that the evidence is inadequate or false may win the day (what was once acceptable evidence loses value as time goes by). Some lack in the account, evidence, or child is discovered and wielded. The story and the child are seen as somehow "tainted" (with falsehood, superstition, credulity, fabrication) and consequently rejected. If the child is living and present "among us," then the limited success or complete failure of attempts to rehabilitate and communicate with him or her may lead to the repudiation of the case as a whole as a mere instance of congenital pathology. In any event, the high hopes of the adults who encounter the wild child – the king's hope to hear wonderful stories about life in the wild, the philosopher's hope to understand the natural state of man, the scientist's hope to ascertain the difference between heredity and environment or uncover the secret of children's language acquisition, the missionary's hope to secure another soul for Christianity, the pedagogue's hope to perform an educational miracle – are not realized. Wild children are children who disappoint. And what happens in the end to the wild children? If they do not escape or do not die soon after being captured, they may be looked after until their death by more or less friendly people, sink into anonymity, or suffer further neglect and abuse.[47]

To what extent does the fascination with wild children arise from (or depend on) the fact that their stories give pleasure *as stories*? Is it ultimately a fascination with narrative, the uses of narrative, and narrative understandings of human experience and subjectivity? Writers of dry theoretical or analytic works (e.g., many twentieth-century authors of psychology and sociology textbooks) "break into story" when dealing with the wild child. But the story-form may be deceptive. The wild child's life is constructed as a single linear story from bits and pieces, fragmentary testimonies, silences, observations, and interpretations. The linear narrative is nothing but a discursive device, a speculative tool and thinking aid. Yet once the story has been put together, it acquires an independent reality as it were and induces the illusion that everything about the child's life is recorded in it and that nothing has been left out. I try to resist this illusion of transparency by refusing to cover up the gaps in the accounts and emphasizing instead that we *do not know* everything about the wild child – and I do not mean any essential or hidden truth but very mundane things like whether he ever smiled or when she shed her first tear.

One last word about classification: in the chapters that follow I trace two major movements: from wild man (*Homo ferus* or *homme sauvage*) to wild child (*enfant sauvage* or feral child), and from the wild child as *exception* with respect to all other children to the wild child as *representative* of children in general. My objective is to show how, when, and why *the child* began to function as a possible prototype for "the savage" and the *wild child* came to be seen as best example of the whole class of children.

PART TWO

Of Savages,
Philosophers, and
Naturalists

CHAPTER THREE

Peter of Hanover and the Wild Girl of Songi

Did [the wild girl] not regret the woods one took her from ... When, after emerging from the hands of nature, one sees our manners, our injustices, etc. if one [cannot] go back into the forest, at least one should be able to lead the life of a good and honest peasant.

Gaspard Guillard de Beaurieu, *Cours d'histoire naturelle*[1]

PETER OF HANOVER and the wild girl of Songi, discovered in the early eighteenth century, excited the attention and curiosity of a large number of people from different stations in life and across national and linguistic borders. They are the first wild children on whom we have dossiers. In texts of very different status, length, quality, and reliability, the wild children's observers and interlocutors recorded what they saw and what they thought about it.

The many accounts of Peter produced during his long life include reports in the British press about his discovery in Hanover and transfer to England; observations and commentaries by people who met him in England in the years following his arrival; German accounts of his capture and its aftermath, and descriptions of Peter in his old age. The earliest British press reports were translations from the foreign press:

Hanover, Dec. 11, 1725. The Intendant of the House of Correction at Zell has brought a Boy hither, suppos'd to be about 15 Years of Age, who was catch'd some time ago in a Forest or Wood near *Hamelen*, where he walk'd upon his Hands and Feet, run up Trees as naturally as a Squirrel, and fed upon Grass and the Moss of Trees. By what strange Fate he came into the Wood is not known, because he cannot speak. He was presented to his Majesty at *Herenhausen* while at Dinner, when the King made him taste of all the several Sorts of Dishes that were serv'd up at Table, in order to bring him by Degrees to human Diet. His Majesty has given special Command that he may have such Provision as he likes best, and that he may have all the Instruction possible to fit him for human Society.[2]

This account corresponds quite closely to the earlier stories of wild children, even though no explicit connection to any of them was made at this time. The boy was captured "some time ago" (the report did not say when, but according to the German sources it had been more than a year earlier, in 1724) alone in a forest near Hameln, walking on all fours, climbing trees like a squirrel, feeding on grass and moss, unable to speak. Following an attempt to escape into the same forest, "he was there catched on a tree, where he thought to hide himself."[3] He became news in England after he was brought to the attention of George I, elector of Hanover and king of Great Britain and Ireland (from 1714 to 1727), who offered him a place at his table and gave orders that he be provided for and educated.

As a result of the king's curiosity and compassion, the "Savage Boy" exchanged the solitude of the forest for the polite society of the court. In January of the following year the British press announced that the king had given the "wild Youth" to the Princess of Wales as a present, "and he is sent for accordingly." In March, readers were informed that he was being "brought over, being a great curiosity."[4] After his arrival in London in early April, he was carried "into the presence of his Majesty, and many of the nobility." The reporters now had a chance to observe and describe the strange phenomenon in greater detail: "He is supposed to be about thirteen years old, and scarce seems to have any idea of things." Whereas in his first encounter with the wild boy the king had introduced him to the civilized pleasures of dinner at court, now the symbolic exchange between savagery and civilization was marked by a glove and a gold watch: "He took most notice of his Majesty, and of the Princess giving him her glove, which he tried to put on his own hand, and seemed much pleased, as also with a gold watch, which was held to strike at his ear." The boy disliked wearing the blue clothes that had been put on him and could not "be brought to lie on a bed, but sits and sleeps in a corner of the room; whence it is conjectured he used to sleep on a tree for security against wild beasts, they having been obliged to saw down one when he was taken."[5] In early 1726 Count Nikolaus Ludwig Zinzendorf (1700–1760), who would become famous as a religious reformer, requested the assistance of Countess Schaumburg-Lippe, lady-in-waiting at the court, to obtain guardianship of the boy to watch the development of his innate ideas, but even though the countess believed that Zinzendorf's care would benefit the boy's soul, she could not comply because the king had already given the boy to the Princess of Wales, who had in turn entrusted him "to the care of a philosopher, in order to make the experiment which your lordship intended."[6] The "philosopher" was Dr John Arbuthnot (1667–1735).

The "Savage Boy" attracted the interest of the court and the learned, that is, of those social groups whose own self-definition most rested on notions of civilization and culture. This is not to say that he did not invite "popular" interest as well; he did, both in Hanover and in England, but more as a freak or monster than as a "savage," to be watched and laughed at rather than studied or made a subject of speculation. His adventures and progress continued to furnish news copy. In April he was "dressed in green lined with red, and ... scarlet stockings" and he sat for his picture. Being "pretty much forwarded in speech," on the evening of 28 June he was baptized at Dr Arbuthnot's house near Burlington Gardens.[7] A reporter who saw the "wild creature" at court declared him "one of the greatest curiosities that has appeared in the world since the time of Adam" because, according to "the accounts they give us of his behaviour" when he was found in the woods of Hameln, he seemed "entirely unacquainted with his own species." Questions about the boy's wild life took up "the conversation of the learned."[8] Yet by the end of the year the initial expectancy was giving way to a certain chagrin (and the first hints that something may have been wrong with the boy himself): "We are told that Dr Arbuthnot has not yet been able, notwithstanding all the pains he has taken, to bring the wild youth, either to the use of speech, or pronunciation of any words, which some impute to his want of understanding, because he still retains the natural wildness in all his actions and behaviour."[9] (There is no extant account of Dr Arbuthnot's work with Peter and thus we do not know how he related to his charge or the methods he used to instruct him.)

The intriguing account of the "most singular creature ... a real savage," included by César de Saussure, a Swiss visitor to London, in a letter home, gives evidence of the public curiosity Peter aroused in his first months in England and the rumours that were circulating about him. Saussure offered an elaborate version of the discovery and capture: "A short time before [the king left] Hanover some huntsmen saw an entirely naked human being in a dense forest. It fled at their approach and disappeared. Surprised at such a sight in an entirely deserted spot, the huntsmen went back several times in the hopes of seeing it again, and were one day lucky enough to do so. They followed the creature, and found it had hidden and taken refuge in the trunk of a big hollow tree. Having seized it, they found it was a youth of from fifteen to sixteen years of age. On being taken prisoner, he gave the most terrible howls, and could not articulate a single word." Saussure's overstated portrait of the boy indicates that the popular imagination was at work: "His hair was matted and bristling, his nails very long, his skin hardened and tanned by the air – in a word he was a perfect savage, probably born, fed, and brought up with the wild beasts of the forest, and speaking no human language." Of special interest is his reaction on seeing the boy in St James's Park: "I was much struck with his appearance ... His eyes were haggard, and did not rest on any object, and he looked so wild and extraordinary I cannot describe the impression he made. He frightened me." An anecdote about Peter's skilful tree climbing prefigures similar ones later told of the wild girl of Songi and Victor: "I am told that the first time he was taken to the park, he showed the greatest joy and pleasure at finding himself in a sort of wood. With surprising agility he climbed up the highest tree, and his keepers had much difficulty in getting him down again." But Saussure's account ends in a startling anticlimax: "Everyone was looking for the savage to speak, to learn his history, but that satisfaction was not to be. The change of food and his new way of living helped no doubt to make him fall ill; he pined away and died about two months after his arrival in England, and just as he was learning to say a word or two." It seems that the legend of Peter's early death was born right at the beginning of his British career as a wild boy.[10]

Besides drawing-room conversations, travellers' correspondence, and excursions to St James's Park, Peter's arrival in England spawned a series of pamphlets, the most notable being those penned by the two greatest authors then writing in English. It is hardly surprising that Daniel Defoe (1660?–1731) and Jonathan Swift (1667–1745) would be attracted to what Saussure called "a real savage" since both of them had already written books in which savages and savagery were prominent: *Robinson Crusoe* (1719) and *Gulliver's Travels* (published anonymously in late 1726 but completed many months before). Defoe may have begun to ponder the wild boy's significance when he reported the discovery in *Applebee's Journal* in December 1725. Swift, who was in London in April 1726, most likely became interested in the boy through his friend Arbuthnot. "This night I saw the wild Boy, whose arrivall here hath been the subject of half our Talk this fortnight," Swift wrote to

Thomas Tickell. "He is in the Keeping of Dr Arthbuthnot, but the King and Court were so entertained with him, that the Princess could not get him till now." He added: "I can hardly think him wild in the Sense they report him."[11]

Two anonymous pamphlets published in 1726 are commonly attributed to Swift or Arbuthnot, possibly both. *The Most Wonderful Wonder that Ever Appeared to the Wonder of the British Nation*, which bore little relation to the known facts of Peter's life, is a satirical dialogue between the boy and his alleged foster mother (a bear), mocking the English obsession with him and criticizing the court and civilized society. The Dutch gentleman Mynheer Veteranus, keeper of a gin shop in Amsterdam, "hearing the kind Reception the wild Boy met with here in *England*, and of the great Care taken for his Instruction in the Principles of the Christian Faith," thought he could do no better service "to this generous Nation" than finding and bringing over "the Bear to whom the Care of his Infant State was committed." A moving reunion ensues, after which the boy tells his old nurse about the character and customs of the "Beast call'd Man."[12]

The second pamphlet, *It cannot Rain but it Pours, or, London strow'd with Rarities*, subtitled *Of the wonderful Wild Man that was nursed in the Woods of Germany by a Wild Beast, hunted and taken in Toyls; how he behaveth himself like a dumb Creature, and is a Christian like one of us, being call'd Peter; and how he was brought to Court all in Green, to the great Astonishment of the Quality and Gentry*, is another incisive satire on the court and contemporary fashion. It also interjects piquant points based on Swift's and Arbuthnot's meetings with Peter and their acquaintance with current opinion. The narrator related Peter to the legendary Romulus and Remus (but not to earlier wild children), and this time gave him a sow for foster mother. Peter had been brought over by a Mr Rotenberg and caused a stir at court, his young age greatly disappointing the ladies "who came to the Drawing-Room in full Expectation of some Attempt upon their Chastity." The boy had very acute senses and "a Father and Mother like one of us" – which decades later Monboddo took to mean that Peter was visibly European, not to be confused with "exotic" savages. Unable to speak any known language, "that Care being left to the ingenious Physician, who is entrusted with his Education," Peter nonetheless knew the language of animals and birds, took "vast Pleasure in Conversation with Horses," and expressed joy "most commonly by Neighing" (according to the narrator, and paralleling Gulliver's views on the Houyhnhnms, the horses he encountered in his fourth voyage, neighing was "a more noble Expression of that Passion than Laughing, which seems to me to have something Silly in it"). Peter had moreover invented a personal language, in which "a young Lady is a Peacock, old Women Magpies and Owls; a Beau with a *Toupee*, a Monkey; Glass, Ice; Blue, Red, and Green Ribbons, he calls Rainbows; an Heap of Gold a Turd." Doubtful that Peter was "wild in the Sense they report him," Swift seemed less concerned with the boy and his putative savagery than with how he made visible his contemporaries' vices and follies.[13]

In *Mere Nature Delineated*, the most important early discussion of Peter and the first book-length work on a wild child, Defoe made an effort to assess whether the "facts" of the case were physically possible and reviewed the available evidence to separate fact from rumour or fiction. Defoe's purpose was to ascertain *who* and *what* Peter was; in his words, to "settle the Point about the Person; as, 1. How it is introduced into the World; what they that found, or caught him, *as they call it*, say of him, or of the Wilderness Posture of his Affairs; and upon what Foot they presented him to the World: And, 2. What is his real Circumstance as he now appears in Life."[14] As the reports were not free from inconsistencies, some people might be inclined to judge the story a "Fable" and proclaim that what "the whole Business" amounts to is that "they have only brought an Ideot upon the Stage, and made a great Something out of Nothing" (4). Defoe dealt in turn with each objection. How could such a young child live alone in a harsh climate, naked, without shelter or food except "Apples and Nuts, Moss and Leaves"? If he lived a long time in this condition, how did he survive the winters and defend himself from wild beasts, bearing in mind that after his capture he did not strike the observer as especially clever or courageous? Besides, how could he have remained undiscovered for a long time? The woods where Peter was found were not "so wild and desolate, such Desarts and Wildernesses" that "such a Creature as this was (for his Way of living) could live many Years there, and be undiscover'd" (15). Conversely, if the boy's wild life had lasted only a short time, "how is it that he cannot speak, and is so meer a Part of wild Species as we still find him?" (9). Defoe rejected outright the idea that Peter was nursed by a wild animal and challenged the claim that he went upon his hands and feet, first, because it was neither likely nor practicable, and second, because when the wild boy was captured he did not show "any Difficulty of standing upright, or of walking erect, as he does now" (11).[15]

Defoe's conclusion was cautious. He did not see "Probability enough" in the story "to make it rational to believe it" but had not found absolute

Mere NATURE *Delineated:*

OR, A

BODY without a *SOUL.*

BEING

OBSERVATIONS

UPON THE

Young FORESTER

Lately brought to Town from

GERMANY.

With Suitable

APPLICATIONS.

ALSO,

A Brief Diſſertation upon the Uſefulneſs
and Neceſſity of *FOOLS*, whether
Political or Natural.

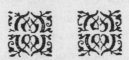

LONDON:

Printed for *T. WARNER*, at the *Black Boy*, in
Pater-Noſter-Row. 1726. [Price 1*s.* 6*d.*]

Mere Nature Delineated, attributed to Daniel Defoe, published in 1726.

grounds for disbelief either: "There may be Mistakes in the relating it, and yet the substance of the Story remains untouch'd" (15–16). Peter was neither a fraud – the man who brought him to the court would not "impose such a Cheat upon his Sovereign" (24) – nor "an *Idiot*, or what we call a *Natural*" – he had "some apparent Capacities of being restored and improved" (25) – yet Defoe could not accept all claims proffered about him. Irrefutable elements of the story were "That there is such a Boy, about 14 or 15 Years of Age, perfectly wild, uninstructed, unform'd, *that is*, uninform'd, and the Image or Exemplification, as I say in my Title, of *Meer Nature* ... that he is like a Body without a Soul; that he was found, or, as they title it, was catch'd in a Wood or Forest about *Hamelen* in *Germany*, and brought to *Zell*; and from thence, as a Curiosity in Nature, for the Rareness of it worth enquiring into, brought to *Hanover*, when the King of *Great Britain* was there, and shew'd to his Majesty; and that he is since brought over to *England*, and every Day to be seen" (16). The wild boy's miserable state was incontrovertible as well: that he was "all wild, brutal, and as Soul-less as he was said to be; acting MERE NATURE, and little more than a vegetative Life; dumb, or mute, without the least Appearance of Cultivation, or of having ever had the least Glympse of Conversation among the rational Part of the World" was evident, because "He is himself so far the miserable Evidence of the Fact" (3). Having thus determined the indisputable facts underlying the reports and rumours, Defoe proceeded to analyze the nature and implications of Peter's condition.

Even if Defoe was convinced that the boy was in a state of mere nature, he was less sure of what had caused this state. Had it been natural defect or lack of education? Was the boy's soul "unfetter'd by Organick Ligatures, at Liberty to act, and not interrupted by the Defects of Nature, only wanting Culture, and Improvements" (18)? Did the wild boy have a human soul? Defoe perceived in him two "Testimonies or Evidences of human Soul" (17): Peter gave some signs of thought, and he could laugh.[16] But if Peter had a soul, why did he shun the company of the men he could not have failed to see while he lived in the forest? Why, despite his *"Leap in the Light"* – "from the Woods to the court; from the forest among Beasts, to the Assembly among the Beauties; from the Correction House at *Zell*, (where, at best, he had convers'd among the meanest of the Creation, *viz.* the Alms-taking Poor, or the Vagabond Poor) to the Society of all the Wits and Beaus of the Age" – was he still averse to human beings, constantly seeking means to escape? Was Peter's silence deliberate, a judgment on the true value of "the present inspir'd Age" (22)? In the end, Defoe resolved that even if "we see very little of the ordinary Powers of a Soul acting in him" beyond what may be discerned "in the more sagacious Brutes," Peter must be granted a human soul (23). To Defoe's mind, no matter how "wild" and strange, the boy was fully human, at least in potential. Still, Peter's humanity appeared condemned to stay sadly limited: he was "but the Appearance or Shadow of a rational Creature, a kind of Spectre or Apparition ... a great Boy in Breeches, that seems likely to be a Boy all his Days" (28). Defoe's words proved prophetic: Peter would be "the Wild Boy" until his death in 1785.

What was to be done with such a creature? Defoe was aware that "Dr. A—tt" was attempting "to make him docile, or willing to learn." He wondered what language the doctor would teach the boy first, whether English or "High Dutch" (German), which some people thought "most proper for him, as being best adapted to his primitive State," and for this reason the one he might learn soonest. But Defoe realized that the wild boy could never benefit as much from his renewed contact with the civilized world as the latter could profit from the discovery: "the Business then is to make his Circumstance useful to the rational Part of the World, whether the World can be made so to him or no" (28–9). Defoe himself made use of the wild boy's circumstance to speculate at length on the relation between thinking and words, deaf-mute education, and education in general, but he insisted that in the final satirical chapter on "fools" the object of laughter and ridicule was not the boy himself (whom he deemed to be an object of pity instead) but "our modern Men of Mode," who "want Teaching as much as he does, and, of the Two, something the more" (iv).[17]

The other anonymous pamphlets printed in 1726 rehearsed some of the same tropes: animal nurses, descriptions of the boy's strangeness, theories about his origin, and the contrast between his natural (or savage) existence and the (polite or depraved) court. In *An Enquiry how the Wild Youth, Lately taken in the Woods near Hanover, (and now brought over to England) could be there left, and by what Creature he could be suckled, nursed, and brought up*, Peter was introduced as "a Creature of a real human Kind and Species, naked and wild," lost in infancy by a "Set of travelling People" and nursed not by a wolf or wild sow but by a bear (depicted in terms that echo Connor's account of the Lithuanian bear boys): "It is not impossible, that some She-Bear, somehow or other deprived of her Cubs, finding this Infant, and being full of a suckling, nursing, tender Temper, finding it a Living-thing, laid her self down to it, and suckled it ... having *thus taken to it*, nourished it 'till it

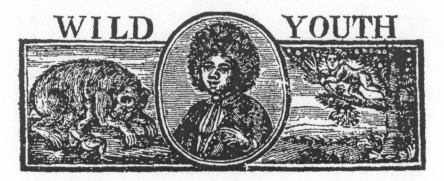

Peter's extraordinary origin and remarkable transformation; *An Enquiry how the Wild Youth, Lately taken in the Woods near Hanover, (and now brought over to England) could be there left, and by what Creature he could be suckled, nursed, and brought up*, published in 1726. Notice the similarity between this representation of Peter being nursed by a bear and the one in Connor's *History of Poland*.

could shift for it self." Empirical confirmation for "the Opinion of his being brought up by that Creature, rather than any other" could be had if, at the sight of a bear, the boy "discover[ed] by some Action or other, that might naturally break out, that that Creature had been no Stranger to him." The boy laughed often and was "strait and upright, & not Hairy, except a bushy Head of dark brown Hair" – that is, he was not *tetrapus* and *hirsutus* as Linnaeus's future *Homo ferus* would be. The reason why he did not speak was not a "Deficiency in Nature" but "*Non-Use*, and want of not having heard People speak about him, and to him." Now "under the Care of proper Persons to make a civilized Creature of him," Peter could repeat monosyllables after his tutor, whom he feared because he corrected the boy's mistakes "by striking his Legs with a broad Leather Strap." But he only learned "by Rote, as any dumb Creature is taught to fetch and carry." In *The Manifesto of Lord Peter*, the wild boy was represented as the son of a philosopher who "from a deep Sense of the Miseries brought upon Mankind by being civiliz'd" conducted an educational experiment (leaving the child in "a desert Forest") to "convince the World, how much a nobler Creature a Wild Man was than a Tame one." Now "Lord Peter" is looking for a suitable (wild) wife. *Vivitur Ingenio*, a collection of observations on love, politics, religion, and history, was not about Peter but allegedly written "in Characters of Chalk, on the

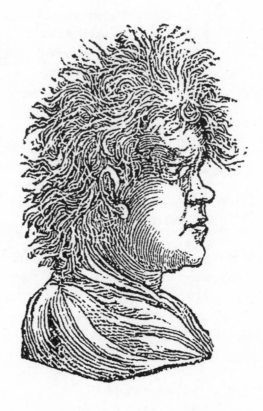

Peter, in *The Manifesto of Lord Peter*, published in 1726.

Boards of the Mall in St. James's Park; for the Edification of the Nobility, Quality and Gentry" by a "Wild Man, who stiles himself *Secretary to the Wilderness there*; and is reputed Father of PETER THE WILD BOY, lately brought from Hanover."[18]

The larger questions raised by Peter's arrival were incisively addressed in the poem "The Savage," which appeared in 1726 as well. What characterizes a savage? What are the marks of civilization? Was it morally right to capture and attempt to civilize the wild boy, that is to say, to remake him in our own image? The first part of the poem lists the advantages Peter could derive from social intercourse and the virtues he could learn from his civilized benefactors:

> Ye Courtiers, who the Blessings know
> From sweet Society that flow ...
> Receive this Youth unform'd, untaught,
> From solitary Desarts brought,
> To brutish Converse long confin'd,
> Wild, and a Stranger to his Kind:
> Receive him, and with tender Care,
> For Reason's Use his Mind prepare;
> Shew him in Words his Thoughts to dress,
> To think, and what he thinks express;
> His Manners form, his Conduct plan,
> And civilize him into Man.

The tone changes as the poem's speaker weighs the dangers and evils of civilization and decides that it is not always preferable to savagery:

> But with false alluring Smile
> If you teach him to beguile;
> If with Language soft and fair
> You instruct him to ensnare,
> If to foul and brutal Vice,
> Envy, Pride, or Avarice,
> Tend the Precepts you impart;
> If you taint his spotless Heart:
> Speechless send him back agen
> To the Woods of *Hamelen*;
> Still in Desarts let him stray,
> As his Choice directs his Way;
> Let him still a Rover be,
> Still be innocent and free.

By the end of the poem, the meaning of savagery has shifted, and "the savage" is no longer – or at least not only – the boy:

> He, whose lustful lawless Mind
> Is to Reason's Guidance blind,
> Ever slavish to obey
> Each imperious Passion's Sway,

Smooth and Courtly tho' he be,
He's the Savage, only He.[19]

The wild boy's presence in London inspired his contemporaries to reflect on the tension between savagery and civilization, innocence and corruption, vice and virtue. As Swift/Arbuthnot put it: "Let us pray the Creator of all beings, wild and tame, that as this wild youth by being brought to court has been made a Christian; so such as are at court, and are no Christians, may lay aside their savage and rapacious nature, and return to the meekness of the Gospel."[20]

Although the British accounts made virtually no reference to the time between Peter's capture and his appearance before the king, a German report furnishes a more complex picture of that period.[21] Peter was first encountered in the fields on 4 May 1724 by a citizen of Hameln. He was running "completely naked" except for the remains of a shirt hanging from his neck. The citizen, who estimated the boy's age to be about thirteen, thought him curious enough to warrant further attention, especially when instead of answering his questions the boy "fell to the ground, kissed him and made the strangest faces and contortions." Dragged to town, the strange child was received by a curious mob and placed by the public authorities in the poorhouse. The people of Hameln noticed that he could hear but not speak and "acted more like a wild man than anything else." The boys in the street made fun of him; the adults were disgusted by his filthiness and "crazy" antics. He was a fast runner, but it was not true, the report's author asserted, that he could climb trees like a cat or squirrel and jump from one tree to another, as later rumour would have it. His muteness was attributed to a malformation of his tongue, which was very thick and attached on both sides. At first the boy did not seem to appreciate the new life that was being imposed on him. Because he constantly sought the means to run away, a guardian was employed to "tame" him. The guardian applied himself to this task so efficiently that, he said, after three days "it sufficed merely to show him the rod" to make the boy obey. The guardian also taught him to eat bread and other ordinary foods (initially he would only eat vegetables), and then "he ate so much that he surpassed two persons."

The report's author drew a two-edged portrait of the boy's personality. On the one hand, the "severe surveillance of his superiors," while restraining his "wild manners," had not completely eliminated the "violent fury" that sometimes prevailed over his fear (once he "bit himself in the arm out of rage"). On the other hand, he was cheerful and peculiarly affectionate: "In the beginning he sometimes kissed, now the walls, now the ground, and then his hands, just as he used to unbutton the clothes of anyone whom he met and kissed them on the chest. He could not stand women, but pushed them away from him with both hands and feet. If someone showed him fruit, particularly nuts, he would fall on the ground and kiss it as well as kiss his own hands and throw kisses to everybody. He did not care much about money, but always threw it away from him, though some say that he very skilfully hid money in his hair." His fondness for music was remarked: he often sang without words, and on hearing music became so happy that he began to dance and jump. But the boy's progress in his new life was limited, and after several citizens tried to teach him a trade without success, the authorities sent him to the orphanage at Zell, where, as we know, a definitive solution to his plight was found once the king's attention was drawn to this "real savage."[22]

Peter never regaled King George with marvellous stories about his wild life. As Countess Schaumburg-Lippe informed Count Zinzendorf, even though "every possible means has been used" to teach him English, in the expectation that "he might give some description of the place and manner in which he had lived before, and if possible, of his notions of things," he had not learned enough to ask "for the most necessary things": "His hearing is good, but the sound of his voice is rather like barking than speaking ... In short: he has very little in him more than the outward form of a human creature; and there is no hope left, that he will ever learn anything."[23] When Arbuthnot gave up his efforts to instruct Peter, he was entrusted to the care of Mr James Fenn, a yeoman farmer at Axter's End, Hertfordshire (the arrangements were made by Mrs Titchbourn, one of the queen's bedchamber women). After James Fenn's death, Peter was transferred to his brother Thomas at the farmhouse Broadway, within a mile of Berkhempstead, also in Hertfordshire, and lived there with the several tenants of the farm – his caretakers received a royal pension for his support and maintenance – until his death, on 22 February 1785. He was about seventy-two years old.[24]

The parish register of Northchurch, Hertfordshire, where Peter was buried, contains an account of his life by a long-time resident in the neighbourhood who knew his story well and had repeated opportunities to observe him.[25] Dismissing the "idle tales" about Peter's "climbing up trees like a squirrel, running upon all fours like a wild beast, &c.," the author recounted colourful anecdotes of the wild boy's later life that in turn gave

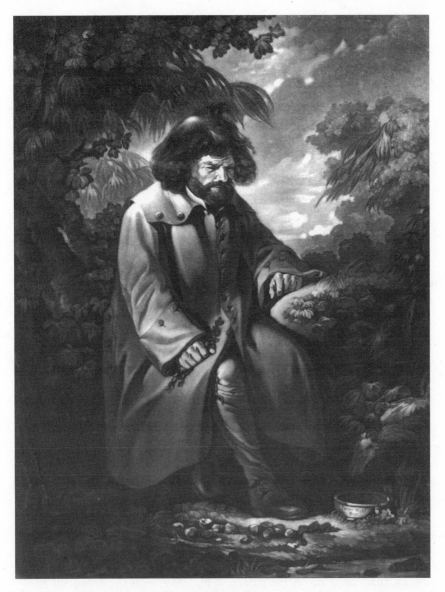

Peter the Wild Boy, by Valentine Green, after Pierre-Etienne Falconet (1767).
Courtesy of the National Portrait Gallery (London).

birth to new legends: "Upon the approach of bad weather he always appeared sullen and uneasy. At particular seasons of the year, he shewed a strange fondness for stealing away into the woods, where he would feed eagerly upon leaves, beech-mast, acorns, and the green bark of trees; which proves evidently that he had subsisted in that manner for a considerable length of time before he was first taken. His keeper therefore at such seasons generally kept a strict eye over him, and sometimes even confined him, because, if he ever rambled to any distance from his home, he could not find his way back again." During one of these flights he went as far as Norfolk, where he was not recognized and was "punished as a sturdy and obstinate vagrant."[26] As a grown man Peter was well made and of middle size, his only physical peculiarity being a web that united two fingers of his left hand up to the middle joint. He was "so exceedingly timid and gentle in his nature, that he would suffer himself to be governed by a child," and apparently had "never discovered any natural passion for women." Yet, the author claimed, notwithstanding the "extraordinary and savage state" in which he was found, the "strange opinions and ill-founded conjectures" published by "men of some eminence in the literary world," and the fact that he did not *look* like one, Peter was "certainly nothing more than a common ideot." The author wished to set the record straight so that "posterity may not ... be hereafter misled upon the subject."[27]

Peter may have been buried and remembered as "a common ideot without the appearance of one," but both before and after his death he continued to elicit curiosity and speculation, and in his later years received visits from important people. In 1763 the author of *Philosophical Survey of Nature* mentioned "an anecdote furnished by a gentleman of veracity in an ingenious private controversial piece" that "in a good measure discredited" the story of Peter. While in Paris, this gentleman had heard from a German acquaintance that Peter was "'nothing more than a poor peasant's child, born an ideot; and that the marvellous part of the story was invented over a bottle, for a jocular purpose, at the palace of H.'" Although the author of *Philosophical Survey* believed that this was "perhaps the most probable account," he went on to recount the "generally received relation" and added that Peter "continues to this day a meer orang-outang": "The people with whom he is boarded, can make him break or cleave wood, draw water, or thresh in the barn, but his rude narrow mind could never be enlarged, owing principally to his never acquiring the habit of speech." In turn, Lord Monboddo, who, we know, was deeply interested in wild children and did not miss any opportunity to meet one in person, went to see Peter in Broadway in early

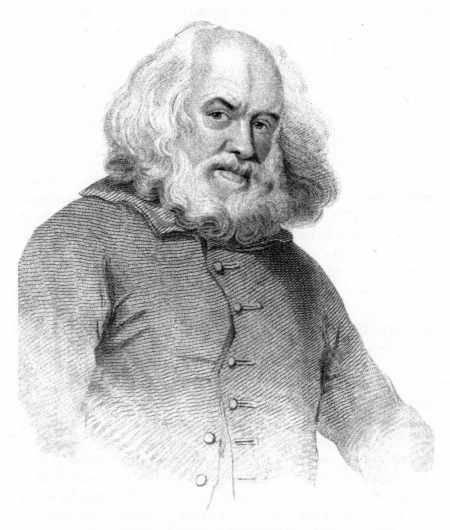

Peter the Wild Boy, stipple engraving published by R. Cooper in 1821, after unknown artist. Courtesy of the National Portrait Gallery (London).

June 1782. What Monboddo found was a man "of low stature, not exceeding five feet three inches," with "a fresh, healthy look" despite his advanced age. Peter's bearded face was "not at all ugly or disagreeable" and his expression appeared "sensible and sagacious for a savage." He did not speak, but, the woman of the house told Monboddo, he "understood every thing that was said to him concerning the common affairs of life." He ate the same food as the farmer and his wife, drank beer and spirits ("of which he inclines to drink more than he can get"), was never mischievous, and could sing many songs. And he still did not care about money: if given any, he took it but gave it to his caretakers. While in the neighbourhood, Monboddo questioned Mrs Callop, an old woman from Hempstead (a larger village about three miles away), who remembered that when Peter first arrived in the area some fifty-five years earlier he had fed mainly on leaves, especially cabbage.[28]

Monboddo must have thought that his visit had not produced all the information that could possibly be extracted from Peter, because he entreated Mr Burgess, "a young gentleman of Oxford," to visit him again and make inquiries in the surrounding farms and villages. Manifestly relishing the assignment, Burgess went to see Peter twice, interviewed the farmer, the master of the inn at Berkhempstead, the people at Two Waters (a small village two miles away), and an old gentleman in Hempstead, and then drew up a lively and detailed account. Peter still retained some of his most distinctive characteristics, such as his passion for fine clothes and bright objects and his taste and talent for music: "If he hears any music, he will clap his hands, and throw his head about in a wild frantic manner ... When he has heard a tune, which is difficult, he continues humming it for a long time, and he is very uneasy till he is master of it. He can sing a great many tunes; and will always change the tune when the *name only* of another tune, with which he is acquainted, is mentioned to him. He does not always hit upon the tune at once which is asked, but he corrects himself easily with the least assistance." Peter was fond of fire, water, onions, and gin. He understood what others said to him and was able to say (but had little or no *desire* to say) quite a few things:

While I was with him, the farmer asked several questions, which he answered rapidly, and not very distinctly, but sufficiently so as to be understood even by a stranger to his manner. Some of the questions were, Who is your father?—King George. What is your name?—Pe-ter; (he always pronounces the two syllables of his name with a short interval between them). What is that?—Bow-wow, (for the dog). What horse will you ride upon?—Cuckow; (This is not the name of any of their horses, but it is a name with which he always answers that question; perhaps it was the name of one of his former master's horses). What will you do with this? (tea, gin, &c.)—He will put his hand to his mouth. If you point to his beard, nose, or mouth, and ask what is that, he will tell you plainly. His answers, I think, never exceed two words; and he never says any thing of his own accord. I forgot to mention, that he has been taught also to say, when he is asked, What are you?—Wild man. Where were you found?—Hannover. Who found you?—King George. If he is told to tell twenty, he will count the number exactly on his fingers, with an indistinct sound at each number; but, after another person, he will say, one, two, three, &c. pretty distinctly.

The wild man's singular reaction to the weather, moon, and stars led Burgess to wonder whether he had, or appeared to have, "any idea of the great Author of all these wonders," but Peter's caretakers told him that he had never shown "any consciousness of a God from his own feelings." Peter had only recently lost his "superior" strength ("he was suddenly taken ill, fell down before the fire, and for a time lost the use of his right side") but his personality was gentle and he was "extremely good tempered." He was never violent (but sometimes became angry), had no sexual feelings for women, and showed a strong attachment to his master.[29]

Burgess related that on one occasion in which Peter was employed by his master in filling a dung-cart, having been left alone for a moment he had not stopped the work once the cart was full: "He saw no reason why he should not be as usefully employed in emptying the dung out as he was in putting it into the cart." Whereas for Burgess and Peter's master this anecdote exposed the wild man's oddness, inability to do useful work without supervision, and perhaps idiocy, Monboddo was quick to affirm that what the story showed was merely that Peter "knew nothing of farming."[30] The Edgeworths (Richard Lovell, 1744–1817, and his daughter Maria, 1767–1849), who for some years lived in Northchurch, Hertfordshire, and knew of Monboddo's interest in Peter, also visited the wild boy. But whereas Monboddo approached Peter as a fascinating object of speculation, the Edgeworths made him the target of some rather pointless "experiments" meant to illustrate that intellectual progress depended on signs and language.

In 1779 we visited him, and tried the following experiment. He was attended to the river by a person who emptied his buckets repeatedly after Peter had repeatedly filled them. A shilling was put before his face into one of the buckets when it was empty; he took no notice of it, but filled it with water and carried it homeward:

his buckets were taken from him before he reached the house and emptied on the ground; the shilling, which had fallen out, was again shewn to him, and put into the bucket. Peter returned to the river again, filled his bucket and went home; and when the bucket was emptied by the maid at the house where he lived, he took the shilling and laid it in a place where he was accustomed to deposit the presents that were made to him by curious strangers, and whence the farmer's wife collected the price of his daily exhibition.

Monboddo believed that Peter was a savage; for the Edgeworths, he was an idiot who "had acquired a few automatic habits of rationality and industry" but "could never be made to work at any continued occupation; he would shut the door of the farm-yard five hundred times a day, but he would not reap or make hay." Monboddo's boundless curiosity spurred Burgess's carefully drafted and endearing account; in contrast, the picture of "Peter the wild boy" that emerges from the Edgeworths' work is flat and disparaging.[31]

When almost a century after Peter was discovered and more than twenty-five years after his death Blumenbach revisited the story and examined the available documents, he found that the many discrepant and contradictory reports made of it "a striking example of the uncertainty of human testimony and historical credibility." In spite of his declaration that Peter was not worthy of the attention he had received from some of the best eighteenth-century minds, Blumenbach conducted a thorough investigation and unearthed many details that add to our knowledge of Peter's life and fate. He reprimanded overly enthusiastic people for having neglected "two little circumstances in the history of his discovery," the fragments of a torn shirt hanging from his neck and the unusual thickness of his tongue, which in Blumenbach's opinion belied the boy's "savagery." Other little-known facts, such as the "singularly superior whiteness" of Peter's thighs compared to his legs (which occasioned a townswoman's remark, on his first appearance in Hameln, that he "must have worn breeches, but no stockings") and the testimony of some boatmen, who had seen several times in the summer a poor naked child on the banks of the Weser and had given him a piece of bread, strengthened Blumenbach's suspicions. He contended that Peter was the dumb child of Krüger, a widower of Lüchtringen, who had first run away to the forest in 1723 and was found the following year, "but meanwhile his father had married a second time, and so he was shortly afterwards thrust out again by his new step-mother." The boy many had taken to be an "ideal of pure human nature" thus turned out to be "nothing more than a dumb imbecile idiot." Ostensible signs of Peter's idiocy were his lack of speech, his lifelong indifference to women (which above all proved his "more than brutish and invincible stupidity"), and the fact that "no one ... ever saw him laugh – that cheerful prerogative of mankind."[32]

Blumenbach purported to settle the matter permanently – concerning both Peter and *Homo ferus*. As we know, he did not, and scholars and commentators continued to debate Peter's condition. Tafel challenged Blumenbach's main objections (for instance, the statement that the boy had been seen by boatmen was unsupported) and maintained that Peter's indifference to women was a clear sign that he was *not* an idiot, since "numerous examples" prove "that natural idiots are very sensuous." Rauber conceded that Peter's mental capacities were limited but cautioned that whether his idiocy was inherited or "acquired through extraordinary neglect and solitude" had yet to be determined. And Zingg both acknowledged Blumenbach's work as a major primary source and discarded its claim "that Wild Peter has no more interest than any 'poor dumb idiot.'"[33] While I abstain from expressing an opinion on Peter's, or any other wild child's, condition, abilities, or nature, I take exception to Blumenbach's characterization of Peter's life as a "vegetatory existence." Whatever he *was*, Peter had the fortune to live a long and, if not happy, at least contented and peaceful life. The same authority that brought him over from Hanover fulfilled its responsibility towards him until his death. The ongoing curiosity he attracted never turned out of control and did not permanently harm his well-being. His caregivers basked in the attention and money they derived from their close relation to him but treated him kindly, and his community granted him a place as an odd but tolerable member. Not many wild children were that lucky. "Peter the Wild Boy" was certainly not "poor Peter."[34]

SEVEN YEARS AFTER Peter's discovery, in September 1731, a wild girl was captured in Songi near Chalôns in Champagne. The wild girl of Songi (christened Marie-Angélique Memmie and later known as Mlle Leblanc) occupies a unique place in the literature on wild children. Despite the rich available evidence, and despite the fact that she was one of the examples in Linnaeus's original list of *homines feri*, most later authors did not know what to make of or do with the wild girl. Scarcely ever discussed at length in later treatments of wild children, she never functioned as "best example" or representative of the whole class, as at various times Peter, Victor, Kaspar, Kamala, or Genie did. To reconstruct her story it is necessary to consider three distinct aspects or stages of her life, which are, in order of increasing uncertainty, the time following her discovery (in turn subdivided into the period of her "taming" and her civilized but difficult later years), the time immediately preceding the discovery, and her early years. Information on each of these aspects may be gleaned from accounts written at the time of the discovery and reports produced by later visitors and investigators.[35]

In many respects the details given in the earliest accounts – two letters printed in the *Mercure de France* in December 1731 – on the discovery and capture of the wild girl and the initial impressions of the people who found her conform to the general pattern of the early stories of wild children. The girl was first seen in the vineyards, skinning frogs and eating them with tree leaves, by the shepherd of Songi, who brought her to the castle of M. d'Epinoy. This lord ordered the shepherd to lodge her and himself took care of her nourishment and other expenses. For "almost two months" M. d'Epinoy allowed her to "spend most of the day in his castle" and let her "fish in his ditches and search for roots in his gardens"; the attention he paid her "attracted many people to his house."[36] A short time after, she was entrusted to the religious authority. The bishop of Châlons placed her in a hospice (Hôpital Général) with the children of the poor, and there "attempts [were] made to humanize and instruct her" (2,986). But in one significant respect the response to the wild girl strikingly departed from any already established pattern. Like the other wild children, she struck observers as strange and "savage," but for some reason, and unlike the others, she was perceived to be not only "wild" but also *exotic*. The physical descriptions we have of the wild girl, admittedly scant, offer no clue to explain this unusual response. According to the *Mercure* correspondents, she appeared to be about eighteen years old; she was of middle size, had a tanned neck and complexion, and blue and lively eyes; she ate raw food and roots, which she dug out of the earth with her thumb and index finger; she drank water on her knees from a bucket, like a cow; she slept on the floor (refusing to do it on a mattress); she climbed trees with unbelievable agility, fished and swam very well, and imitated the songs of the birds "of her country" (2,986).[37] Whereas the people who encountered Peter thought he was born of "a father and mother like one of us" (i.e., European) and became a savage due to his lack of contact with other human beings (or was no "savage" but an "idiot" who did not look like one), those who encountered the wild girl advanced a different explanation for her strangeness. They were convinced that she was a savage because she had come *from another country* and they interpreted her behaviour and progress accordingly.

Because the girl changed dramatically and made great intellectual advances in the space of a few weeks only, it is difficult from these letters to assess exactly what she was like and did at first, and in particular to what extent she could already speak. It is said that, having had little contact with the world, she knew "only a few badly-articulated French words" (2,983), and some remarkable examples of the wild girl's language were transcribed: "She calls a Fillet *Debily*, in her Country's dialect; to say good morning, Girl, one said, according to her, *Yas yas, fioul*, and to call her, they said *Riam riam, fioul*; this shows that she begins to understand the meaning of French words, interpreting them in relation to those of her Country" (2,987). The spectacular transformation and religious conversion the wild girl underwent in these first weeks was not painless: it provoked a serious deterioration in her health and a sharp decrease of her fearsome strength (Mlle Leblanc told Racine that she had once prevented six men from entering her room by holding the door shut). But the *Mercure* letters state that she submitted voluntarily and appreciated the efforts of her benefactors. She began to eat bread to please her caretakers, even though it made her ill, and stopped climbing trees after being told that it was inappropriate in one of her sex. She expressed the wish to be baptized into the "Earthly Paradise," as she called the churches, and having heard that she was to be taken to court, when someone went to visit her in the hospice "she does not dare appear, cries and worries, fearing she will be taken away, because she is very happy there, and well taken-care-of" (2,988). The girl's utter ignorance of the value and use of money, her imperviousness to threats or caresses, and her frightful screams at the approach of any man were all seen as evidence of her unwavering "wisdom." Persuaded that "she must obey to see one day her Mother the Holy Virgin" (2,990), she gaily did her share of housework. She nevertheless retained some of her wildness and displayed it for the benefit of others' curiosity. When the archbishop of Vienna, passing through the village, asked to see her, witnesses watched, "with a kind of horror, how this Girl ate more than a pound and a half of raw Beef" (2,990).

Right before arriving in Châlons the wild girl had been seen beyond Vitry-le-François in the company of another girl, "a Negress" (a "Moresse," in the second letter), from whom she parted after the two girls fought over a rosary. The "Negress" was later spotted in the nearby village of Cheppe and then disappeared. The wild girl's foreignness was taken for granted, but in view of her lack of knowledge of French and unfamiliarity with the world her "country of birth" could not be identified with precision. This difficulty was circumvented by means of an experiment whose outcome led the author of the first letter to conclude that she came not from Norway, as had been said, but from the French Antilles: "a Person from Châlons, who has been to Guadeloupe, having shown her a *Cassava*, or *Manioc*, which is a Bread eaten by the Savages of the Antilles, she screamed with joy" (2,984). As additional proof, she had a similar reaction when shown other objects from the same country. Two further points about her past had been learned "by dint of making her speak" (2,984): she had crossed the sea and she had lived for a while with a lady of quality who had given her clothes (until then she had been covered only in skins) and taught her to embroider and do tapestry, but she could not say where that had been because the lady did not allow her to see anyone else or go out, and she eventually had to leave because the lady's husband could not stand her presence. The wild girl's baptism record (she was baptized on 16 June 1732, her godfather and godmother being M. Memmie le Moine, administrator of the hospice, and Marie-Nicole d'Halle, superior of the same hospice) indicates that she was about eleven years old, had been "born in or transported at a very young age to some Island in America," and did not know or remember her parents.[38] Inasmuch as she was taken to be exotic, the central question evoked by her strange presence was not how she had survived in the (nearby) wild but rather where she had come from. Contemporary views of her "wild" condition were not merely predicated on lack (of culture, of language, of ideas) but hinted at *another* culture and *another* language – but still not at ideas. What puzzled the girl's interlocutors and observers was that she remembered practically nothing of her early life and that her few lasting memories seemed vague and confused. They devised experiments to stimulate her memory and made conjectures to solve the mystery of her past.

Parisians reacted to the discovery of the wild girl in the same way the British had reacted to the discovery of Peter: with curiosity followed by indifference. "When the news reached Paris," wrote the Jansenist poet Louis Racine (1692–1763), son of the playwright, "people talked about nothing but the Wild Girl and how she should be brought to court; but since news are quickly forgotten when something else becomes the topic of conversation, people stopped talking about the Savage."[39] In later years Marie-Angélique was interviewed, in Champagne, Versailles, and Paris, by members of the nobility, the clergy, and the republic of letters, some of whom wrote and published long accounts. Charles Philippe d'Albert, duc de Luynes (1695–1758), recounted, in his *Mémoires*, her visit to Versailles in September 1753.[40]

The wild girl's biography, *Histoire d'une jeune fille sauvage, Trouvée dans les Bois à l'âge de dix ans* (1755), was attributed to Madame Hecquet or to Charles-Marie de La Condamine (1701–1774), a traveller and philosopher with a longstanding interest in "exotic" savages. It was based on conversations with Mlle Leblanc and the testimony of other persons who knew her, and the author hoped it would encourage further investigation of the girl's past: "This is one of the reasons why I wrote it."[41] The *Eclaircissement sur la fille sauvage*, Racine's "clarification" of his earlier reference to the wild girl in "Epître II sur l'homme" (1747), was also based on conversations with Mlle Leblanc and testimonies of people who knew her in Châlons. Monboddo saw the former wild girl during a stay in France in 1765. He made a trip to Songi expecting to recover the objects she carried when she was found but met with no success. Upon his return to Edinburgh Monboddo commissioned his clerk William Robertson to prepare a translation of the *Histoire*, to which he contributed a preface tackling the story's significance. By then copies of the original *Histoire* were hard to find, but Mlle Leblanc sold them for a small profit. Monboddo printed her address so that readers could buy it and verify his allegations if they so wished.[42]

The degree to which Marie-Angélique achieved "civilization" (language, manners, religion, manual skills, work habits) was unequalled by any other wild child, yet her achievements came at great cost to her health and spirit and did not prevent her later life from being a series of misadventures. Her change of life and diet, as well as the frequent bleedings administered to reduce her strength and tame her wildness, caused serious illnesses, pains in her stomach and throat, nervous contractions, and melancholy. Moreover, she was unable to secure a permanent patron, occupation, or income. Her first protector, M. d'Epinoy, having disappeared from her life before long (Madame H...t surmised that since he was not listed among those in attendance at her baptism he may have been dead by then), she lived for a while in a religious community in Châlons. In 1737 she had a chance to replay her earlier wildness for the queen of Poland (the mother of Marie Leszczynska, Louis XV's wife), who was passing through Châlons. She hunted rabbits and uttered piercing cries. When one of the queen's officers, having heard that Marie-Angélique never let any man touch her, "wanted to make the experiment," the promptitude with which she repelled him and "the fury in her eyes" convinced him that it was true.[43] Mlle Leblanc told Madame H...t that even though "she had been tame for several years ... her moods, her manners, and even her voice and her speech appeared to be ... those of a little girl of four or five." Charmed, the queen made known her desire to take the wild girl with her to Lorraine and place her in a convent in Nancy, but Marie-Angélique's caretakers dissuaded her from accepting the queen's offer.[44]

For a while Marie-Angélique found a new protector in the duc d'Orléans, who met her in Châlons "on his return from Metz in 1744" and after that paid a pension for her upkeep. In time she became increasingly uncomfortable living where everyone remembered her savage state and arranged a transfer to a convent in Ste Menehould. On her arrival there in September 1747 she chanced upon La Condamine at the inn: "He had dinner with her and the Hostess, and spoke to Mlle le Blanc, without her knowing that he was looking for her nor that she was the object of his curiosity." Hearing that Mlle Leblanc regretted not having followed the duc d'Orléans's proposal to have her enter a convent in Paris, La Condamine informed her protector, who found her a place with the Nouvelles Catholiques, in the rue Sainte Anne, in Paris, and went to see her there. She had her first communion and confirmation and projected to become a nun at the Visitation in Chaillot, but her plans were thwarted, first by a severe head injury and then by the duke's death while she was recovering at the Hospitaliers of the Faubourg St Marceau.[45] Her protector dead, her pension reduced by the new duke (from six hundred to two hundred livres, not enough to cover her expenses in the convent), she was neglected and forgotten.[46]

Madame H...t made Mlle Leblanc's acquaintance "under such sad circumstances" in November 1752. During the meetings that provided the material for the *Histoire*, the author requested a demonstration of the wild girl's savagery, witnessing with the greatest astonishment what remained of her "agility and speed" ("it cannot be conceived without having seen it, so swift and singular is her way of running") and "inconceivable eye mobility," now performed only on demand, "because the rest of the time her eyes are like ours; fortunately, she says, because many efforts were made to cease them from so moving, and often people despaired of succeeding." Despite unrelenting pecuniary difficulties, which had forced her to move to a small room put at her disposal by a charitable person, Mlle Leblanc's trust in God was intact: "Why, said she, with a confidence that astonished me, would God have come to seek me and take me from among the wild beasts, and make me a Christian? Could it be to abandon me when I have become a Christian, and let me starve to death? That is impossible. I know no one but him; he is my father; the Blessed Virgin is my mother: they will take care of me." With these words the narrative reached its climax. The "pleasure" with which the author reported them "pays me with interest for all the effort I put into the composition of what has just been read."[47]

The wild girl's humanization and conversion were complete, and her faith and confidence may have been admirable, but her situation remained dismal. Her visit to Versailles, during which the queen attentively listened to her story, resulted in a one-time gift of "3 or 4 louis." When Racine and his daughter visited her, she was melancholic and solitary – but as she related her story her eyes seemed to recover something of their singular movement. Racine's faith matched Mlle Leblanc's: "I ignore where she is now: but I am assured that she lacks nothing."[48] When Monboddo sought her out in 1765, he most likely anticipated another astonishing exhibition of savagery, and he therefore deplored that Mlle Leblanc was in poor health and had lost her extraordinary physical faculties (she would have been in her mid-forties or early fifties, depending on whether she was nine, ten, or eighteen when she was found in 1731). All that was left of her original state was a certain wildness in her look. Monboddo nevertheless treasured the meeting, because "this Girl, who had been born and bred a savage, and could give so good an account of that state by her speaking the French language," was "the greatest curiosity I had ever seen."[49] He questioned Mlle Leblanc intensively about her early savage ways but said very little about her adult life in France.

The *Histoire* supplemented the sketchy depiction of the wild girl's discovery, capture, and taming in the *Mercure* letters. Her first appearance in Songi, "barefoot, the body covered with rags and animal skins, the hair under a crown of calabash, black face and hands, like a Negress," was a memorable scene. The people who saw her thought she was the devil – soon afterwards they would call her "the Shepherd's beast." They watched with shock as she killed with her short and thick club the ferocious dog someone threw at her and "full of joy at her victory she jumped many times over the dog's carcass." Then she climbed a tree and went to sleep. The vicomte d'Epinoy sent orders that the strange creature who had arrived in his lands be captured, but it was necessary to resort to tricks to make her come down the tree. Someone guessed that she must be thirsty, "a very simple conjecture which nonetheless reveals great knowledge of the ways and customs of the Savages," but the wild girl fooled her captors: she drank the water they offered her and climbed straight up the tree. The same "expert" had another idea: to place a woman and some children close by ("because ordinarily the Savages did not run away from them like they did from men") and to have them show "a cheerful appearance and smiling face." The wild girl succumbed to these displays of sympathy. She was captured and brought to the kitchen of the castle, where she startled witnesses by quickly devouring some poultry and a rabbit. She tried to escape many times, but each time she was followed and recaptured. The most persistent, and in her caretakers' view offensive, of her "wild" habits was her love of raw meats and blood, but she was known to eat the leaves, branches, and roots of trees too. In the course of a sumptuous dinner at M. d'Epinoy's, realizing that none of her preferred dainties was available, she ran like a flash to the pond and filled her apron with frogs, which she happily distributed to the guests, saying *"Tien man man, donc tien."* She could not understand why the others did not appreciate her gift. Underneath her savage behaviour and looks, she was eager to please. As she became tamer she evinced "a very happy temperament and a gentle and humane character that the savage and ferocious habits necessary for the preservation of her life had not entirely effaced."[50]

Mlle Leblanc's visitors endeavoured to find out more (or, when there was nothing to be found, to make conjectures) about her earlier tribulations and displacements. The wild girl and her companion had been sighted in the region a few days before Marie-Angélique's capture. She was later told, and informed Madame H...t in turn, that M. de St Martin, a gentleman of the neighbourhood, saw the girls swimming in the Marne and taking them for moorhens shot at them (and missed). The wild girl came out of the water with a fish in each hand and an eel between her teeth. It was after cleaning and devouring the fish that she found the rosary over which the girls quarrelled. Our girl beat her companion with her weapon but then felt compassion, "that movement of nature which leads us to assist our fellow creatures."[51] According to the *Histoire*, she dressed the wound and the girls separated, "the wounded one taking the path to the river, and the victorious one towards Songi." According to the *Eclaircissement*, when she returned with the unguent to dress her companion's wound, the latter had disappeared. Some travellers found the wounded girl and took her to a village, where she died.[52] Of the time preceding the girls' arrival in Champagne, Mlle Leblanc retained "only remote and confused memories." Madame H...t was deeply aware of the problems involved in the attempt to reconstruct the girl's early story. Mlle Leblanc had "confessed" that "during all the time she spent in the forests, she had almost no other ideas than the feeling of her needs, and the desire to satisfy them," and only began to reflect "after having received some education." To complicate matters, at present she could not discriminate between what she genuinely remembered and what she thought later or heard others say: "There are many things, in what she has told me in several occasions, about which she could not affirm having retained a distinct memory without admixture of facts and ideas acquired after she began to reflect on the questions posed to her then and afterwards."[53] Madame H...t distrusted the account of the girl's early life in the *Mercure* letters (how could she have communicated such a detailed story shortly after she was found, when her command of the French language was so poor?); however, the narrative that resulted from her own research and speculation did not considerably deviate from those early rumours.

From diverse clues, Madame H...t inferred that the wild girl was born an Eskimo of Labrador in northern Canada. Her white skin, "similar to ours," proved that she was not originally from Africa or the warmer zones of America but from the Arctic regions. Her only childhood memory was of seeing in the sea or a river (she could not say which) a great beast swimming with two feet like a dog, which to Madame H...t's mind was a seal. To elicit recognition and memories Madame H...t conducted experiments modelled on those reported in the *Mercure* letters. She first compared Mlle Leblanc's description of the weapons and other implements the girls supposedly carried on their arrival in Champagne (clubs; a kind of billhook to disembowel animals and defend themselves; a sack or pouch for the weapons, attached to a large skin belt that reached to their knees; a necklace and earrings) with Eskimo figures. Always willing to help, Mlle Leblanc interpolated that the inscriptions in the weapons might assist in the identification of her nation, but, as ill luck would have it, they had been taken away from her at M. d'Epinoy's and kept as curiosities. Madame H...t then showed Mlle Leblanc dolls representing different kinds of savages from Canada in their typical dress, and even though, Madame H...t noted, the Eskimo dolls were not the prettiest, they were the ones upon which Mlle Leblanc fixed her attention, "considering them one after the other in silence, not as something new and extraordinary, but as something already seen, without knowing where, which she now tried to recognize." Seeking verbal confirmation, Madame H...t asked Mlle Leblanc to provide details of the dolls' dress, but the latter said that "such remote ideas ... did not count for much."[54] All the inquisitive biographer had to fall back on was what she perceived as Mlle Leblanc's first, as if instinctive, focus on the Eskimo figures.

Madame H...t's answer to the riddle of the wild girl's past was that she (and perhaps her companion as well) was kidnapped by a European captain and taken to one of the colonies in the Antilles to be sold as a slave, artificially painted black as a joke or fraud (to pass her as an African), and then transported by sea to France by her new masters (the lady who taught her to embroider and the man who mistreated her). Neither Racine nor Monboddo disapproved of this account of the girl's origin and foreignness. Racine proposed more embellishments: the two girls were either brought from America in a ship that wrecked or born in a ship and abandoned in a forest, "where they might have been nurtured by animals until they could have themselves found their nourishment." Less interested in reconstructing Mlle Leblanc's life history than in learning, through her, about the condition of her people and their place in his grand scheme of human progress, Monboddo managed to draw out a wealth of detail about her country and culture. He learned that the wild girl's country was "very cold" and "covered with snow a great part of the year"; that the children learned to swim and climb trees "as soon as they can walk"; that her people subsisted by fishing, wore skins, did not use fire, and had elaborate funerals:

She says that she remembers the custom of funerals in her country; that the defunct is carried to a place where there is a great deal of snow, where he is set upon his breech in a sort of case, not unlike an easy chair. That his relations approach him with many reverences and prostrations, and the nearest relation makes a speech to him, which she repeats in her own language, importing that he has eyes, ears, hands, arms, &c. yet is no more, but is gone above to the most high; and then the ceremony is concluded with what she calls *un cri de tristesse*, which is a cry that they also use upon occasion of any danger or distress, and which she remembers to have used upon a particular occasion to the terror and astonishment of the whole neighbourhood.

From the fact that the few words Mlle Leblanc remembered were "chiefly French words, spoken in the tone and manner of her own country," Monboddo inferred that her native language was "little better than inarticulate sounds from the throat, in the formation of which the organs of the mouth have very little share." He corrected Madame H...t's conjecture: the wild girl was "originally of a white race of people, living somewhere upon the coast of Hudson's Bay," either the "*Huron* race" or "a nation speaking the Huron language."[55]

The accounts of the wild girl of Songi are unique and puzzling for several reasons. First, the wild girl could speak. It is true that we do not have her story in her own words; even so, we know that, unlike Peter, who was only observed and spoken or written about, she participated in the production of all the accounts by answering questions and supplying information. The assumption, and the hope, had been that when and if wild children learned to speak they would not only tell wonderful stories about their early lives but also offer enough certain facts to settle all disputes regarding their condition and its cause. The wild girl of Songi spoke distinctly, but what she said did not solve any controversy, did not dispel the mystery of her past, and brought about more confusion, suspicions, and disappointment.

Second, the wild girl spoke but lacked clear memories. She did not remember clearly even the events of her most recent past, and those memories she did have might have been the product of later reflection and hearing others tell her story. Tinland's explanation for the wild girl's lack of memories of her country of birth and exotic adventures is simply that there was nothing to remember. He argues that the wild girl was just another case of *ensauvagement* ("wildness" caused by isolation) and that the story put together by Mlle Leblanc was a false memory fabricated in response to her interlocutors' pressing questions.[56] The relation between memory, identity, and story making and the difficulties encountered in trying to separate "true" from "false" memories are urgent topics of debate in our own time. The story of the wild girl unquestionably constitutes a superb example of the intricacies and traps of memory and its role in the construction of personal narrative. Still, as we have seen, Madame H...t, and Mlle Leblanc herself, were aware of these problems and deliberately strove to sift original impressions and later additions or distortions. For instance, Mlle Leblanc's repeated claim that "she twice crossed the sea" was taken as authentic, but what she once said about being in the sea for a long time because the ship made stops in different islands "could not be but the repetition of some comment that she overheard about her adventures."[57] A more delicate question is why the account Mlle Leblanc gave Monboddo in 1765 was so much more elaborate than the earlier ones. Had she been able to remember more incidents and details about her early life in the years between the *Histoire* and Monboddo's visit? Was she imagining more? Were her memory or imagination triggered in any way by Monboddo's questions and the direction of his interrogation?[58] Half a century before Tinland re-edited the *Histoire*, and knowing very little about the wild girl, Maurice Halbwachs advanced a different explanation for her inability to remember: the social character of memory. Suddenly deprived of her social context, abruptly separated from family and group and transported to a place with a different language, people, and customs, the girl could not hold on to the many memories she originally possessed of her first years. In general, a child that is transplanted from one society to another "will have lost the ability to remember in the second society all that he did and all that impressed him, which he used to recall without difficulty, in the first." In contrast to Tinland's condescending reaction to Madame H...t's experiments and inferences, Halbwachs implicitly applauded the means she employed to stimulate Mlle Leblanc's memory as the right ones: to "retrieve" some of the child's "uncertain and incomplete memories" he must be shown, "in the new society of which he is part," images of his original group and milieu.[59]

Third, even though all the wild children gave rise to conjectures about their unknown (and unknowable) pasts, the theories about the wild girl's origin were distinct and singular. Her status is ambiguous: she was perceived, alternatively or simultaneously, as a member of one of the "savage nations" that so interested her contemporaries and as the *Puella Campanica*, an example of Linnaeus's *Homo ferus*. Her "wild" appearance and habits could be interpreted either as the expression of a different (savage) culture or as the effects of early deprivation of human contact. Reviewing the *Histoire* for *Nouvelles littéraires*, the abbé Guillaume-Thomas Raynal (1713–1796) weighed both alternatives, suggesting that the girl's epistemic value would rise if she were indeed an isolated wild child like the boy found among bears in Lithuania in 1669: "If this girl was really born in the country of the Eskimos, all she did was to preserve the customs of her nation, and there would be nothing marvellous in that. But it would be interesting for the philosophers if this child had been born in France, if she had been abandoned by whatever accident in a forest as it happens sometimes, and if nature alone taught her all she could do."[60] In the recent literature on wild children, the story of Marie-Angélique is often reinscribed as a "typical" case of isolation and her purported exoticism dismissed as a figment of her interlocutors' wild imaginations. But if this were the case, then why do we find such agreement in all the testimonies of people who met the wild girl, and not a single dissenting view? Why is there no record of similar conjectures being concocted in response to any other wild child? None of the accounts contains a detailed physical description of the wild girl, as a child or as an adult, nor do we have portraits of her as we do of Peter. What did her European observers see in her? Was their certainty that she was foreign motivated by something distinctive in the way she looked?

Fourth, the wild girl is one of the very few wild children who fully "recovered," and thus her initial strangeness cannot be reduced to congenital idiocy or some other defect. Supporters of the view that she was a case of isolation commonly ascribe her recovery to the presence of a companion, that is, to the fact that her "isolation" was not complete. Yet despite her full recovery the experts on wild children approach her with extreme caution, granting her less attention than other cases and never viewing, or using, her as best example of the class. One reason that is given is the low quality of the evidence. Itard, recalling the wild girl as an antecedent of his own savage, admitted that her story was "one of the most detailed" but "so badly told, that if we extract first what is insignificant and then what is incredible in it, it offers but very few particulars worthy of notice." Zingg laments that the sources on the *Puella Campanica* are "inadequate and especially incommensurate with the importance of this case ... marred by fantastic theories of her origin."[61] Another reason is that, whatever else they do say, the accounts do not dwell on the wild girl's *isolation*, which would in the future be seen as the wild child's most defining characteristic. As Rauber put it, "the extent to which the girl was previously deprived of human companionship remains uncertain." Julia Douthwaite suggests a third reason: it may have been precisely the wild girl's exceptional recovery, in combination with her gender, that confounded later writers.[62]

Whatever her origin and the reasons for her initial strangeness and eventual integration may have been, Mlle Leblanc's end was quite unlike Peter's. They were both called "savages," but each child's wildness was interpreted differently and provoked different responses. The old "Wild Boy," always strange and always silent, benefited until the last day of his long life from governmental protection and support, gentle care and supervision, enough curiosity to keep him interesting, and a rural and free setting. Mlle Leblanc, fully "Frenchified," urbanized, and converted to Catholicism, was destitute already in her thirties, and nobody seems to have cared to record her whereabouts after 1765 or even her death. She spoke; she told and retold her story; for a while she attracted the attention of powerful and learned people – but her interlocutors still did not know what to make of or how to provide for her.[63]

CHAPTER FOUR

The
Debates

Let us delineate his Condition, if we can: He seems to be
the very Creature which the learned World have, for
many Years past, pretended to wish for.

D. Defoe, *Mere Nature Delineated*

WILD CHILDREN'S extraordinary condition offered Enlightenment philosophers a motive for reflection as well as empirical evidence to support or illustrate a variety of views and theories in epistemology, natural history, and anthropology. The most consequential seventeenth-century accounts of wild children, such as Digby's (Jean of Liège), Tulp's (the *Juvenis balans*), and Connor's (the Lithuanian boys), had been embedded in philosophical or medical discussions. The intense concern with wild children evinced throughout the eighteenth century partly built upon these earlier accounts and problems. It was also linked to three other sources of cultural and intellectual concern: the longstanding myth of the "wild man," the encounters with "savage" peoples, and the growing curiosity about the anthropoid apes. The figures of the mythical wild man, the savage, and the ape impinged on the reception of wild children in the eighteenth century, infiltrating, as it were, the conceptual frameworks through which they were grasped, the expectations they raised, and the speculations they inspired.[1]

In this chapter I review the Enlightenment debates featuring wild children. The main themes and questions on which wild children were expected to shed light are innate ideas and sensationist epistemology; the "forbidden experiment"; the state of nature; the definition (or essential characteristics) of man; the place of man in the system of nature; the origin and implications of human diversity; and conjectural and progressive histories of man. In the last section of the chapter I discuss intimations and survivals: how some eighteenth-century debates prefigured problems that would be fully formulated in the next century and how some questions posed and positions taken by Enlightenment philosophers and naturalists may still be discerned in more recent discussions in anthropology and social theory.

The first significant debate in which wild children played a central role was the dispute concerning the existence of *innate ideas*, associated with the names of René Descartes (1596–1650) and John Locke (1632–1704). How could the existence of innate ideas be proved or refuted? One way to do it was to determine whether children who grew up in isolation from other human beings or among animals had any ideas – in particular those of God, the soul, and morality – before their return to society. Philosophers opposed to innate ideas were the ones who most exploited the available reports of wild children to champion empiricism (knowledge comes from experience), sensationism (knowledge and ideas derive from the senses), materialism (the soul is not a separate substance), and even atheism. The most frequently cited case was that of the Lithuanian boys, and it was almost invariably linked to the account, published by the permanent secretary of the Parisian Academy of Sciences, Bernard le Bovier de Fontenelle (1657–1757), of a young deaf-mute of Chartres who suddenly recovered his hearing and a few weeks later began to speak. Questioned by theologians on his earlier state, the youth admitted having until then lived "a purely animal life" with no knowledge of God, the soul, or the goodness and evil of actions. The account ended with a declaration that would be repeated verbatim by Condillac and at the turn of the century by Bonnaterre and Itard: "The greatest source of ideas among men is in their dealings with each other."[2]

Wild children made an appearance in influential works by La Mettrie and Condillac. In the last chapter of *Histoire naturelle de l'ame* (1745), titled "Stories Confirming That All Ideas Come from the Senses," the notorious Julien Offray de La Mettrie (1709–1751) furnished five cases as empirical corroboration for his sensationist and materialist argument against innate ideas: the deaf-mute of Chartres; a man without moral ideas; Cheselden's blind man; the method of teaching deaf-mutes developed by Johann Conrad Amman (1669–1724) in Amsterdam; a child found among bears; and the wild men, called "Satyres." These cases are a compendium of figures interesting to eighteenth-century philosophers by virtue of their extraordinary, defective, primitive, or quasi-human nature. If individuals with impaired sensory input, negligible experience of other people, or no education had no ideas of God and morality, it could be inferred that these ideas were not innate. La Mettrie recounted the story of the Lithuanian boys and, like Defoe, he read the wild child's dislike and avoidance of other human beings as a sign of lack of reason: the proof that Connor's "poor child" had no reason at all was "that he ignored the misery of his condition; and that instead of seeking commerce with men, he ran away from them, and desired only to return with his bears." For years he "lived mechanically," his intellect resembling that of "a beast, a newborn child, or a man who is asleep, in a state of lethargy or apoplexy." La Mettrie returned to the wild children in the section on "Satyres," where he described these "*Hommes sauvages*" (the great apes) and contrasted them with other cases of "*Sauvages*" (isolated children). Since wild children do not think during their savage existence, which passes "like a dream," they are unaware of the wretchedness of their condition ("their wild life, however long, does not bother them, since for them it has lasted only an instant") and retain no memory of it. The examples in this section are the boy exhibited in Holland, who had been found "in the desert among goats" and preserved "the same inclinations, the same sound of the voice, the same imbecility portrayed in his physiognomy," and the recent case, much talked about in Parisian circles, of the wild girl of Châlons in Champagne. La Mettrie brought the individual wild children together (before Linnaeus) and reduced them to the status of useful examples. By 1751, when he revised this work for inclusion in *Œuvres philosophiques* (as *Traité de l'ame*), La Mettrie had heard "many particulars" about the wild girl "who had eaten her sister" from "Mgr. the Marshal of Saxe," but he did not repeat them as they were "more curious than necessary to understand and explain what is most surprising about these cases." Construed as equivalent and interchangeable ("Only one suffices and provides the key to all others; at bottom they are all alike"), wild children were on their way to becoming a class, their particularities understated or overlooked so that every case fit the type.[3]

The sensationist philosophy expounded by Étienne Bonnot, abbé de Condillac (1714–1780), was an extension of Locke's empiricism. In *Essai sur l'origine des connaissances humaines* (1746) Condillac argued that to have ideas it is necessary to have signs (gestures or language) with which to express them. Like La Mettrie, Condillac followed his theoretical exposition with a chapter presenting "facts" to support the theory – the stories of the deaf-mute of Chartres and the boy found in Lithuania in 1694. But

Condillac's approach to these cases was novel, his philosophical objective being not to find out whether the ideas of God, the soul, and morality are innate (he was already convinced that they are not) but rather to ascertain the origin of ideas in general and the order of their formation. He wished that the young man of Chartres had been asked questions of epistemological rather than theological import, namely what ideas he had first acquired after his recovery. Furthermore, Condillac formulated the first fully developed psychological explanation of the wild child's destitution. If an individual with "healthy and well-constituted organs" were raised among bears, the demands posed by his extraordinary circumstances (to provide for his physical needs and satisfy his passions) would not suffice to develop his intellectual faculties. Only the weakest traces of the operations of the soul would be perceptible in him:

Almost without recollection, he would frequently go through the same state without recognizing that he has already experienced it. Without memory, he would have no signs to make up for the absence of things. Only possessed of an imagination which he is unable to have at his disposal, his perceptions would not be aroused except when chance presents him with an object to which he would have been connected by circumstances; finally, without reflection, he would receive the impressions that things make upon his senses, and obey them by instinct only. He would imitate the bears in everything, have a cry resembling theirs, and drag himself about on his hands and feet. We are so inclined to imitation, that perhaps even a Descartes in his place would not attempt to walk on his feet only.

Of the three kinds of signs postulated by Condillac – accidental, natural, and established (conventional or arbitrary) – only the first would be accessible to "a child raised among the bears." Only through contact with other human beings can a child acquire arbitrary signs and attain the full development of the soul's faculties. It is in this sense that Condillac understood Fontenelle's claim about the importance of human interaction: "A consequence of the fact that men cannot make up signs unless they live together is that the source of their ideas, when their mind begins to form, is only in their dealings with each other. I say *when their mind begins to form* because it is evident that, once it has made some progress, it knows the art of making up signs and can acquire ideas without any assistance from others." Condillac's *Essai* set forth a philosophical account of wild children's condition with reference to an epistemological framework for which the stories of wild children were simultaneously wielded as confirmation. This text was crucial in turning wild children (and, potentially, children in general) into privileged objects of knowledge and intervention.[4]

In *Traité des sensations* (1754) Condillac considered the extent to which knowledge could be acquired through sensation alone without the aid of signs. To find out which ideas we owe to each of our senses he imagined a statue, "inwardly organized like us, and animated by a spirit deprived of any kind of ideas," to which he gave use of one sense at a time, beginning with smell. In due course Condillac explored the amount and kinds of knowledge the statue could have if she (in French, "statue" is female) were to have the use of her five senses but no contact with any other (human) being. The statue's natural needs (to feed herself, protect and defend herself against accidents, and satisfy her curiosity) and the accidents to which she might be exposed would determine the development of her knowledge and faculties. Since, Condillac argued, knowledge arises from experience, experience from need, and need from the alternative between pleasure and pain, it could be rightly concluded that "with the aid of sense only" the statue would acquire all kinds of knowledge. The theoretical discussion was backed once again with the example of Connor's Lithuanian boy: if, like him, the statue were occupied exclusively with the need to find food, she would live a purely animal life with no time left to study other objects. Her intellectual faculties dulled, she would learn from animals, just as the Lithuanian boy had done. The *Traité*'s conclusion that "all our knowledge comes from the senses, and particularly the sense of touch," which "instructs the others," should not make us forget that in the *Essai* Condillac granted signs an indispensable part in the formation of ideas and the progress of the mind.[5] Indeed, Condillac was not alone in relating wild children's apparent lack of reason to their lack of conventional signs. Defoe, having noticed that Peter's senses seemed to be in perfect condition but that his impressions were not accompanied by any discrimination or ideas ("When a Batallion of Soldiers, exercising in the Park, fired their Volleys, the Horses, the Dogs, the Deer, all discovered an Emotion, but he none at all"), reasoned, like Condillac in the *Essai*, that sensations alone do not lead to ideas. "Words are to us, the Medium of Thought," Defoe wrote; "we cannot conceive of Things, but by their Names, and in the very Use of their Names." Christian Wolff (1679–1754) also brought up the Lithuanian boys (and, predictably, the deaf-mute of Chartres) to strengthen his argument in *Psychologia rationalis* (1734) that reason cannot be actualized without language.[6]

Condillac put forward his famous statue as a definitive refutation of inn-atism. The statue, he wrote, "is nothing except what she has acquired. Why would it not be the same in the case of man?" The statue stood for "man" – thus the passage just cited appeared under the subheading "Man is nothing except what he has acquired" – but in a special way: it was both a fictive rep-resentation of man-still-unformed and a narrative-epistemological strategy designed to reveal the process of formation of a human being. Philosophers interested in origins (of ideas, knowledge, language, morality, inequal-ity, society, and so on) had to resort to speculative devices like Condillac's statue because certain kinds of claims about human beings seemed other-wise impossible to prove. In fact, Enlightenment philosophers believed that there *was* a way: if children were raised in isolation *on purpose*, as part of a controlled experiment, these questions could be investigated empirically.[7]

Two old stories in which history and legend are intertwined tell of attempts to conduct such an experiment. According to Herodotus, the Egyptian king Psammetichus (664–610 BCE) had two ordinary children raised in isolation. A similar experiment was reported in Salimbene's *Chronicle* as having been performed by Holy Roman Emperor Frederick II (1194–1250). In both cases the children were provided with everything they needed but prevented from hearing any word. The purpose was to find out what language the isolated children would speak when they reached the right age. Since Psammetichus assumed this would be the original language (the language spoken by the most ancient people) he believed the experiment would disclose whether the Egyptians were indeed the oldest nation, as they held. Frederick II was just interested in knowing what language the children would speak. Neither ruler doubted that there *would* be a language. The outcome of the experi-ment was different in each case. In Herodotus's story, it was a success. The children spoke a Phrygian word, and it was determined (and accepted) that the Phrygians were the oldest nation. Psammetichus found the answer he was looking for and the children apparently did not suffer any harmful con-sequence. In contrast, Frederick's attempt was a disastrous failure: all the children died. To Salimbene at least, the experiment did reveal something: without interaction with others, more than language fails to thrive. The children "could not live without clappings of the hands, and gestures, and gladness of countenance, and blandishments."[8]

In these early versions the "forbidden experiment" was hazarded by pow-erful rulers, yet the ones who revived it in the eighteenth century were phi-losophers and scientists. At first, it functioned as a speculative aid. Pierre

Bayle (1647–1706) recalled the earlier attempts in his polemic against innate ideas and religious intolerance: "You may perhaps remember ... that certain Princes were curious to discover the first language, or the language that Nature left to itself would teach us. They gave orders that some children not be taught to speak. A Great Mongol had another purpose: this was to embrace the religion of the country whose language was the one spoken by such a child; but the child spoke none. What a standard of truth for choosing a religion!"[9] La Mettrie closed the *Traité de l'ame* with a paraphrase of "one of the most beautiful passages from Antiquity," Arnobe's hypothetical description of a single child kept from birth in an underground hole "shaped like a bed," dark, and noiseless, so that his senses would receive as few impressions as possible. The child is cared for by a silent woman and released when he reaches adulthood. What would his ideas be then? La Mettrie painted a sad picture: "More stupid than a beast, he will have no more feeling than a piece of wood or a stone." The thought experiment led him to three conclusions: that there is no divine and immortal soul; that there are no innate ideas, and that man owes everything to education: "There you see man! If he lived eternally separated from society he would not acquire a single idea. But let us polish this rough diamond, let us send this old child to school, *quantum mutatus ab illo* [how changed from what he was]? The Animal becomes a man, learned and wise." In Arnobe's conjecture, the "old child" would not suffer irreversible effects from his unusual upbringing, and even belated education would turn him into "a man, learned and wise" after all. Still, La Mettrie did not go so far as to recommend that the experiment be conducted in reality.[10]

Other philosophers did – or at least they expressed the desire, in writing or before a scientific society, to try such an experiment, also indicating what they expected to learn from it. In *Lettre sur le progrès des sciences* (1752), Pierre-Louis Moreau de Maupertuis (1698–1759) advised that several groups of children be raised in isolation, a "metaphysical experiment" that would "not merely instruct us on the origin of languages" but also "teach us many other things about the origin of ideas themselves, and about the fundamental notions of the human mind." In the paper on "the principal means employed to discover the origin of the language, ideas, and knowledge of men" that Jean-Henri-Samuel Formey (1711–1797) read in 1762 to the Berlin Academy of Sciences (of which he was perpetual secretary, and Maupertuis had been president), he argued as well that an isolation experiment would settle the question. The observation of children and savages, of children found in forests, of the deaf-mute of Chartres, only exposes what we already know: "that we are what the situation in which we are born and in which we live make of us." Formey held that language was not an invention of the early human beings but had been taught to the first man by God. To prove it, he proposed that a group of children be separated from human society, looked after by silent nurses, and then allowed to live together in conditions similar to those of the first human groups. Formey predicted that the children would not invent language even if the experiment lasted several generations. Montesquieu (1689–1755) consigned yet another rendition of the forbidden experiment to his notebooks: "A prince could do a beautiful experiment. Raise three or four children like animals, with goats or with deaf-mute nurses. They would make a language for themselves. Examine this language. See nature in itself, and freed from the prejudices of education; learn from them, after they are instructed, what they had thought; exercise their mind by giving them all the things necessary to invent; finally, write the history of the experiment." Unlike Formey, Montesquieu imagined that the children would invent a language and have thoughts (but he did not predict what their language or thoughts might be). Although they did not foresee any adverse effects on the children, Formey and Montesquieu supposed that a prince, not a philosopher, was called upon to carry out (and authorize) the "beautiful experiment." Montesquieu's articulation of the experiment's reach is pregnant: "See nature in itself, and freed from the prejudices of education." The forbidden experiment was envisioned as that which would (artificially) "protect" the child from any kind of human influence or interference and in so doing permit the experimenter to screen the natural and the artificial or acquired, that is to say, to observe and study human nature.[11]

The stakes were high. Yet despite the many proposals and expressions of desire, we have no evidence that the experiment was performed in reality in the eighteenth century. All the same, the inordinate expectations tied to the imagined isolation experiment largely account for the intensified interest in wild children throughout the Enlightenment. Wild children were perceived, and welcomed, as fortuitous or natural instances of the forbidden experiment. Hence it was hoped that when – and if – the silent and unformed wild child was instructed she or he would provide the priceless information, insights, and answers philosophers expected to derive from this experiment. The encounters with wild children raised but did not satisfy these expectations because the children did not speak; spoke very little or seemed to have nothing of consequence to say (the Lithuanian boys and Peter); or spoke but what they said was puzzling (Marie-Angélique). On the one hand, each wild child was received *as if* he or she were the ultimate embodiment of the desired experiment; on the other, the child never yielded the hoped-for answers and the desire to conduct the experiment persisted. The fraught but inextricable relation between wild children and the forbidden experiment clarifies why time, money, and energy were spent so liberally – and would be spent even more liberally in the future – on efforts to educate wild children, especially to teach them language. At the same time, the rise of sensationist philosophy and its practical corollary (that the formation of ideas and the progress of the faculties depend upon our dealings with others) gradually eroded the certainty that a controlled isolation experiment would lead to anything but a disastrous outcome. Still, at this point curiosity and expectations prevailed over anticipations of disaster.

Enlightenment philosophers approached wild children to elucidate another of their pressing concerns: the question of the "state of nature," a notion that, as Sergio Landucci indicates, was used in three different senses. In a theological sense, the state of nature was opposed to the state of grace; in a juridical sense, to the civil state; and in an ethnological sense, to civilized life. Racine portrayed the wild girl of Songi as a representative of the state of nature in its first (theological) aspect:

> In earlier times scattered, fierce, and mute,
> Men wandered through the forests, we are told,
> Even though they still had only their nails as weapons,
> They filled them with cries, murders and dangers;
> And what our savage forebears were then,
> A girl in our time allows us to see with our own eyes.
> What her mouth articulated were not words,
> But from it only came out a sound, a piercing and fierce cry.
> Of the living animals her hand tore open,
> Quivering pieces assuaged her hunger.
> From childhood she wandered from mountain to mountain
> And she soiled her deserts with the blood of her companion.
> Why did she sacrifice her to her fury?
> What interest could have been so great to separate two hearts

United by their forests, their age and their misery?
Let us recognize the morals of our ancestors.

As a kind of living fossil, the wild girl made visible the savage, irrational, violent, and aimless condition of our ancestors and exemplified "the misery of man abandoned to himself." Lacking religion and morals, Racine's state of nature was a miserable, undesirable state from which men, like the wild girl, were saved through "the omnipotence of grace." But the Jansenist Racine was an exception. Most other eighteenth-century thinkers conceived wild children in relation to the third meaning of state of nature, the state of man outside (or before) society.[12]

Philosophers intent on investigating the state of nature faced a serious problem in that this state was by definition inaccessible to the enlightened member of civilized society. Wild children were interrogated to see if the condition in which they were found was equivalent or comparable to that state. Could the wild child, for better or worse untouched by society and civilization, offer the student of human nature a glimpse of (real, past, or potential) "natural man"? Defoe thought so: Peter's condition, assimilated to the forbidden experiment, was the answer to the philosopher's quest for natural man and the original language. Because Peter was "in a State of Meer Nature, and that, indeed, in the literal Sense of it ... He seems to be the very Creature which the learned World have, for many Years past, pretended to wish for, *viz.* one that being kept entirely from human Society, so as never to have heard any one speak, must therefore either not speak at all, or, if he did form any Speech to himself, then they should know what Language Nature would first form for Mankind." Among those who saw in the wild child a vision of the state of nature and drew lessons from it were Montesquieu and the abbé Raynal. At the beginning of *De l'esprit des loix* (1748) Montesquieu considered whether in the state of nature man is affected by any natural laws. Arguing that the first ideas of natural man would be concrete and connected with self-preservation and that all he would feel at first would be "weakness" and excessive "timidity," he offered as proof the known instances of "savages found in forests; trembling at everything, fleeing from everything." A footnote referred readers to the story of "the savage found in the forests of Hanover." Raynal's natural-man-in-the-guise-of-a-wild-child was the girl of Songi, whose fight with her companion showed that "the state of nature would be the despotism of the passions." The lesson was clear: we must not presume that "men free to follow only the movements of nature" would be better than contemporary civilized men, since "they would have had the same passions in the heart" without "the same motives to subdue them." Thus, Raynal affirmed, "the savage nations have always been barbarous nations."[13]

If wild children's condition was indeed equivalent to the state of nature, the picture they presented of it was, in Raynal's words, "quite humiliating for poor humanity." It is therefore understandable that proponents of a different, more optimistic view of natural man were reluctant to see him in wild children. For the main referent in the debate on the state of nature in the second half of the eighteenth century, the philosopher widely identified with the idea of the "noble savage," wild children did not exemplify this state. While in the second *Discours* Rousseau posed the fundamental philosophical problem of natural man as a question of "experiments" and "means" – "*What experiments would be necessary to achieve knowledge of natural man? And what are the means of carrying out these experiments in the midst of society?*" – he bypassed the possibility that wild children might *be* the means, as other philosophers thought. Rousseau did address the stories of wild children in the same *Discours*, as we know, but in a note, to argue that far from representing his (also isolated) natural man, they were *un*natural and monstrous. In adopting the quadruped position, in imitation of the animals with which they lived, wild children contradicted the most essential demand of man's physical organization. Their unusual skills were not the result of nature but of habit. Rousseau interpreted wild children as an extreme illustration of the perfectibility separating man from the animals.[14] But observers of wild children were often reminded of Rousseau, whether, like Tomko's guardian, to identify wild child and noble savage ("Rousseau should have seen and watched him. How much Rousseau's fiery imagination would have made him envy Tomko, had he described the fate of this pupil of nature!") or, like Frobenius confronting the wild boy of Kronstadt, to challenge Jean-Jacques to revise his views ("You state that those are the happy individuals who remove themselves from the social life into the woods. If you could look at this miserable man, you would see how much happier is your state than his").[15]

The celebrated director of the Jardin du Roi (Royal Botanical Garden) and author of the best-selling *Histoire naturelle, générale et particulière*, Georges-Louis Leclerc de Buffon (1707–1788), referred to wild children in two separate discussions of the state of nature. In *Histoire naturelle de l'homme* (1749) Buffon conceded that "wild man [*l'homme sauvage*]" was, of all animals, "the most singular, the least known, and the most difficult to describe" because we do not possess a reliable means to distinguish what we owe to nature from "what has been communicated to us through education, imitation, art and example." He continued: "An absolutely wild savage [*Un sauvage absolument sauvage*], such as the boy raised among bears, mentioned by Connor, the youth found in the forests of Hanover, or the little girl found in the woods in France," would be "a curious spectacle to a philosopher," who "could, by observing his savage, ascertain precisely the force of the appetites of nature; he would see the soul exposed, distinguish all its natural movements, and perhaps recognize in it more gentleness, more serenity and peace than in his own; perhaps he would see clearly that virtue belongs more to the wild man than to the civilized man, and that vice owes its birth to society." Buffon linked natural man and the known wild children, but rather than drawing, like Raynal and Montesquieu, pessimistic conclusions about the state of nature from the wild child's reported destitution, Buffon estimated that the careful study of such a savage was an important task that remained to be done. Moreover, he foretold that the observation of natural (or wild) man would uncover the moral superiority of nature over civilization.[16]

When Buffon reconsidered the "state of pure nature" almost ten years later, in his treatise on carnivorous animals, he seemed to have changed his mind. He now engaged directly with Rousseau – who had relied heavily on Buffon's natural history of man in the second *Discours* and would do so again in *Émile* (1762) – challenging the notion that an "ideal state of innocence, of high temperance, of complete abstinence from meat, of perfect tranquility" had ever existed. Rousseau's solitary savages were nowhere to be found, since all known human beings, including the savages met by travellers in remote corners of the world, lived in organized communities. Besides, unlike newborn animals, who "do not need their mother for more than a few months," children "perish" unless "assisted and cared for during many years." Buffon here defended a view of natural man that was diametrically opposed to Rousseau's conception of a noble but isolated savage, and he used *children* as proof that human beings could never have lived and thrived in complete isolation: "Therefore the state of pure nature is a known state; it is the Savage living in the wilderness, but living in a family, knowing his children, known by them, using speech and making himself understood." But then of course Buffon had somehow to account for the *known* cases of solitary savages who neither spoke nor formed families:

The wild girl caught in the woods of Champagne, the man found in the forests of Hanover, do not prove the opposite; they had lived in absolute solitude, they could have no idea of society, no use of signs or speech; but had they only encountered one another, the inclination of nature would have brought them together, and pleasure would have united them; attached one to the other, they would soon have understood each other, they would have first spoken the language of love between them, and then that of tenderness between them and their children; and moreover these two savages had been born of men in society and had no doubt been abandoned in the woods, not in the first age, because they would have perished, but at four, five or six years, at the age, in a word, when they were already strong enough in body to provide for their own subsistence, and yet too weak in mind to retain the ideas that had been communicated to them.

Against the confusion of natural man with the isolated wild children, Buffon proffered two arguments. If only Peter and Marie-Angélique had met, they would have discovered in each other their real (social, familial) nature. Perhaps realizing that some readers might shrink from the imaginative stretch required by this romantic scenario, Buffon reminded them that even the wild children were born within a social group. Their own origin was social, and their "wildness" a result of chance or criminal action, not nature.[17]

In the later part of the century the opposed positions on the relation between wild children and the state of nature were rearticulated by Monboddo and Blumenbach. To Monboddo's claim that wild children were living examples of natural man and proof of the real existence of the state of nature Blumenbach retorted that there was nothing *natural* about wild children's condition: "No condition can be conceived more different to that which nature has designed for man, than that of those wretched children alluded to; for we might just as well take some monstrous birth as the normal idea of human conformation, as take advantage of those wild children to demonstrate the natural method of man's gait and life." Blumenbach brandished the reported differences between the so-called wild children as evidence that they were "altogether unnatural deformed creatures" and that man has no natural state: "They had no originally wild species to degenerate into, for such a race of mankind ... no where exists, nor is there any position, any mode of life, or even climate which would be suitable for it." In Monboddo's and Blumenbach's works, which resume and encapsulate the Enlightenment debate on the state of nature and the related questions it raised, we see that the authors' positions on this state may not be dissociated from their stand on wild children. The wild child was imagined as either natural (original) man, the starting point of humanity's progress towards civilization, or as the pitiable result of an individual process of degradation or degeneration, in Tinland's words, "the extreme downward limit of human existence." Thus "wildness" denoted either *lack* of civilization or *loss* of (fall from) civilization.[18]

The eighteenth century is the one in which the study of man emerged as a scientific field of inquiry separate from theology. The Enlightenment "science of man," natural history of man, or anthropology investigated human beings in their relation not to God but to the rest of nature. A unified area of research (not yet subdivided into specialized sciences such as physical anthropology, cultural or social anthropology, psychology, linguistics, and sociology), it was also part of the general science of nature. At first the emerging science set itself the task of defining human nature. But students of man seeking to delineate what is universal in and essential to him confronted two problems: the problem of *boundaries* (between human beings and animals) and the problem of *human diversity*. Following the realization that a scientific definition of man could not be arrived at except by classification and comparison, the tasks of human science were reformulated as 1) to ascertain the place of man within the system of nature and analyze the differences between human beings and other animals, above all the anthropoid apes, and 2) to scrutinize and explain the varieties within the human species. Wild children played a key role in these debates, together with a host of other figures, creatures and kinds of people: apes, "savage" nations, deaf-mutes, "idiots," and children in general.[19]

A universal definition of man would have to specify the necessary and satisfactory criteria that would allow us to recognize a human being from among all other living creatures. The essential characteristic (or characteristics) of man would have to be found in all human beings, and in human beings only. Philosophers and naturalists, no longer content with *a priori* attributes like the rational soul, faced mounting difficulties in their search for suitable defining criteria whose universality and exclusivity could be unwaveringly upheld.

One widely held criterion was man's upright position, but how did this square with reports that wild children walked on all fours? Was biped locomotion natural to man, determined by his physical structure, or an acquired (cultural) trait? It was in order to defend the naturalness of man's biped gait that Rousseau deciphered the quadruped locomotion of wild children as a

deviant response to their unnatural, extreme circumstances: "A child abandoned in a forest before he is able to walk, and nourished by some beast,
will have followed the example of his nurse in training himself to walk like
her. Habit could have given him capabilities he did not have from nature,
and just as one-armed men are successful, by dint of exercise, at doing with
their feet whatever we do with our hands, he will finally have succeeded
in using his hands as feet." Rousseau disqualified the example of children
because "their natural strength is not yet developed nor the limbs toned
up"; in other words, children could not stand for "man." Johann Gottfried
von Herder (1744–1803) and Blumenbach reaffirmed Rousseau's view. In the
chapter on organic differences between "Man and Beasts" of *Ideen zur Philosophie der Geschichte der Menschheit* (1784) Herder argued that the upright
position was not only exclusive to man but also the cause of his superiority over all the other animals. Herder admitted that children "brought up
among beasts" (he mentioned Tulp's boy, the girl of Songi, and the "flemish
maiden" who "retained so much of the feminine nature as to bedeck herself
with a straw apron") empirically demonstrate that biped locomotion is not
"so essential to man, that it's opposite is as impossible for him as to fly."
In acquiring "the gait of quadrupeds," wild children underwent striking
physical alterations, strong proof that "the pliable nature of a human being"
could, in a few years, "habituate itself ... to the inferiour mode of life of the
beasts." Less compromising, Blumenbach proclaimed that man is "the only
biped" and neutralized the example of wild children: "Hard necessity, perhaps too imitation, taught these wretches to go on their hands and feet at
the same time that they were obliged to creep through woods and fruit-
bearing copses, and even into the dens and receptacles of wild beasts." It
was not even certain, Blumenbach added, that all the so-called wild children were quadrupeds. Some of them, like the girl of Zell, the girl of Champagne, and the boy of Hameln, went upright, while others, like the Hessian
boy, "*sometimes* only walked as a quadruped." As for infants, as "must be
very well known to any one who has observed them," they rarely crawl as
quadrupeds and indeed "squat upon their buttocks, rest upon their hands,
and as it were row with their feet." Monboddo, however, insisted that wild
children and infants prove that man's erect posture is learned: "After what I
have related of Peter the Wild Boy, and other solitary savages that have been
found in Europe, the reader will not be surprised when I tell him that my
opinion is, that walking upright is likewise an acquired habit. When we are

in the most natural state of any, that is, when we are born, we certainly go upon all four."[20]

Similarly, wild children's speechlessness undercut the efforts of the many defenders of language as the criterion supposedly distinguishing man from the other animals. The accounts of wild children disturbingly intimated that speech could not be the condition that defined humanity. Monboddo took advantage of this fact to ground his theory that language is not natural but was invented at a certain point in human history. British readers who doubted that men ever existed without the use of speech could convince themselves "without going out of their own country, and without trusting to the reports of historians or travellers, antient or modern, foreign or domestic," simply by visiting Peter. For Monboddo, wild children's lack of speech confirmed that articulation was "the work of art, at least of a habit acquired by custom and exercise." Because the challenge of learning to articulate can be successfully met only in childhood, Monboddo was not alarmed by Peter's speechlessness: "The wonder would have been, and indeed I should have thought it a miracle, if either Peter had spoken when he was first catched, or if the Orang Outangs had the use of language in the state in which they live."[21]

In addition, a wild child, the wild girl of Songi, cropped up in philosophical discussions of the moral law. In "Poëme sur la loi naturelle" Voltaire (1694–1778) tried to establish the existence of a natural and universal morality independent of revealed religion. In the preface to the poem he stated that remorse is not a weakness instilled by education but a natural feeling. "If the ardour of passion makes us commit a fault," he wrote, "nature, left to itself, feels that fault." The wild girl bore out this claim: "The savage girl found near Châlons confessed that, in her anger, she gave her companion a blow from which the unfortunate girl died in her arms. As soon as she saw the blood flow, she repented, she cried, she tried to stop the blood, she put herbs on the wound. Those who say that this return of humanity is nothing but a form of our self-esteem do great honour to self-esteem. Call them what you will, reason and remorse exist, and they are the foundation of the natural law." Voltaire's natural law was inscribed by God in our hearts, a stamp of man's special place in the order of things. Despite his adamant opposition to innate ideas, La Mettrie accepted the existence of a similar kind of natural law, a universal feeling that teaches us what we must not do because we do not want the same thing done to us. This law did not stem from revelation or education and was shared by human beings and animals: "One cannot destroy the Natural Law. The Impression is so strong in all the Animals, that I do not even doubt that the most wild and most fierce among them do not have some moments of regret. I believe that the Wild-Girl of Châlons in Champagne would have felt sorry for her crime, if it is true that she ate her sister. I think the same of all those who commit crimes ..." La Mettrie was as impressed by the wild girl's remorse as Voltaire and Racine. But it is doubtful that thus sandwiched between ferocious animals and violent criminals Mlle Leblanc had anything to gain from her notoriety.[22]

By mid-century it was becoming clear that human beings could not be distinguished from the other animals, in particular the great apes, using strictly physical (or natural) criteria. Philosophers and naturalists could not reach a consensus regarding a definitive characterization of man's specific difference. The formulation of three new, more flexible criteria implied a rethinking of the concept of human nature and the relation between the natural and the social (or civilized) state. The most important of these criteria was Rousseau's notion of perfectibility, the idea that man's essence is his capacity to learn, to become something else than what he is. Perfectibility must not be understood as a tendency towards (and even less a guarantee of) perfection but as the set of faculties that predispose human beings to develop a wide range of skills and qualities, both good and bad. It entailed the promise of reason and intellectual attainment but also the danger of barbarism and stupidity, the possibility of increasing virtue but also the risk of vice, the ability to benefit from education but also the absence of a predetermined, instinctually based form of life, the potential for happiness and unhappiness at the same time. Inseparable from perfectibility, its flip side, was the recognition of man's natural destitution. Bereft of instincts, natural man is a creature even lower than the animals, as the stories of wild children poignantly put in evidence and as Defoe wrote of Peter: "A *Man* is no more fit to be a *Beast*, than a *Beast* is to be a *Man*; the rational Part being taken away from him, his Carcass, left utterly destitute, is unqualified to live."[23] Finally, human perfectibility could only find expression in social existence. The paradox evoked by eighteenth-century human science is that man's "nature" is not *nature* but *society*. Man could only rise from his natural destitution and fulfill the promise of his perfectibility within society and among his fellow men. Perfectibility, natural destitution, and sociability were advanced as dynamic criteria that could account for the special and superior abilities of human beings as a *potential* and explain the limitations of wild children as well. Reinterpreted in terms of these notions, the stories of wild children shifted meaning, making visible the sad condition of isolated (or "natural") man while highlighting the superiority of man elevated above the other animals through perfectibility. In this sense, if man was by nature destined to live a social existence, wild children were somehow *not human*. Accidentally deprived of contact with others, they could not *acquire* human nature.[24]

The figure of the savage haunted philosophico-scientific attempts to study humanity and specify the place of man in nature. But "savage" could mean several things. Besides wild children (isolated or solitary savages), two other candidates for the appellation were the great apes (or Orang-Outangs) and the exotic savages (or savage nations). Like wild children, apes and savages inhabited that fluid boundary between human and non-human that philosophers and naturalists were intent on solidifying. The great minds of Europe pondered the disquieting implications of the resemblance between human beings and apes and the visible savagery of some human groups. "At the sight of the Orang-Outang," Jean-Baptiste Robinet (1735–1820) noted, "one is tempted to ask: what does he lack to be a man? Seeing certain races of men, one would almost dare ask: what kind of animals are those?"[25] The Enlightenment approach to the savage (broadly understood) took place in several registers of experience and discourse: the remnants of ancient myth, legend, and popular ritual; face-to-face encounters; and reports of the encounters (travellers' accounts, anatomical and medical treatises, anthropological inventories of bones and skulls, interviews with former wild children). Reported observations fuelled the search for more evidence – new encounters with wild children, new voyages of discovery and scientific observation, new ape specimens transported to Europe to be described and dissected. During the eighteenth century the anthropoid apes were collectively known as "Orang-Outangs" or "wild men." Knowledge of their anatomy and physiology being very limited, there was no clear sense of their precise relation to man. In a letter to Johann Georg Gmelin, Linnaeus confessed that he could not find a strict natural criterion to differentiate apes from men: "I demand of you, and of the whole world, that you show me a generic character – one that is according to generally accepted principles of classification – by which to distinguish between Man and Ape. I myself most assuredly know of none."[26] Working with scant factual information and within conceptual frameworks and taxonomic systems in process of formation, some thinkers entertained the idea that the apes were just another kind of human being. The apparent "inhumanity" of wild children and their lack of most characteristics traditionally assumed to define man lent weight to their arguments.

The anonymous and scandalous pamphlet L'âme matérielle defended the absolute equality of man and animal, human and animal intelligence, pronouncing that animals' reason is less perfect than ours only insofar as ours is perfected through education and study, which animals do not have. Some men whose humanity was unchallenged, like the deaf-mute of Chartres, the Lithuanian boy, and the members of some savage tribes, lived like the stupidest of animals. If lack of education was all that separated "the man of Chartres and the man of Poland, ... the Savage of the island of Borneo, and the savages of Africa and America" from civilized men, then the same could be claimed of the apes, "who, when dressed and instructed, perfectly imitate the actions of the most sensible men." La Mettrie agreed: inasmuch as children who spent their lives isolated in the forests had neither speech nor ideas when they were found "and yet everyone agrees that they are human beings," it was legitimate to question the prevalent opinion that "Satyrs" were "nothing but animals." Likening apes to congenital deaf-mutes, La Mettrie propounded that with the proper method an ape could be taught to articulate and understand language. No longer "wild" or "defective," the talking ape would be "a perfect Man, a little Gentleman, with as much matter or muscle as we have, to think and profit by his education."[27]

Like the author of L'âme materielle, La Mettrie reduced the intellectual distance between man and animal to attack the concept of man's uniqueness. While Monboddo's purpose was different, his aim being to explain the historical origin of man's distinctive characteristics rather than to dissolve the boundary between man and animal, his views coincided in so many points with La Mettrie's that their effect was equally offensive to eighteenth-century readers. Monboddo was convinced that the Orang-Outangs were unidentified men, every bit as human as Peter, who looked human but lacked the most essential human traits. With "proper pains" the Orang-Outang could be taught to speak, "which will convince the most credulous of his humanity." In reaction to these outrageous proposals Cornelius de Pauw (1739–1799) denied that wild children's mutism, attributable to isolation, portended that the Orang-Outangs might one day speak (with our help). Unlike the "mute Savages" found in the woods of Hanover and the solitary regions of Lithuania and the Pyrenees, for whom speech was "both impossible and useless," apes lived in groups, and had they had the faculty of speech they would have been able to develop it on their own.[28]

The confusion surrounding savages and apes crystallized in Linnaeus's complex and changing classification of man in *Systema naturae*. In the first edition (1735), the first class, *Quadrupedia*, contained the genus *Homo* under the order *Anthropomorpha*, which also included *Simia* and *Bradypus* (sloth). *Homo* was succinctly characterized as "*Nosce te ipsum*" (know thyself). In the second edition (1740) *Homo* was subdivided into four varieties based on geographical location and skin colour: *Europaeus albus* (white European), *Americanus rubescens* (reddish American), *Asiaticus fuscus* (dark Asian) and *Africanus niger* (black African). Later revisions to the *Systema*, published after Linnaeus's appointment, in 1741, as professor of medicine at the University of Uppsala, reflected his shifting conceptualization of man's relation to the animals most resembling him and of the internal divisions within the genus *Homo*. Whereas in the sixth edition (1748) *Homo* remained intact (*Simia* was enlarged to include sixteen species of apes), the tenth edition (1758) constituted a major rethinking of man's place in the system. Not only was the order *Anthropomorpha* replaced by *Primates* (and the class *Quadrupedia* by *Mammalia*) but the subdivisions of the genus *Homo* were reworked: *Homo* was now composed of two main subgroups, *Homo sapiens* and *Homo troglodytes* ("nocturnal" man), and to the four earlier varieties of *Homo*, now listed under *Homo sapiens*, were added two more, our *Homo ferus* and *Homo monstrosus* (*Alpini, Patagonici, Monorchides, Macrocephali, Plagiocephali*, and so on). The importance of Linnaeus's taxonomic work for anthropology and human science in general cannot be overemphasized. For the first time human beings were included *as animals* in a systematic, comprehensive, and cohesive scientific classification of nature. The inclusion of man within the system of nature was expected to settle questions arising from external ambiguities (the boundary between man and ape) and internal distinctions (the different varieties of man). However, the shifting classes and classifications throughout the twelve editions of his magnum opus reveal that Linnaeus could not make up his mind as to where exactly the boundary lay nor how many varieties could be identified (and according to what principles). For our own purposes, let us note that, by creating the class *Homo ferus* as a variety of man, Linnaeus both gave scientific legitimacy to the stories of wild children and called forth criticisms and objections to the class.[29]

Theologians and traditionalist scientists questioned Linnaeus's classification not only for envisioning man as an animal but also for introducing divisions within humankind. The Judeo-Christian creation story held that human beings have a single origin because they derive from a single act of divine creation. Scientists understood this to mean that all human beings belong to one species. But Enlightenment philosophers and natural historians, befuddled before the unprecedented wealth of data on the physical and cultural diversity of people gleaned by the explorers, were revaluating this received belief. What was the origin of human diversity? Was the belief in a single human species with a common origin merely another item of religious doctrine that enlightened thinkers had a duty to challenge and replace with a sounder scientific and empirically grounded theory? The reports about some "savage" tribes, like the Hottentots, whose appearance and habits seemed especially repulsive to Western sensibilities, troubled European classifiers. Three responses were possible: a) that all human beings, savage and civilized alike, belong to the same species (but then how did the striking differences between them arise?); b) that there is more than one species of human being, and that the different species have separate origins; and c) that the lowest groups of savages are not human beings at all. (Other options were to reject the reports or reinterpret the savages' alleged inferiority as neutral difference or special nobility.) These questions and positions inaugurated two controversies: the debate on human origins, opposing monogenists and polygenists (defenders of single or multiple origins respectively), and the debate on the existence, proper characterization, and significance of human races.

Within Linnaeus's conception of fixed species marked by different morphology, human diversity seemed to lead inevitably to multiplicity (of species and origins). Buffon's new definition of species as "a constant succession of similar individuals who can reproduce" expanded the range of variation possible within a species by adding the temporal dimension: what makes a species is "the constant succession and the uninterrupted renewal of these individuals that constitute it." On this *scientific* basis, Buffon embraced the view that human beings belong to one species with several varieties. To account for the differences, Buffon proposed that some groups had "degenerated" from humankind's original character due to the diversifying effect of climate and geography. Blumenbach's anthropology brought together elements from Linnaeus's and Buffon's theories. While acknowledging the pioneering nature of Linnaeus's taxonomy, Blumenbach declared that his "division of mankind could no longer be adhered to" and put forth an amended classification in which the first two of ten natural orders comprised in *Mammalia* were *Bimanus* (*Homo*) and *Quadrumana* (*Simia, Papio, Cercopithecus, Lemur*). Blumenbach discerned five varieties of humanity (Caucasian, Mongolian, Ethiopian, American, and Malay) delimited partly by colour but primarily by the conformation of the head. After many years of study and observation, Blumenbach had no doubt that all the varieties (or races) were part of a single human species and, like Buffon, he resorted to the idea of degeneration to explain their origin. Blumenbach's reformulated classification had no use for a class dependent on accidental circumstance and individual example such as Linnaeus's *Homo ferus*. Because he was concerned with "the varieties of whole nations," he believed himself "quite justified in making no mention here of those unfortunate children, who have been now and then found amongst wild beasts." Rare and anomalous, wild children did not warrant a separate class. Indeed for Blumenbach there could be no such thing as a *wild* child (or wild man) because man is "a domestic animal" with no "wild condition": "Other domestic animals were first brought to that state of perfection *through him*. He is the only one who brought *himself* to perfection." Variability and degeneration were the underside of perfectibility, consequent upon the fact that "nature has limited [man] in no wise, but has created him for every mode of life, for every climate, and every sort of aliment."[30]

The earlier view of human nature was static, as evinced in Voltaire's conviction that there was no reason to believe that human beings had ever changed: "Man in general has always been what he is ... he has always had the same instinct that leads him to love himself in himself, in the companion of his pleasures, in his children, in his grandchildren, in the works of his hands."[31] A more fluid concept of human nature was needed to account for the diversity within the human species and phenomena such as the wild child. Buffon and Blumenbach accepted that human nature could change and had changed but, as noted above, they conceived of this change as degeneration, a decline or loss of qualities evident in some varieties of humanity and unfortunate individuals. But other philosophers and naturalists reversed the direction of change and envisaged it as *progress*. In their view, *all* human beings began in a state of destitution (or savagery) and slowly acquired what we now see as man's distinctive characteristics. The theory that "human nature" is the outcome of a historical process of transformation was first advanced as a conjecture or hypothesis, most eminently by

Rousseau in the second *Discours*. In the last decades of the eighteenth century it was further developed by Lord Monboddo, whom we have already often encountered and whose ideas it is time to explore in more depth.

Although, as we have seen, wild children inspired, assisted, and resisted the thinking of many Enlightenment philosophers and naturalists, in no other case were they so crucial to the very foundation of a philosophico-scientific universe as in Monboddo's. That wild children were intimately connected to Monboddo's views becomes clear when one considers his preface to the English translation of Madame H...t's *Histoire d'une jeune fille sauvage*, published several years before his major works, *Of the Origin and Progress of Language* (1773–1792) and *Antient Metaphysics* (1779–1799). In it he formulated in brief all his anthropological ideas: a) that the primary task of human science is to investigate the state of nature; b) that in his progress (or history) man passed through different stages; c) that the traits and skills that now characterize man are not natural but latent potentialities that had to be realized (invented or acquired) historically; d) that the only characteristic that properly distinguishes man is the capacity to perfect his mental faculties, and for this reason man must be defined not as rational but as *capable of rationality*; and e) that the wild girl's story proved these claims and epitomized man's progress from wild animality to the civilized state.[32]

In his later anthropological works Monboddo did not modify his basic arguments, but he elaborated them and furnished additional evidence. The state of nature could be understood in two different senses, as *telos* (man's "most perfect state, to which his nature tends, and towards which he either is or ought to be always advancing") and as *origin* ("the state from which this progression begins ... before societies were formed, or arts invented"). The natural history of man must be concerned with the state of nature in this second sense, as the original state, "the ground-work and foundation of every other through which he has passed." Whereas for Rousseau the (original) state of nature was a hypothesis, a demand of thought but not necessarily a condition to be found in past or present reality, and for other anthropologists, like Blumenbach, there was no such thing as a natural state of man, Monboddo argued that the state of nature had real existence both as the original or primitive condition of all of humankind and as the present condition of some human groups and individuals. His core contention was that "men are not, nor have not been always the same, in all ages, and all nations, such as we see them at present in Europe." The historical progress of man was not a linear and inevitable change for the better but a necessary

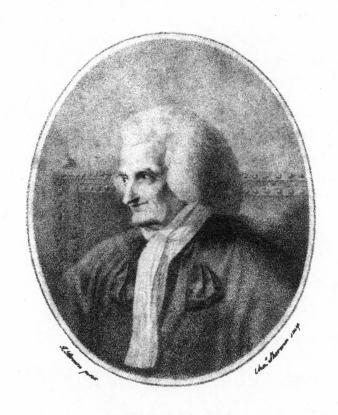

JAMES BURNET,

Lord Monboddo,

James Burnett, Lord Monboddo, in *Of the Origin and Progress of Language*, vol. 1, 2d edition (1774).

A N

ACCOUNT

OF A

SAVAGE GIRL,

CAUGHT WILD

IN THE WOODS OF *CHAMPAGNE.*

TRANSLATED

FROM THE FRENCH OF MADAM *H——T.*

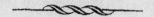

WITH

A PREFACE,

CONTAINING

SEVERAL PARTICULARS OMITTED IN THE ORIGINAL ACCOUNT.

BY THE HON. LORD MONBODDO.

𝔄𝔟𝔢𝔯𝔡𝔢𝔢𝔫 :

PRINTED BY BURNETT AND RETTIE,

AND SOLD BY

JOHN BURNETT, BOOKSELLER.

1796.

*An Account of a Savage Girl Caught Wild in the Woods of
Champagne,* with a preface by Monboddo (1796), first published
in 1768. Courtesy of Northern Illinois University Libraries.

correlate of his potential to become, improve, invent, and adapt – in other words, perfectibility.[33]

What specific roles did wild children play in Monboddo's philosophy? Firstly, they demonstrated that human beings could and did exist who lacked some or all of the traits believed to be natural or essential to man, like speech, the upright position and biped gait, sociability, religion, and so on. The wild girl's cries and her description of the language of her country confirmed that before inventing speech human beings "conversed together by signs and inarticulate cries." The fact that wild children lived alone and ran away from other people proved that in the natural state man has "no instinct or inclination which prompts him to associate with his fellow creatures." Peter's example showed that in the natural state man cannot "form any idea at all, much less an idea so noble and exalted as that of God." Many faculties of the body, like swimming, were not natural to man either. In the wild girl's country adults took great pains to accustom children to the water and teach them to swim. Her remarkable swimming skills were therefore learned and later partly lost through lack of practice. Secondly, wild children's condition suggested that speech, the upright position, and even reason not being natural and universal human attributes, they could not be part of the definition of man except as capacities. If human beings were characterized by "*the capacity of intellect and science*," it was perfectly possible that "an animal may be a *man*, without being actually intelligent or scientific, though he be not in the state of infancy but full grown." Availing himself of his broadened definition of humanity as *potential*, and with the help of wild children, whose membership in the human species was not in question, Monboddo proclaimed that the Orang-Outangs were human beings too. Lastly, wild children allowed Monboddo to reconstruct empirically the earlier stages of man's "wonderful progress" from capacity to actuality. With obvious pride, he asserted that he had "seen with mine own eyes ... which I believe is what very few now living can say," three of these stages: Peter the Wild Boy, representing "the pure natural state"; the Orang-Outang or "Man of the Woods," so called "by the people of Africa ... who do not appear to have the least doubt that he is a man; which, as they live in the country with him, they should know better than we can do"; and the wild girl, "who came from a country where the people had learned to articulate very imperfectly indeed, but sufficiently to communicate their wants and desires."[34]

Monboddo's belief in the Orang-Outang's humanity exposed him to the ridicule of his contemporaries. James Boswell (1740–1795) reported Dr Johnson's sneering comment that unlike Rousseau, who "*knows* he is talking nonsense, and laughs at the world for staring at him ... Monboddo does *not* know that he is talking nonsense." Chauncey B. Tinker carried on the tradition of sarcastic and condescending assaults on Monboddo, contending that he had "the credulity of a child," "believed nearly everything he was told and all that he found in print" and "must have been deliberately gulled by practical jokers, returned travellers, and yarn-spinning sailors."[35] There may be some truth in this. But Monboddo knew that the main reason why his theories were laughed at was his conception of humanity's origin. Any man who snubbed his views suffered "from a ridiculous vanity, which makes him scorn to be a race who were once Orang Outangs; and he might as well be ashamed that he himself was once an embryo in the womb, and then an infant, very much weaker, and every way more despicable, than the infant of an Orang Outang." And yet who is laughing now? As Alan Barnard observes, Monboddo's Orang-Outang "seems closer to that of biological science now than at any time since the eighteenth century." His books may have brimmed with bizarre examples and his eccentricities may have been legion, but with the passing of time Monboddo's main ideas, in some form or another, became the founding premises of biological evolutionism and of every field of inquiry that interrogates the process of becoming human in historical, social, and cultural terms.[36]

Herder took Monboddo seriously enough to introduce his work to German readers and write the preface to the German translation of *Origin and Progress*. Still, Herder's version of human origins was a critical (or defensive) reaction to Monboddo's radical anthropology. Herder refused to accept that there was any relation of consequence between human beings and apes, stating that human perfectibility acts as an insuperable barrier between them. The distinctive attributes and faculties of man could not have originated in a historical process:

How much trouble has it cost, to habituate the wild men, who have been found, to our food and manner of living! yet these were not originally wild, but had become so only by being a few years among the brutes. The eskimaux maiden had some ideas of her former state, and remains of the language and instincts of her native country: yet her reason lay bound up in brutality; she had no remembrance of her journey, or of the whole of her wild state. The others were not only destitute of language, but were in some measure for ever lost to human speech.—And would the human beast, had he been ages of ages in this abject state, and formed to it by totally different proportions a quadruped in his mother's womb, have left of his own accord, and raised himself to an erect posture? From the powers of a beast, eternally pulling him back, would he have made himself man, and, before he became a man, invented human speech?

Herder reinstated the thesis that the erect position and language were natural to man, adding that the latter presupposed the former: "Men, who have been accidentally brought up among beasts, not only lose the use of speech, but in some measure the power of acquiring it: an evident proof, that their throats are deformed, and that human speech is consistent only with an erect gait."[37] In many respects Herder's views ran counter to Monboddo's, yet this time too the burden of proof rested with wild children – more precisely, with the meaning given to wild children's strangeness.[38]

IN THE EIGHTEENTH CENTURY, as we have seen, Peter of Hanover and the wild girl of Songi occasioned a number of observations, speculations, interviews, and reports. Philosophers and naturalists relied on them, and on earlier wild children, to advance, confirm, test, or refute a variety of opinions, conjectures, theories, and systems. Beginning in the nineteenth century there was a major shift in interpretations and uses of the wild child that both reflected and contributed to a new social and scientific interest in childhood and in technologies of formation and transformation of people. In some eighteenth-century discussions inspired by wild children intimations of this new interest may be detected.

From Locke's empiricism to La Mettrie's materialism and Condillac's sensationist epistemology, the critique of innate ideas lent a new urgency to education and inaugurated a sustained reflection on learning. The wild child made visible the dire effects of educational deprivation. Peter thus motivated Defoe's verdict that education is "the only specifick Remedy for all the Imperfections of Nature." Human beings need "the Guidance of an Instructor" not only to learn how to "speak, read, write, dance, swim, fence, or perform some of the best and most necessary Actions of Life" but also to "know, think, retain, judge, discern, distinguish, determine, or any of those Operations, in which the Soul is wholly the Operator." The differences between people, when not due to natural or accidental infirmity, could be imputed to differences in instruction. Defoe's sense of the reach and value of education was unqualified: "an untaught Man, a Creature in human Shape, but intirely neglected and uninstructed, is ten thousand times more miserable than a Brute."[39]

The notion of perfectibility reinforced the need for education because it implied, on the one hand, that human beings have the capacity to learn and an unlimited potential to improve their intellectual, moral, and even physical achievement, and on the other, that unless human beings develop this potential and acquire the characteristics that elevate man above the rest of the animals, they remain miserable and inferior creatures. But how does a human being *become a human being*? And when? Through a process of learning, and during childhood, of course. Perfectibility directed attention to the deliberate and rational intervention of adults in the lives of children. For the author of *Philosophical Survey of Nature*, the "well known story of Peter the wild boy" revealed "what [man] owes to the experience of former ages, carefully instilled into him by proper education, as his faculties open" and "of what importance the cultivation of our infant faculties is." Herder noted that "man must learn every thing, it being his instinct and destination to learn all, even to his mode of walking ... Even children, whom chance has thrown among beasts, have acquired some human cultivation, when they have lived for a time among men, as most instances show; while a child, brought up from the moment of his birth by a brute, would be the only uncultivated man upon Earth." To persuade her friend Sophie that education alone caused the "infinite differences" between people, Manon Roland (1754–1793) resorted to a child abandoned in a forest in words that recall Buffon's: "What is a man when he leaves his mother's womb? As limited and as ignorant as all the other animals, he is even the weakest among them. If he is abandoned in solitude in a forest when he is three or four years old, age at which he will be strong enough in body to seek the satisfaction of his needs but too weak in mind to keep the impression of the ideas he will have already received, what will become of him morally and intellectually? And what difference would remain between him and the other animals? If he is found many years later, he will be like that savage of Hanover and this little girl caught in the woods of Champagne: without language, without signs, and in all likelihood without ideas." The wild child validates fervent defences of education as the exclusive means through which the capacities with which human beings are born may be fully realized. "We are born with the principle of knowledge and the seed of instruction," wrote Mme Roland, "but only communication and society can develop one and fertilize the other."[40]

Eighteenth-century observers of wild children surmised that the power of education was not limitless. If certain types of learning did not take place during childhood, catching up became extremely arduous. Defoe claimed that Peter would experience much greater difficulty learning to speak at his age than he would have as a young child: "the Soul being left unpolished, and not able to shine, and having lost the Seasons in which it should have been taught and enur'd to its proper Functions, the Organs being grown firm and solid, without being put into a Capacity by due Exercise, are not so easily disposed for the necessary Motion and Application; and so the Difficulty will be the greater to bring it to work, and may not, in a long Time, if ever, be overcome." Peter verified "the Necessity of early Education of Children," because in them "not the Soul only, but the organick Powers are, as a Lump of soft Wax, which is always ready to receive any Impression." Defoe associated the decrease in learning ability with organic growth: with time, the child's "organick Powers" became hardened, and "like what we call Sealing-Wax, obstinately refuse the Impression of the Seal, unless melted, and reduced by Force of Fire." Like twentieth-century proponents of "critical periods" for learning, Herder connected the decline in children's learning capacity with the growth of the brain. In young creatures the brain is "more soft and tender" and possesses "that delicate humectation for all the vital functions, and internal operations" that allows the creature to "acquire capacities." As time goes by, "the brain grows more firm and dry" and "the animal, whether man or brute, is no longer susceptible of such light, agreeable, fugacious impressions."[41]

Another issue that would take centre stage in the future and to which some attention was paid in eighteenth-century writings on wild children was the question of sensory and intellectual defects – their cause, the relation between "defective" and "full" humanity, and the prospects for treatment, amelioration, or cure. Two figures are relevant here: the deaf-mute and the idiot. Attempts to instruct deaf-mutes using specially designed methods fired eighteenth-century imaginations and suggested the idea that these methods could be used to teach wild children (and apes) to speak. For Defoe, it would require "almost as much Art" to teach Peter to speak "as to teach one deaf and dumb from his Birth," and who was in a better position to try it than a deaf-mute educator? Defoe recommended Mr Henry Baker (who married one of his daughters); La Mettrie, Amman of Amsterdam, and Monboddo, Mr Braidwood of Edinburgh. And the idiot was the wild child's foil. Was idiocy a better explanation than savagery (social deprivation) for the wild child's peculiarities? Monboddo tenaciously denied it: "It is evident that [Peter] is not an idiot, not only from his appearance, as I have described it, and from his actions, but from all the accounts that we have of him, both those printed, and those attested by persons yet living." He was rather "such a man as one should expect a mere savage to be, that is, a man that has not the use of speech, and is entirely uninstructed in all our arts and sciences."[42]

Finally, the progressive view of human history reoriented the relation between savages and Europeans by introducing the suspicion that the contemporary savage might be merely *backward*. The distance between savage and civilized took on a new, temporal meaning. Consequently, the present of savage nations (and savage individuals) might afford the means to contemplate and study "our" own past. In turn, an analogy was drawn between the progress from savagery to civilization and the transformations in the life of a human individual, from unformed, animal-like child to rational man. To persuade sceptics that man had undergone changes throughout history, Monboddo reminded them of their own process of formation. Anybody could see the "progress in our children, from the mere Animal to the Intellectual Being"; what could be "more natural than to suppose the same progress in the species"? He developed the analogy: "In the womb, man is no better than a vegetable; and, when born, he is at first more imperfect, I believe, than any other animal in the same state, wanting almost altogether that comparative faculty, which the brutes, young and old, possess. If, therefore, there be such a progress in the individual, it is not to be wondered that there should be a progress also in the species, from the mere animal up to the intellectual creature ... for the species, with respect to the genus, is to be considered as an individual."[43] The correlation between the progress of the human species and the progress of a single human being – which in the nineteenth century would give rise to the concept of recapitulation – once again brought attention to bear on the child as a figure of origins.

Some eighteenth-century problems and concerns related to wild children survived in the work of later anthropologists, sociologists and social psychologists. What lessons can we learn from these stories about the relation between nature and culture? For anthropologist Ruth Benedict, the wild children found in Europe in the past corroborate the view that, unlike ants, human beings do not inherit culture biologically. They were "all so much alike" that Linnaeus, unable to accept "that these half-witted brutes were born human," invented for them the classification *Homo ferus* "and supposed that they were a kind of gnome that man seldom ran across." Wild children were not gnomes but "children abandoned in infancy" who had lacked "association with their kind, through which alone man's faculties are sharpened and given form." Benedict believed that such children would no longer be found "in our more humane civilization." Considering by what means it would be possible to find out where nature ends and culture begins, another influential twentieth-century anthropologist, Claude Lévi-Strauss, pointed out that the first means that comes to mind, "to isolate a new-born child and to observe its reactions to various stimuli during the first hours or days after birth" (the forbidden experiment), is inadequate because, for the findings to be valid, the experiment would have to last several months or even years, and then the experimental environment would be "no less artificial than the cultural environment it purports to replace." Wild children, chance occurrences of the isolation experiment, would appear to be another means to probe the precise limit between nature and culture and as such were greatly valued by eighteenth-century philosophers, but Lévi-Strauss warned that they are equally inadequate because, firstly, most of them were "congenital defectives," and secondly, as Blumenbach taught us, man has no wild state. Wild children "may be cultural monstrosities, but under no circumstances can they provide reliable evidence of an earlier state" nor unveil the natural state of man. Malson disagreed with Lévi-Strauss: far from being congenital idiots, hence valueless for science, wild children must be regarded as key examples supporting the thesis that "man has no nature but has – or rather *is* – a history." According to Malson, believers in human nature question the existence and refuse the implications of wild children due to their reluctance to "allow such backwardness any cause other than physical abnormality." Malson's own characterization of human "nature" (or history) as the "absence of particular determinations ... perfectly synonymous with the presence of indefinite possibilities" reiterates the Enlightenment notion of perfectibility. Indeed, regardless of their disparate positions on the cause of wild children's strangeness and their exact relation to nature, culture, and history, these human scientists share the view that wild children were somehow less than human. In Malson's words, "children deprived too early of all social contact ... remain so destitute in their solitude that they appear to be pathetic beasts, lower animals."[44]

During the Enlightenment wild children were linked to the anthropoid apes as figures of difference lurking at the borders of humanity. In the twentieth century they continued to be associated with apes in interesting ways. Piqued by the widely publicized reports of Indian wolf children in the 1920s and 1930s, Winthrop N. Kellogg, professor of psychology at Indiana University, conceived the idea that the forbidden experiment might be reversed. To ascertain the effect of environment on human development one would need to know what the outcome would be "if a human infant, the child of civilized parents, were placed in the environment of the jungle or in some similar situation, and allowed to mature in these surroundings, without language, without clothes, and without the association of other humans." It was impossible to draw firm conclusions from the historical examples of wild children because the accounts were unreliable (Kellogg nevertheless hypothesized that their condition was due not to "congenital feeble-mindedness" but to their unusual circumstances). Moreover, the experimental production of isolated children for purposes of rigorous study, however desirable (and, in theory, conclusive), would be "legally dangerous and morally outrageous." What Kellogg proposed was to conduct the inverse experiment: "Suppose an anthropoid were taken into a typical human family at the day of birth and reared as a child." Kellogg and his coresearcher wife Luella reared the young female chimpanzee Gua in their home for nine months. They meticulously compared Gua's development with that of their son Donald and communicated their observations, measurements, and results in *The Ape and the Child* (1933). The Donald-Gua experiment would merit full treatment on another occasion; what I want to stress here is how it was inspired by the stories of wild children, in effect springing from the same desire these children both elicit and frustrate.[45]

Why is it that, since their inception in the eighteenth century, the human sciences seem unable to free themselves from the shadow cast on them by wild children? From the Enlightenment debates we distil two reasons (there are more, which will appear in later chapters). First, wild children are inseparable from any attempt to define the human or to delineate the boundaries between human and non-human. This problem has an epistemological and a moral aspect, having to do both with the grounds upon which we practice human science and professions engaged in forming and transforming people, and with the way we relate to and care for others who are different from us. Second, wild children are irrevocably attached to that particular form of the desire to "know ourselves" that I have been calling the forbidden experiment. Human scientists are still haunted by the forbidden experiment, convinced that it, and it only, would definitively reveal ourselves to ourselves. But whereas during the Enlightenment the idea that the experiment might be conducted one day was sometimes entertained, twentieth-century scientists seemed to have given up that hope altogether. They insistently conjured it up only to reject it right away as ethically unacceptable. And as protestations against real attempts to perform a controlled isolation experiment increased in intensity, the relation to wild children became more overt. Besides the examples of Lévi-Strauss and the Kelloggs mentioned above, consider the following:

No scientist would dream of an actual experiment with a human subject under any such rigorous control as removing all human association and contact. Cases of feral man, and certainly the recent one of the Wolf-children of Midnapore, offer objective data, subject to this control, of fundamental importance to theories of human studies. Thus we may say that we have satisfactory evidence from far-away India of a crucial experiment made by a mother-wolf.

What ... a zoologist can do, we as sociologists cannot. Any deprivation experiment on a human infant would be a criminal act in the narrowest sense of the word. Besides, even if the required cruelty were present, it would not be easy to carry out ... We must be satisfied with what the French call a *pis aller*, a second best – with the observation of conditions of isolation or semi-isolation which come about by accident or malfeasance.

What would children be like if, somehow, they were raised without the influence of human adults? Obviously, no humane person could bring up a child away from human influence as an experiment. There have been, however, a number of much-discussed cases of children who spent their early years away from normal human contact.[46]

The discovery of a new wild child, the long-awaited substitute for the forbidden experiment, excites ambivalent responses. Since the wild child was created by nature (or criminal parents) the scientist is allowed to exploit the child's miserable condition to produce knowledge without having to feel any guilt or moral responsibility. Besides, since the reason why the wild child is scientifically desirable is that he or she has endured unspeakable deprivation, the scientist feels compelled to seize the opportunity to study the child. By forcing the wild child to provide answers and reveal secrets, by producing something useful, indeed precious, out of the child's suffering and wretchedness, the scientist may be seen as justifying the wild child's existence. However, since the wild child does not reveal any secret or answer any question after all, the scientist's expectations turn to disappointment: was that all?

Wild children frustrate the desire to know and mark the insuperable limit of certain scientific aspirations. For the human sciences, they stand both as the ultimate object of desire and the ultimate object of embarrassment.

PART THREE Civilizing the Savage, Educating the Child

CHAPTER FIVE

The Wild Boy of Aveyron

Shew him in Words his Thoughts to dress,
To think, and what he thinks express;
His Manners form, his Conduct plan,
And civilize him into Man.

"The Savage" (1726)[1]

IN THE EIGHTEENTH CENTURY, as we have seen, wild children attracted the attention of philosophers and naturalists who saw in them a means to address a wide range of themes and problems. Wild children thus became involuntary participants in the gradual formation and consolidation of human science. In this process, *speculation* and *observation* were the methods employed to produce knowledge, and the wild child was understood (and sought) primarily as a *savage*. The early nineteenth century witnessed the rise of a new way of producing knowledge about people and a new way of understanding the wild child. Knowledge was reformulated as *intervention*, and the wild child was approached as *child*. My purpose in these next two chapters is to show that the new attitude to the wild child signals the historical emergence of "the child" as a privileged object of knowledge and intervention, and with it the inauguration of a space of inquiry and practice that is still our own.

What will now come to the fore is the fourth moment of the story-form or narrative prototype of wild children: response, care, treatment. The response to the wild child depends on the questions brought to bear at the moment of the encounter and the knowledge the adults in charge possess or seek. In virtually every case, this response takes the form of an attempt to transform the wild children – tame, humanize, civilize, normalize, educate, cure, or rehabilitate them. The earliest accounts mention the training wild children received (to stand on two feet, walk, speak) only briefly and vaguely, and even though both Peter of Hanover and the wild girl of Songi were subjected to at least some systematic instruction, it seems that those efforts were not deemed significant enough to be recorded in detail. While hitherto the training of the wild child had been instrumental, its significance restricted to its actual success or failure, beginning with Victor, the wild boy of Aveyron, training acquired an additional purpose. As a new body of knowledge about human beings was being elaborated, and, more important, as new techniques to extract knowledge from human beings were invented (and, we will see, Victor himself played a crucial role in the constitution of this knowledge and these techniques), the wild child's training came to be explicitly designed as a medical and pedagogical experiment. The wild child's transformation, and the methods through which it was attained, became the object of attention, observation, and controversy.

The wild boy of Aveyron is the most famous wild child and his story the most consequential in the history of the human sciences. My approach to his story, so often told and retold, is twofold. On the one hand, by discussing it as one among many other stories of wild children, I intend to make possible a more accurate assessment of the ways in which it both overlaps with and departs from them. Only by grasping the story of Victor against the background of the wild children who preceded and followed him, who prepared his reception and trod on his shadow, may we fully appreciate what makes this story so special and powerful. On the other hand, by presenting a more complex account of Victor's life and the responses it evoked, I hope to unsettle the reductive and unilateral readings that persist as founding myths of various sciences of childhood. Any identification of a historical change with a particular century risks oversimplification, but in this case it may be unavoidable: Victor's definitive capture took place in early January 1800. Straddling two centuries, he appeared when one way of formulating questions about people was dissolving and another one was taking shape. More specifically, he literally embodied the moment when, borrowing Hacking's wording, the organizing concept of human nature, characteristic of the eighteenth century, was giving way to that of "normal people."[2] Although Victor's significance ultimately lies in his unwitting contribution to the rise of the new conceptual framework (which is still our own), to make sense of his fate we must attend to the temporary coexistence, clashes, and confusion between the two.

For several years after his capture, the wild boy inspired a steady stream of writings, which make up the largest and most diverse dossier of first-hand accounts of a wild child to date. The dossier was reconstructed slowly, though, and until quite recently the story was known mainly through Itard's reports of 1801 and 1806, which tell only a partial version of it. Despite the large number of recovered documents many gaps in the story remain, and each scholar fills them in his or her own way, with varying success and openness. Moreover, most historical and interpretive studies of Victor's life are written from the perspective of a specific science or profession (psycho-linguistics, deaf education, special education, child psychiatry, and so forth) and subordinate the story to disciplinary or professional aims, questions, and methods. In what follows, I propose both to do justice to the sources as the only surviving trace of past events without covering up the linger-ing gaps between sources and events and to approach the story from the perspective of the child and his relations with the adults around him rather than the concerns of future experts.[3]

Let me first outline the bare facts. A naked and speechless boy was cap-tured in the vicinity of the town of Saint-Sernin, Aveyron, on 9 January 1800 (19 nivôse of the eighth year of the French Republic), just weeks after the Brumaire coup that installed Napoleon at the head of the French nation. The local government commissioner, Constans-Saint-Estève, placed him in the neighbouring hospice of Saint-Affrique. Many times the wild boy tried to escape, and every time he was chased and recaptured. Inquiries revealed that he had been sighted in the region in the preceding months and twice seized and briefly confined in Lacaune, Tarn, but his origin and family remained a mystery. As the news spread, the strange boy was claimed by Randon, central commissioner of Aveyron (Constans's superior), and by Jauffret, secretary of the newly founded Society of Observers of Man, backed by Lucien Bonaparte, minister of the interior and brother of the First Consul. At first Randon prevailed, and in early February the boy was sent to Rodez, Aveyron's capital, where he was studied by the naturalist abbé Bonnaterre and looked after by the servant Clair Saussol and a woman who prepared his meals. A few months later he was escorted to Paris by Bonnaterre and Clair. On his arrival in the capital on 6 August, following a long and troubled trip and a bout of smallpox in Moulins, the wild boy faced great expectations and intense public curiosity. He was admitted to the Institute for Deaf-Mutes, directed by the abbé Sicard (who had returned to his position in January after a period in hiding), and a commission appointed by the Society of Observers of Man examined him to ascertain his condition and prospects.

But after heated controversies in the press and a few inconclusive reports (by Bonnaterre, the alienist Pinel, and the natural historian Virey), the Parisians grew tired of the wild boy and he suffered temporary neglect. At the end of the year Itard was appointed resident physician at the Institute, and he began to work with the boy at some point before or after that (the date is uncertain) with the assistance of Mme Guérin, who was primarily entrusted with the boy's care. At the request of the Observers of Man, and to convince the new minister of the interior, Chaptal, to continue funding the boy's education and paying Mme Guérin's wages, Itard composed his first report. Its immediate success secured the support of the scientific and institutional authorities for Itard's endeavours and made him famous. The following years were marked by disagreements and negotiations with Chaptal, some progress on the boy's part and high hopes on his teacher's, and more observations and reports. Still, when in 1806, entreated by yet another minister of the interior, Champagny, Itard wrote his second report on the boy he had named Victor, the training had already stopped (we do not know exactly when). Victor's overall progress did not meet anyone's expectations, but Itard's work was favourably evaluated by the third class of the National Institute of Sciences and Arts and widely praised. Itard went on to become a well-respected doctor. Victor stayed at the Institute for Deaf-Mutes with Mme Guérin until in 1810 the administrators requested that they move out. From 1811 until his death in early 1828 Victor lived with Mme Guérin in a house very near the Institute, his expenses covered by a government pension – but about those years we know nothing.

The wild boy elicited reactions at different levels: the level of general public concern (the people of Tarn, Aveyron, and Paris; enlightened Parisian and provincial elites; newspaper correspondents and foreign visitors; playwrights, novelists, and poets); the level of government (a long series of authorities and officials, ministers, and administrators); the level of science (Bonnaterre in Rodez; Mouton-Fontenille in Lyon; the Observers of Man, Sicard, Pinel, Virey, Itard, the National Institute, and so on in Paris). The general public was driven mostly by curiosity and love of the strange and sensational, but occasionally some people displayed genuine interest in and compassion for the wild boy. From Constans onward, the French authorities took charge of the boy and decided his fate, not without a measure of tension between the different governmental jurisdictions (local, departmental, and central), the capital and the provinces, the welfare institutions and the

ministers to which they were accountable, regarding the rights and responsibilities of each party (the boy, science, society, humanity). From Constans
onward too, concern for the boy was inextricable from the desire to study
him. The story unfolded against the intellectual and scientific background
of the ascendancy of the *idéologues* (concentrated in the second class of the
National Institute), innovations in medicine and psychiatry (notably Pinel's
moral treatment of insanity), and the institutionalization of deaf education
in the Institute for Deaf-Mutes.[4] There is a fourth level as well: that of silent
or silenced characters, comprising the peasants of Tarn and Aveyron, Clair
and Mme Guérin, and all those other relations and incidents that must have
transpired in Victor's life of which no written trace exists or has been found.
The wild boy's fate was to a great degree determined by the juggling between
governing authorities, welfare administrators, and scientific institutions
and the hierarchical pairing of authorized and unauthorized observers and
caretakers (Bonnaterre and Clair, Itard and Mme Guérin).

Whereas most philosophers and naturalists interested in Peter and
Marie-Angélique had to be content with visiting and observing them many
years after they were found, the wild boy of Aveyron was examined, studied,
and described almost constantly from the day of his definitive capture until
1806, and with singular intensity in the first two years. Rather than striving
to reconcile all the descriptions in a single portrait, I retain the different
observers' outlooks and judgments because they shed light on fundamental questions concerning the epistemology and ethics of descriptions and
diagnoses of others. Some issues I want to bring attention to are the difference between scientific and non-scientific portrayals of the boy; the relation
between diagnosis (what the boy *was*) and prescription (what was to be *done*
to and with him); the distinctive way each description invokes notions of
savagery and civilization, human and animal, what is natural and what is
(or seems) disgusting, and singles out disparate aspects of his appearance,
behaviour, progress, or limitations depending on its goals (to stir up expectations, obtain funding, discourage hopes); the many anecdotes that pepper
scientific and official accounts of the boy to illustrate his savagery (or peculiarities, or progress) or simply to entertain; the limitations of the available
descriptions in view of the fact that key witnesses (the peasants, Clair, Mme
Guérin, the deaf-mute children at the Institute) did not write down their
impressions of the boy.

The first to encounter the wild boy were the peasants and farmers of the
departments of Tarn and Aveyron, in southern France. Some woodcutters
met a naked boy who ran away from them in a part of the forest of Lacaune

called La Bassine, in Tarn, sometime between 1797 and 1799 (the date varies depending on the source). It is said that they took him for a strange animal – or the wild man of legend: "They expected to find behind this child other individuals of the same species ready to defend and protect him from any attack. Fear of such an eventual apparition, however imaginary, paralyzed them."[5] But not for long: they captured the strange boy and brought him to Lacaune, where he excited so much curiosity that he had to be put on display in the public square. Curiosity was followed by indifference; his captors momentarily relaxing their vigilance, the child took advantage of their inattention to steal away. The peasants could sight him in the field bordering the forest, digging out turnips and potatoes to eat. They found some rudimentary shelters with beds of leaves and moss in remote corners of the forest, behind a tree, at the foot of a rock, and attributed them to the boy. In June or July 1799 (again the dates vary) three hunters spotted him in the same forest, and even though he climbed a tree to elude them they managed to capture him by force and bring him back to Lacaune. The poor widow who was paid to look after him took very good care of him, or mistreated him, or perhaps both (the sources differ here too).[6] She clothed and fed the boy, noticing that he smelled the food before eating it and refused meat regardless of whether it was cooked or raw. (From the wild boy's dislike of meat some observers inferred that man is not carnivorous by nature.[7]) His hunger satisfied, the wild boy wanted to recover his freedom and looked for ways to leave the house until, realizing that he was locked up "like a bird in a cage," he "resigned himself to the destiny of a recluse and crouched down in a corner of the house where he fell into a long and deep sleep."[8] In the end, after eight days, he attained his purpose.

This time he did not go back to the forest but reached the higher mountains of the region separating Lacaune and the village of Roquecezière, in Aveyron. Details about this period may be gleaned from a report by the government commissioner for Saint-Affrique, Guiraud, who was later in charge of the local inquiry into the boy's origin:

During the day he approached farms, entered the houses with confidence, and unsuspectingly waited to be given something to eat. The compassion he inspired and the hospitable customs of the inhabitants of these mountains were amply manifested. Everywhere people offered him the foods he preferred. Then he went away again to find refuge in the most desert places. For a long time he was seen wandering about Roquecezière. Many times he would go to a farm near this village where he had become used to encountering the warmest hospitality. He threw the potatoes he was given into the embers and, not waiting for them to cook completely, took them out burning hot and ate them avidly. He was thus getting used to the company of people and through these contacts his intellectual faculties were progressively developing. Often, during the day, he approached the peasants' fields and, carefree, occupied himself near them seeking the roots and bulbs that were his nourishment. He frequented in particular the streams to drink or swim, he climbed trees with astonishing agility, and sometimes was seen running away at great speed, aiding himself with his hands, like the quadrupeds.

Guiraud suggests that for a few months the wild boy entered into some kind of relation – if always from a distance and not entirely friendly, at least not forced or overtly hostile – with the people of the region. He was known to them (he no longer excited their curiosity) but they were not indifferent to him; they offered hospitality but respected his wish, or need, to stay essentially unattached (or free). During this time the boy seems to have exhibited a great deal of initiative and activity, losing his earlier fear of people and beginning to learn some skills from them ("his intellectual faculties were progressively developing"). For a moment, the boy's wildness turns epic. Impassible before lightning and thunder, he reacted to the south wind with muscular contractions and contortions that kindled the imagination: "Full of agitation and anxiety he then turned toward the south roaring with laughter and looking at the sky. He seemed to be hearing aerial symphonies, wandering in thought among the clouds. An ironic smile gently touched his lips, but people never understood the nature of the feeling that pervaded his soul in those moments." The physicians later ascribed this reaction to rheumatic pains linked to a slight deformity in his right leg, but Guiraud did not find this prosaic explanation satisfying: "Whatever the reason, under the influence of this wind his face came to life and his thought seemed to awaken. One would have said that he loved to hear the rumbling of the winds and torrents in solitude."[9]

The wild boy's fate changed dramatically on 9 January 1800. Three weeks later Constans recounted his first meeting with him in a letter to J.-P. Randon. Informed at dawn of the appearance of "an unknown child said to be a savage" in the home of Citizen Vidal, a tanner, in Pousthomy, a short distance from Saint-Sernin – where he sought refuge during a particularly cold night of a very harsh winter – Constans went immediately to verify the news. First turning point: this time, unlike all others when the boy had approached or entered a village, the authority was alerted. Constans stated that the boy was "unknown." We may presume that he had never seen or heard about him before, but were all the inhabitants of Saint-Sernin like-wise unfamiliar with the strange boy who had been wandering around the region for some time?[10] Constans found the child, who looked between twelve and fifteen years old (others said that his age was between ten and twelve), "seated in front of a fire that appeared to give him great pleasure," even though he also showed disquiet at the sight of the many curious people who turned up at the tanner's to watch him. The boy aroused Constans's interest: "I took him affectionately by the hand to lead him to my home; he resisted vigorously; but repeated caresses and in particular two kisses I gave him with a friendly smile decided him on the spot and he trusted me a good deal from then on." Constans wished to confirm the rumours he had heard concerning the boy's food preferences. Presented with different kinds of food, he only ate the potatoes, throwing them in the fire and picking them up right away: "There was no way to make him wait until they had cooled off a bit; he burned himself, and expressed his pain with loud inarticulate sounds, which were however not plaintive." When he was thirsty he made his need known: "spotting a pitcher, without making the least sign he took my hand in his and led me to the pitcher, striking it with his left hand to ask me for a drink." After his meal he "got up and ran through the door" but Constans chased him back. Second turning point: from this moment the boy was no longer allowed to carry on his errant existence in forests and mountains, walking in and out of farms and peasants' homes. Apprehended once and for all, he was put under constant official surveillance.

How did Constans explain his action? He pitied the "hapless child." Because the boy did not answer his questions Constans concluded that he was deaf from birth. He wanted to "offer him permanent shelter from the wild beasts that sooner or later would devour him" and "entrust him to the generous care of the government that would allow him to find an adoptive father in the revered abbé Sicard." But Constans was also filled with "sur-prise and curiosity." The boy's odd behaviour made him suspect that he was close to the state of nature. (To back his supposition he told how, to dry his hands, the boy refused the cloth tendered by Constans and used a hand-ful of ashes, all the while smiling "as if saying that his way was better than mine.") He must have been abandoned by cruel parents owing to his deaf-ness and "lived in the forest since early childhood, a stranger to social needs and practices." Deaf, savage, and abandoned to boot, the boy was bound to incite both pity and curiosity. Indeed, Constans declared that compassion and intellectual curiosity need not be in conflict with each other: the only way to ensure that the boy would not end up spending his whole life in a hospice, deprived of "the limitless freedom he found in the fields and forests," was to bring him to the attention of "philosophers and naturalists." Constans let Randon know that he had called the boy St Sernin – an equivocal gesture (and the third turning point): by giving him the name of the village, Constans simultaneously granted the boy a place in the community and recognized his right to it, yet he did so just as he was recommending that the boy be handed over to the central government and transferred to Paris to be placed under Sicard's care. While he awaited a decision bearing on the boy's future, Constans sent him to Saint-Affrique, advising the administrators of the hospice to take good care of him and guard him to prevent his escape: "In every respect, this interesting and unfortunate being invites the care of humanity." In Constans's view, the boy's strangeness did not detract from his intelligence and his "naturalness" was not equivalent to bestiality. The boy's enforced captivity was warranted as the only means to protect him from danger and give him an education suited to his double condition as savage and deaf-mute.[11]

The impressions of three witnesses give us an inkling of what the wild boy was like and what he did during the weeks he spent in Saint-Affrique. Rinaldis Nougairoles, an administrator at the hospice, noticed that he was "nice-looking" and had dark and lively eyes, "pretty little hands" and "a very pleasing laugh." Guiraud pointed out that "in shape this child does not differ at all from other men" but "one cannot say the same of his tastes, his habits, and his behaviour," while for D. Bourgougnon his manners had "more of the savage than of civilized man." In many respects the boy did not change. He had not reconciled himself to his new circumstances and incessantly looked for a way to escape (he twice ran away to the woods and was recaptured). When his will was thwarted he became angry and sometimes bit people. Nougairoles related that upon his arrival he had been given "a gown of grey linen" which he did not know how to take off but "annoys him greatly"; according to Guiraud, in early February he still abhorred clothes, caps, and shoes. But in other respects the boy's "tastes, habits and behaviour" were changing to conform to his new environment: he got used to sleeping in a bed and betrayed great joy at the sight of clean sheets; he had begun to eat soup and was learning to relieve himself outside instead of wherever he happened to be. The most interesting details are those concerning the boy's hearing, speech, and intelligence. Nougairoles found out right away that even though he did not speak, the boy was not deaf as Constans thought. Bourgougnon went further: he not only "hears very well" but "loves to hear others speak." He "lets slip a few words" and "seems very intelligent." For this observer the boy's silence might have been deliberate, stemming not from "ignorance of the language" but "thoughtful obstinacy." Guiraud confirmed that the boy was beginning to "articulate certain syllables," which led him to presume that "with effort he could be made to adjust to a social existence."[12]

What do we know about the wild boy's origins and early life? Besides the earlier sightings and captures, which came to light right away, nothing. All attempts to locate his family were unsuccessful. The few parents who went to see if he was their own lost child did not recognize him. When in June 1801 Itard contacted the prefect of Aveyron soliciting more details about the boy's life in the forest to insert them in his first report, the prefect admitted that neither he nor Constans could add any to those already made public in Bonnaterre's *Notice historique*.[13] What can we make of this informational vacuum that has persisted for two hundred years? If, as most people think, the boy was originally from the Tarn-Aveyron region, it is possible that the local people knew more about him and his family than they chose to tell at the time. While we can only conjecture that the peasants may have withheld information from the authorities (but why?), it is certain that the latter often evinced a dismissive attitude towards the peasants' word and knowledge and resented having to rely on their testimony. For instance, when Randon wrote to the central commissioner of Tarn requesting particulars on the boy's origin so that he could relay them to Lucien Bonaparte, his request was framed in terms of an opposition between the desired "positive and plausible" information (gathered by authorized observers) and the undesirable and plainly insufficient "rumours" and "tales" then in circulation: "Everything that has been said so far about this boy is somewhat fabulous and above all exaggerated."[14]

In the absence of solid facts about the boy's origin, diverse hypotheses were proposed. It was generally believed that he had lived alone in the forest since early infancy after being abandoned by inhumane or poor parents, but Guiraud surmised that he might have run away instead. Seeing that the boy appeared happy when treated kindly and responded to caresses and kisses, yet became sad and anxious at the first show of harshness, Guiraud reasoned that his first years must have been "painful," and that "it was to escape from the undeserved punishments of atrocious parents that he went to the forest seeking an asylum that would guarantee the freedom of his being." Guiraud took the fact that "every time one shows him a string he himself raises his arms and presents his body to be tied" as evidence that his savage habits were "an effect of extreme rigour." A scar in the boy's neck, seemingly made with a cutting instrument, was also conducive to speculation. As Bonnaterre put it: "Did some barbaric hand, having led the child into the wilds, strike him with a death-dealing blade to render his loss more certain and more complete?" The ominous scar underlay a local legend, a tragic tale of money, jealousy, murder, and remorse, which attests to the soul-stirring power of the boy's mysterious presence. A young woman was married against her will to a rich neighbour whom she found repulsive. Obsessed with suspicions, the husband saw in the birth of her first child the embodiment of his shame and paid a neighbour known for his cruelty to put the unfortunate baby to death. After wounding the baby in the neck, the would-be murderer lost courage and ran away. Some time later the villagers of Roquecezière witnessed the arrival of a man consumed by a secret remorse, who climbed the rock after which the village is named and on reaching its highest point jumped to his death. When the wild boy was found, people associated the two occurrences.[15]

If Constans's intentions were to be carried out, it was necessary to let the rest of the nation, and especially the capital, know about the unusual find. On 25 January the *Journal des Débats* published Nougairoles's letter (dated 11 January) divulging the phenomenon "which has preoccupied all the residents of this community since this morning." Like Constans, Nougairoles closed his letter with a statement of interest and concern: "I leave to scholars the task of explaining this phenomenon and of drawing conclusions. But I desire strongly that this interesting child receive the beneficent attention of the government." Two days earlier Randon had dispatched a letter to his subordinates Constans and Guiraud rebuking them for having kept him in the dark regarding a discovery that was both "a police matter" and "a matter of potentially greater interest to scientific observers and naturalists." Randon knew very well what was at stake: if the boy was truly a savage ("a stranger to society") it was crucial "that his first tendencies be observed before he acquires specific ideas in this respect, either by habit or by instruction." This should be done by a professor of natural history in the provincial capital.[16] Thus the boy's transfer to Rodez (to be studied by Bonnaterre at the Central School) was arranged before the Parisians even had a chance to react to the news. As the Aveyron authorities had expressed great concern for the boy, Randon reassured them that he would do "everything in my power to ensure that this poor child has a happy existence" and that the care he would be given would compensate at least in part for the discomforts he experienced in his new life. But Randon also told Constans that he wished the boy's stay in Saint-Affrique, where he seemed to have been "made to lose some of his habits and behaviours," had been shorter.[17]

In Rodez, the authorities recognized that the boy was valuable insofar as he was a savage and that any increase in his civilization diminished his value. On those grounds, they found a way to keep him for a few months and afford Bonnaterre sufficient time to examine him even though already on 1 February Lucien Bonaparte had written to reclaim "the young man who only utters vague cries and who does not speak any language." To justify the delay in carrying out the minister's command, the Rodez government not only appealed to the need to obtain more information and perhaps find the boy's parents (Bonaparte had said that the boy should be handed over to him only if all hopes of finding his parents were lost) but, to deflate expectations, proclaimed that he was *not* "a true savage": "He is at the most an abandoned child who has lived in isolation in the woods or who at least has not had habitual contact with society."[18] After a few months of silence (on Bonaparte's part) and diligent study (on Bonnaterre's), Sainthorent, the new prefect of Aveyron, reminded the minister that the wild boy was still in Rodez. Apparently having no more use for him and ready to deliver him into the hands of another authority, Sainthorent spared no effort to make him sound enticing. The prefect resolutely professed that the boy retained all his "savage habits" but it was premature to infer from this that his intellectual faculties were impaired; it was to be assumed instead that with the right attention he would make great progress. The nation must adopt this child who did not yet have a name and would "henceforth be known under the designation you will be so kind to give him."[19]

The "general public" manifested interest in the wild boy in several ways. Crowds of curious people turned up to see him every time he was captured, on his arrival in Saint-Affrique, Rodez, and Paris (and at each stop during the trip to Paris), and at the Institute for Deaf-Mutes. The boy did not willingly submit to the attention and scrutiny, at least initially, and sometimes became violent and bit in all directions. In late 1802 Chaptal let the administrators of the Institute know his displeasure with the way the boy was being daily exposed to visitors as "an object of spectacle." As late as July 1810 the welfare administrators claimed as one of the reasons why Victor had to be removed from the Institute the disruptive visits he continued to receive from curious people. In order to become Victor's permanent guardian in 1811, Mme Guérin first had to accept the condition that she would under no circumstance expose him to public curiosity or make a spectacle of him. She was warned that, should she fail to comply, Victor would be taken away from her and placed in a hospice.[20] Some accounts describe encounters between the wild boy and "ordinary" (curious) people. On 30 August 1800, after appearing before Lucien Bonaparte with Bonnaterre and Clair, the boy was presented to a lady who had asked to see him. The lady was still in bed and the boy at once lay down beside her. His reluctance to leave this "voluptuous bed" made everybody laugh. And according to the baronne de V ... 's account of the visit Victor and Itard paid Mme Récamier at her château in Clichy-la-Garenne, the boy delighted the elegant and enlightened guests with a flawless performance that had nothing to fear from comparison with the wildest exploits of Peter or Marie-Angélique: unmoved by his hostess's beauty and charm, he ate voraciously, left the table halfway through dinner, tore off his clothes, and climbed the trees of the garden, frustrating "M. Yzard"'s efforts to retrieve him by jumping from branch to branch and tree to tree. Once calm was restored and the chagrined teacher left the party with his unreliable pupil, the guests drew a "useful comparison between the perfection of civilized life and the distressing picture of savage nature." The conservative critic and poet Jean-François de La Harpe (1739–1803) seized the occasion to discredit Rousseau's views.[21]

Lay observers and visitors recorded their impressions of the boy. R. Vaysse of Aveyron wrote to the editor of *Journal de Paris* stating his surprise at the temporary oblivion into which the child had fallen and reminding readers of the opportunity they were missing. The boy's fear of people proved "that he had never known them, or had last seen them before attaining the age of understanding"; yet despite many indications of "the most characteristic savagery and an entire life spent in the forests," his skin "retained a whiteness that seems to contrast greatly with that state," an astounding fact deserving investigation by naturalists. He had "a pretty face, a gentle and interesting physiognomy," and a gentle and shy character. His initial apathy and insensibility had been replaced by surprise and wonder at the novelties he was being exposed to, and having lately become used to his clothes, he refused to part with them or with the cord used to tie him, which he viewed as part of his dress.[22] British visitors to Paris, who routinely attended the public demonstrations of Sicard's deaf-mutes, described in letters and journals their meetings with the child already well known in Europe as "the young savage of Aveyron." One of them noticed that he was "dressed like another boy" and "kept his eye constantly on the door." Another reported that "as soon as the door was opened [the boy] showed an inclination to get out." Although the Parisian savants took him for "man in his primeval state before he had acquired the use of language," to this observer he seemed "a stupid boy neatly dressed ... one of our species either not completely formed or whose faculties had been injured by accident."[23] Also in disagreement with savants and philosophers was the journalist and pamphleteer Gabriel Feydel (1755–1840), who soon after the boy arrived in Paris started a polemic in *Journal de Paris* with an open letter betting that the "alleged Savage of Aveyron" was "nothing but a little actor who plays his role fairly well," followed by a series of satirical articles under the general title "Qu'est-ce que le Sauvage de l'Aveyron?" Many readers took up Feydel's challenge, some defending the boy's "wildness," some claiming that he was "an imbecile deprived of any kind of intelligence and guided only by instinct," and others merely hoping to win some easy money regardless of the boy's condition.[24] Although these accounts and descriptions may be classed at the level of general popular interest because their authors were not directly aligned with either science or government, all of them bespeak some familiarity with the scientific-philosophical issues that made the boy potentially relevant and valuable. The central question, which had already been raised by the Aveyron authorities in the early days of January 1800, was whether he was *truly* a savage, hence the representative of the state of nature awaited by philosophers and naturalists for more than a century.

Artists appropriated the wild boy's plight and interpreted it in keeping with the rising Romantic sensibility. In an undated "Romance du Sauvage de l'Aveyron" the boy reproaches the men who snatched him away "from the cradle of nature." A benevolent nature that "protected my childhood" and "fulfilled my needs and my tastes," a paternal God who "had pity on my misery," and wild but innocent and well-meaning animals are juxtaposed to the boy's infanticidal parents:

> And you who in my tastes seek
> The habits of primitive man,
> Cease from your frivolous studies;
> Come, let us live among the wolves;

> Their friendship is not treacherous: ...
> The wolf does not murder his children.

Nature is represented in its alternative Romantic form – not nurturing but sublime, "dreary," "dark," and "thorny" – in "The Savage of Aveyron," written by Mary Darby Robinson (1758–1800) shortly before her death. The poem's speaker meets the wild boy in the "mazy woods of Aveyron" and learns that his solitude dates from his mother's murder in the same forest. From his dying mother he learned the only word he now perpetually shrieks: "Alone! alone!"

> And could a wretch more wretched be,
> More wild, or fancy-fraught than he,
> Whose melancholy tale would pierce AN HEART OF STONE.

In this poem the child's destitution is emotional and spiritual, and his solitude mirrors the poet's own melancholy. At the other end of the spectrum, in the comedy *Le Sauvage de l'Aveyron ou il ne faut jurer de rien* by Citizens Emmanuel Dupaty, Maurice, and Chazet, the young Russian officer Polinsky, a prisoner of war in love with Mme Nina de Senanges, learning that a savage captured in Aveyron was to be presented to her beloved, pretends to be the savage to get close to her. The play, which opened at the Paris Vaudeville Theatre on 28 March 1800, was a great success, and the audience cheered the couplets sung at the savage's capture:

> Without knowing all these rights,
> One is never truly free,
> And in the woods our ignoramus,
> Didn't know that he was free,
> But as it has been decided,
> That every man must be free,
> We have arrested him on purpose,
> To inform him that he was free.

Like the individual who refused to obey the general will in Rousseau's *Du contrat social* (1762) but for different reasons (ignorance rather than wilful resistance), the wild boy is "forced to be free." Revolutionary notions of freedom and rights are here complicated by their fraught relations with knowledge and ignorance and with the state's power to enforce them – through captivity, if necessary. Who is "truly free," the savage in the forest or the citizen aware of his rights? And how does one transform the one into the other?[25]

But it is now time to turn our attention to the scientific accounts of the wild boy. The unprecedented character of Bonnaterre's *Notice historique* needs to be emphasized once more: for the first time a naturalist had the opportunity to study a wild child at length shortly after the child was found. Having heard rumours about the finding, the abbé Bonnaterre went to see Randon in late January and offered to go to Saint-Affrique to examine the boy, thus prompting Randon's order to transfer him to Rodez. Bonnaterre understood full well the kind of phenomenon he was confronting due to his acquaintance with the Enlightenment debates on wild children. The *Notice historique* combined observation and description (based on Condillac's sensationist philosophy) and classification (based on Linnaeus's taxonomy, by way of Schreber). It paid particular attention to the boy's "primitive state" and the progress of "his first sensations and his first ideas" while integrating him as a true savage into "the table Linnaeus offered us." The wild boy was "no different from any other" child and had "an agreeable physiognomy and a pleasant smile." He could hear, but his hearing was selective: he seemed insensible to piercing cries and the sound of musical instruments, but if someone softly cracked a walnut behind him he turned to grab it. Bonnaterre estimated that the order of importance of his senses (smell, taste, sight, hearing, and touch) was the inverse of that in men who enjoyed full use of their intellectual faculties. The boy's first response to his reflection in a mirror was to look behind it, "thinking he would find there the child whose image he perceived." Fire gave him great pleasure – "he shakes his hands as a sign of joy; he roars with laughter; he draws up his gown as far as his belt, the better to feel the heat" – but extreme cold did not affect him. Even in winter he went barefoot and covered himself with a single sheet to sleep. To relieve himself, "he generally signals to have the door opened; he goes out; and he goes in a courtyard or in some other spot provided for this purpose." Whereas the Saint-Affrique reports alluded to his beginning to articulate a few syllables (or words), Bonnaterre contended that he only uttered cries and inarticulate sounds. Still, he communicated all his needs through the signs he had learned "since his return to society." He was in good health, growing and getting stronger, but showed no sexual impulses yet.[26]

To avoid the adverse effects of a drastic change of life like that imposed on the girl of Songi, which damaged her health, Bonnaterre allowed his charge to follow "his inclinations and his tastes." But the professor's permissiveness had a limit: the boy's most ardent "inclination" – to recover his freedom – was unswervingly frustrated. He ran away four or five times while at the Central School, but "fortunately he was always retaken, sometimes at considerable distance from the town." In these circumstances he had little else to do than to pursue the two other pleasures he knew: eating and sleeping. He woke up at dawn and rocked back and forth to pass the time; around nine he went into his caretaker's room to have breakfast and returned to his room until lunchtime; in the afternoon he went for a walk or stayed by the fire, then ate some more, rocked back and forth some more, and when bedtime came "nothing can stop him; he takes a torch; he points to the key to his room; and he becomes furious if one refuses to obey him." His bed, made of bundles of straw, was in a dry room with windows covered with linen (because he had broken the panes). During sleep he "presses his two closed fists over his eyes and his face against his knees." Predictably, Bonnaterre itemized the boy's changing food preferences: he relished green peas, beans, and walnuts, and in the spring he developed "such a taste for meat that he ate it raw or cooked." Bonnaterre supported his argument that the boy's intelligence manifested itself almost exclusively in the sphere of food and eating with anecdotes that tell as much about his gaze and methods as about the boy's cleverness. The professor noticed the boy's concentration and dexterity in shelling beans for his own consumption. If he felt like eating fried potatoes, "he would choose the largest ones, bring them to the first person he found in the kitchen, tender a knife to cut them into slices, find a frying pan, and point out the cupboard where the cooking oil was stored." At a certain point he got into the habit of going to the kitchen, lifting the covers of all the pots, and dipping a piece of bread to taste the food they contained. After the woman who cooked his meals severely reprimanded him, he was seen (by an amused Bonnaterre) waiting patiently for the moment when she would be otherwise occupied to dip his bread quickly many times without being caught. On one occasion he hid and buried what was left of a meal, undoubtedly to save it for later. And during the long trip to Paris he would not lose sight of the bag which he knew carried his food.[27]

To construe the boy's significance and explain his condition Bonnaterre relied on Enlightenment notions of the state of nature and the origin of knowledge. Deprived of contact with other men, and hence of signs and chances to multiply his needs and ideas, he had been reduced to a state close to that of animals. His needs and desires revolved around food, freedom, and rest, beyond which he had no ideas, reason, or memory: "Consigned by nature to instinct alone, this child performs only purely animal functions ... his desires do not exceed his physical needs." For Bonnaterre, the boy's character was essentially self-centred: "His affections are as limited as his knowledge; he loves no one; he is attached to no one." The preference he showed for his caretaker was "an expression of need and not the sentiment of gratitude." Although with the help of Condillac's epistemology Bonnaterre could account for the boy's deficiencies as an effect of his previous isolation, he did not rule out the possibility that the boy might be an "imbecile." His conclusion was ambiguous: "Such an astonishing phenomenon will furnish philosophy and natural history with important notions about the primitive constitution of man and the development of his intellectual faculties, provided that the state of imbecility we have remarked in this child places no obstacle in the way of his instruction."[28] The abbé Bonnaterre did not subject the boy to methodical instruction; his attitude was one of detached observation, benign and well-meaning but abstaining from any closer involvement. Historians of the wild boy have upheld the *Notice historique* as an important supplement (or corrective) to Itard's representation of his progress, underscoring the advances in socialization the boy made during his sojourn at the Central School in response to a stable and warm human environment.[29] I am nevertheless puzzled by the disparity between the earlier representations of the boy as full of activity, initiative, and in some peculiar way intelligence, and Bonnaterre's portrayal of the same child as a selfish, instinctive, apathetic, and conceivably imbecile creature. Should we ascribe this disparity to the fact that Bonnaterre, the first skilled observer to come in contact with the boy, grasped his true character and saw what others could not or did not see? Is the divergence between the boy who roamed the forests and mountains of Tarn and Aveyron, who was captured at the tanner Vidal's and taken to Saint-Affrique, and the boy who lived with Bonnaterre in Rodez, due to more accurate and objective observation or to a different attitude on the part of the observers? Or to a change in the boy himself? Conceding that the length of time Bonnaterre had to conduct his study may indeed have permitted him to see more and better, we must also acknowledge, first, that the naturalist was prone to see in the boy a destitute creature comparable to Condillac's statue and Linnaeus's *Homo ferus*, and second, that the life he arranged for the boy, however gentle, was still one of captivity. Set against his former existence – outdoors, in constant movement, having to provide for his own needs and watch out for every potential danger – the urban, sedentary, sequestered, and indoor life the boy was forced to lead in Rodez must have been distressful, extremely uneventful, and plainly *boring*.[30]

Just as the reason behind the wild boy's transfer to Rodez was Bonnaterre's desire to examine him, Lucien Bonaparte's request to have him transported to Paris was spurred by the scientific curiosity of the members of the Society of Observers of Man, founded shortly before the boy's capture. The society's secretary, Louis-François Jauffret (1770–1850), wrote to the administrators of the Saint-Affrique hospice: "it would be very important for the progress of human knowledge that a zealous and sincere observer, taking charge of [the young Savage] and retarding his civilization for a while, ascertain the sum of his acquired ideas, study his manner of expressing them, and see whether the condition of man abandoned to himself is altogether contrary to the development of intelligence." These critical observations, which could only be performed in Paris, by Sicard and "under the eyes of several other Observers of Man," would benefit the boy by "bringing public attention to bear on him and securing an advantageous future for him." A month later Jauffret informed the editors and readers of *Journal de Paris* that the minister was organizing the boy's transfer to Paris and confirmed that he was functionally deaf (three days later Vaysse clarified that he was not deaf but appeared so at first due to a stupidity or stupor from which he was coming out: he was beginning to respond to Bonnaterre's voice and utter some inarticulate words). Jauffret implicitly conjured up memories of the Chartres deaf-mute and the Lithuanian boys: "I ignore what the metaphysicians will conclude from the responses of the deaf-mute savage once Sicard and Massieu have taught him the theory and practice of sign language." Like Constans, Jauffret believed that the boy's right place was in Paris and with Sicard, and that scientific attention would guarantee him a bright future; like Randon, he worried that some of his value might already be lost: "the observers of man will always regret that the most precious month for the observation of this singular creature was lost to science."[31]

An anonymous article in *Gazette de France* that marked the boy's arrival in Paris and recounted his reception by Sicard rehearsed the same issues. The wild boy was expected "with justifiable impatience excited by the memory of the Leblanc girl, another savage, and several events of the same kind, recorded in the proceedings of various academies." Reminding readers that philosophers and naturalists had long dreamed of raising a child in isolation to study the natural development of ideas and language, the author assuredly declared: "This child has been found." Furthermore, the author maintained that the boy, who would from then on be "the object of the observations of true philosophers," was no more civilized then than when first found, Bonnaterre having kept him in the same state in which he was delivered to him. Exhausted after the trip, he would be given a few days' rest.[32] In early September Clair returned to Aveyron, followed a month later by Bonnaterre. There is no record that Sicard ever attempted to instruct the wild boy, as he had been expected to do. A servant looked after him, and when he was not being exposed to the public (or taunted by the other deaf-mutes) he was left alone to wander about the building and garden or confined in a small room in the attic. If life in Rodez had not been particularly appealing, the combination of ravenous curiosity and neglect the boy must have endured during these first months in Paris was no improvement.

Among those who visited the wild boy was Julien-Joseph Virey, who wrote a long report evaluating his condition in relation to the "primordial state of our species," upon which "the whole social edifice rests" but about which so little was known. Many details in Virey's description betray the extent to which his observations, and the questions he asked Clair, concerned traits that could be anticipated by someone acquainted with the earlier accounts of wild children: the boy's skin, originally darker, turned lighter as an effect of domestic life and frequent baths; his thumbs were proportionally larger than those of other children and his fingers very skilful and flexible; he was not hairy, did not swim, and had not been seen climbing trees or walking on all fours lately (this was only right, said Virey, since nature made us to stand erect and walk on two feet). Other details were more specific: the boy, extremely thin when found, had gained weight and lost part of his agility; his sexual organs were less developed than those of children his age living in the city; he had no sense of shame and used to defecate anywhere, but never in his bed ("It is curious that he always squats to urinate, and stands erect to defecate"); he slept more than usual (which Virey imputed to the boredom of captivity) and sometimes had agitated dreams, especially after receiving many visitors; he had begun to drink milk (which he at first rejected) and learned some conventional signs; he loved to be tickled and had a pleasant laugh; he was indifferent to children's toys, games, and amusements but "likes to run bits of straw between his teeth, sucking the lightly sweetened marrow they might contain"; he detested children his age and ran away from them.[33]

But what exactly was this boy? Virey reasoned that, while it was inaccurate to say that he was utterly savage, as he must have been raised in society up to a certain age, he was much closer to the state of nature than us. Neither fearful like Montesquieu's natural man nor brave like Hobbes's, Virey's wild boy approached Rousseau's noble savage: gentle, innocent, a lover of solitude, ignorant of evil and incapable of causing intentional harm. In his lack of ideas and reason Virey did not see a sign of idiocy but "the dark ignorance of a simple soul," one which could be known right away because it had no imposture or hypocrisy. Virey was perplexed by the boy's selfishness ("he has no idea of property, he seeks to possess everything himself, because he considers only himself") and by his lack of gratitude and pity. He perceived no connection at all between the boy and other people and predicted that his puberty would be late and detached from feelings of love. The boy's emotional independence and intellectual vacancy prompted a dramatic statement: "If it were not for his human figure, what would distinguish him from the ape?" The "Dissertation" ended on a lyrical note: "Go, unlucky youth, on this unhappy earth, to lose in civil relations your primitive and simple roughness. You lived in the bosom of the ancient forests; you found your subsistence at the foot of oaks and beeches; you quenched your thirst at crystal springs; and content with your poor fate, limited in your simple desires, satisfied with your way of life beyond which you knew nothing, this usufruct was your sole domain. Now you have nothing except by the beneficence of man; you are at his mercy, without property, without power, and you pass from freedom to dependence." And a prediction: "The path of your education will be watered with your tears."[34]

Another anonymous article, printed in the *Décade philosophique*, also took up the question of the wild boy's relation to the state of nature. Was he an example of natural man or merely a defective being (deaf or imbecile)? And how would the definition of man be affected if he were indeed equivalent to natural man? After distinguishing three views of natural man – man untouched by any external influence or education; man isolated from other people (modified by physical circumstances but not by the moral order); and the ideal or model for human existence – the author claimed that the first and third definitions did not apply to the Savage of Aveyron: "The man who lived in the forests has received, like the others, an education, even if undoubtedly not the most perfect," and the man who fulfills "the destiny of Nature" should be looked for not in an isolated man but in "a family of honest and industrious farmers." The second definition might correspond to the wild boy's condition, but then it was consistent with the notion of perfectibility as man's essential characteristic. Thus the boy's destitution, far from detracting from man's dignity or unsettling our ideas of his origin and destiny, furnished "a new and striking proof" that *"Man is made for society"* and "a new reason to devote ourselves unreservedly to the good of this society, to which we owe everything we are." The article did something else, and more original: it raised the epistemological problem of the proper method to study the wild boy. The author spent many hours with him "and the only result I have obtained so far has been to know how great is the flimsiness, the presumption of those who pretend to have passed judgment; and how difficult it is in fact to form an exact and certain opinion in this regard." No conclusion about the boy's condition could be drawn from his present situation as a captive besieged and upset by curious people. To observe the natural state of such an individual one must spend time in his natural environment, sharing his life in liberty; moreover, to relate effects and causes, one would need to know everything pertaining to his origin and past life.[35]

These suggestions were not heeded – or came too late. The Observers of Man appointed a commission to study the boy and decide what was to be done with him. At the 29 November meeting Jauffret read the first part of the report prepared by Philippe Pinel (1745–1826) but withheld the conclusions to give the other members of the commission time to write their own separate reports (the *Mercure de France* noted a few days later that Pinel's conclusions could be easily foreseen, "and his listeners have already concluded that we have not found natural man this time either"). The second part was read in May 1801. The full report offered an account of the "current state of the organic functions and moral faculties of the child known as the Savage of Aveyron"; accounts of several children and adults, patients at Bicêtre and the Salpêtrière, "whose intellectual or affective faculties are more or less damaged"; a comparison between the boy's physical and moral faculties and those of idiot or insane children, and the "inductions" resulting from the comparison. Its significance was threefold. First, Pinel stressed the boy's defects and deficiencies (as *symptoms*) and invariably interpreted them in the worst possible light. The boy depicted by Pinel was not "wild" but filthy and disgusting, apathetic, insensible, inferior to men and animals alike: "He is entirely insensitive to any kind of music, and on this point he is considerably below many individuals confined in our hospices. Should we be afraid to say that in this respect even elephants have a marked advantage over him?" Pinel did not see a single redeeming or endearing quality in the boy: "One might attribute to a vivid memory, or to the impulse of a lively imagination, these outbursts, these immoderate peals of laughter, which suddenly occur from time to time, with no known cause, and which sometimes animate his features; but I can assure you that these quick transports of vague and delirious hilarity are observed most often in children or adults fallen into idiocy and confined in our hospices." Pinel – who, unlike the author of the *Décade* article, had no qualms about studying the savage in captivity – gave no indication regarding the production of his report and the observations and examinations on which it was based. (Only once did he point to his presence as an observer: "His gaze wanders, and he generally turns towards the window or the most brightly lit part of the room. This is what I noticed repeatedly during the time his portrait was being sketched.") He elided his own relation to the boy by forging a disembodied eye that *fixed* the child outside any context, history, or situation. Pinel's uncaring portrayal of the wild boy has often been rebuked; however, none was more consequential, because Itard, even though he disagreed with Pinel's *conclusions*, retained (to his own advantage) Pinel's *characterization*. Second, Pinel's report detached the boy from the Enlightenment problematic of natural man and inserted him into a different domain, that of mental pathology. Bonnaterre's comparison of the wild boy with other savages was useless because the other cases were drawn from unreliable fragments and lacked detail and precision. In contrast, Pinel argued, his own objects of comparison (idiot and insane children) were there for anyone to observe. He concluded that there was "the greatest degree of probability" that the boy should be classed with the insane or idiot. Third, Pinel's diagnosis led to a prognosis. During the months he had spent at the Institute for Deaf-Mutes the boy had made "no visible progress" or given "any sign of perfectibility," and thus "however circumspect we must be in our predictions, nothing seems to indicate that the future will be brighter." If, as Pinel surmised, the boy was an idiot, there was "no well-grounded hope of obtaining any success from a methodical and further prolonged instruction." For this reason, he must be confined in a hospice "with the other unfortunate victims of an incomplete and mutilated organization."[36]

Pinel's report had two immediate consequences: it provided scientific justification for the disappointment and indifference that had supplanted the great hopes aroused by the wild boy's discovery, and it inspired the young

Jean-Marc-Gaspard Itard to undertake the boy's moral treatment in defiance of his eminent teacher's judgment. A letter to the editors of the *Décade philosophique* printed a year after the boy's arrival in Paris corroborated that he was "utterly forgotten." The author berated the Parisians' unjust indifference (which some people had tried to justify "by proclaiming that he was an imbecile, and that the impairment of his organs is opposed to his ever acquiring the use of reason") and criticized Pinel's method of reasoning from similar effects to similar causes for overlooking the fact that the appearance of idiocy could be due to "moral causes." Fortunately "the poor child of Aveyron" had escaped the severe sentence that condemned him to "expiate in the depth of a hospice ... the misfortune of having seemingly usurped for an instant the place of natural man" through the timely intervention of "C. Ytard, enlightened physician and philosopher" under whose care the boy was making slow but certain progress.[37] We do not know when Itard began to work with (or even first met) the wild boy. He was present at the reading of at least one part of Pinel's report. Did he conceive the idea of training the boy then, or was the training already under way? Sicard introduced Itard to the Observers of Man on 17 June 1801. After Itard informed them that the boy's progress gave him reason to entertain hopes and proposed to write a full report, the Observers invited him to share his observations with the commissioners so that they could repeat them and thus have new elements for their own report. In a letter to the *Mercure de France* that appeared three days later, Itard imparted the favourable changes discernible since the boy had been in his care (and, he was careful to add, since Pinel had stopped seeing him). He announced the imminent publication of his report communicating the "new facts" relative to "the history of the first developments of this child's thought" and the grounds of his belief that the boy was endowed with all the faculties of thinking beings. When Itard read them the report on 26 August, the Observers received it with great applause – yet reminded the inexperienced but daring doctor-philosopher that what they had solicited were not his conclusions on the condition of the boy's faculties but his observations, to aid the commissioners in reaching *their own* conclusions.[38]

It is useful to contrast Itard's approach with those advocated by the anonymous writer of the *Décade* and put into practice by Pinel. Whereas Pinel diagnosed the boy in his present situation (captivity) and the *Décade* writer argued that to study the savage one had to share his savage life, Itard, assuming that what the boy *was* hinged on what he could *become* (that is, on

the extent of his perfectibility), arrived at a conception of knowledge production that depended on direct intervention. To know the wild boy, it was
necessary to instruct him, to treat him, to *develop* his faculties. Departing
from all earlier accounts (of the wild boy and of other wild children), Itard's
report centred on his effort to transform the child, a work he designed and
conducted as an experiment. The report opened with a strong sensationist statement: "Cast upon this globe, without physical strength and without
innate ideas, incapable of obeying by himself the constitutional laws of his
organization, which call him to the first rank in the system of beings, man
can only find in the heart of society the eminent place that was marked
for him in nature, and would be, without civilization, one of the weakest
and least intelligent of animals." Itard acknowledged the immense epistemological import of wild children in the investigation of the origin of ideas.
Even though all the earlier studies of wild children had produced uncertain
results, the recent achievements of metaphysics and medicine enlightened
by analysis gave reason to think that now the outcome would be different.
Confronted with *"such an astonishing being,"* a philosopher and physician
would be able to *"deploy all the resources of present knowledge for his physical and moral development."* Only insofar as the boy's faculties developed
could a certain diagnosis of his condition be issued. If this development
proved impossible or unsuccessful, careful observations would permit us to
*"determine what he is, and deduce from what he lacks, the hitherto uncalcu-
lated sum of knowledge and of ideas that man owes to his education."* Itard's
designs and assumptions by and large emanated from eighteenth-century
themes; however (and this is the novelty of his work), what he envisioned
was not just the (passive) observation of the development of the wild boy's
ideas but an active, medico-pedagogical development of his faculties.[39]

What allowed Itard to undertake his work was his disagreement with
Pinel's view of the cause and (potential) curability of the boy's condition.
Itard did not deny that the state of the boy's faculties was that of an idiot,
but he argued that this idiocy was not congenital (due to organic lesion)
and therefore incurable but contingent or acquired, caused by long years of
isolation and by lack of education and social intercourse. For this reason, it
would respond to the proper training or treatment. Itard's program for the
wild boy of Aveyron, which was medical and pedagogical at the same time,
had five aims: 1) to attach him to social life by making it gentler than the
one he was leading and more similar to the one he had been forced to abandon; 2) to awaken his nervous sensibility through energetic stimulation and

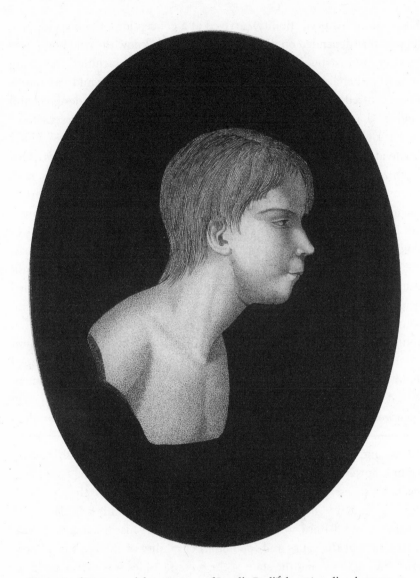

Portrait of Victor and frontispiece of Itard's *De l'Éducation d'un homme sauvage, ou des premiers développemens physiques et moraux du jeune sauvage de l'Aveyron*, published in 1801. Courtesy of the History of Medicine Division, National Library of Medicine.

DE L'ÉDUCATION

D'UN HOMME SAUVAGE,

OU

DES PREMIERS DÉVELOPPEMENS
PHYSIQUES ET MORAUX

DU

JEUNE SAUVAGE DE L'AVEYRON.

Par E. M. ITARD, Médecin de l'Institution
Nationale des Sourds-Muets, Membre de la
Société Médicale de Paris, etc.

Quand on dit que cet enfant ne donnait aucun signe de
raison, ce n'est pas qu'il ne raisonnât suffisamment pour
veiller à sa conservation; mais c'est que sa réflexion, jusqu'alors
appliquée à ce seul objet, n'avait point eu occasion de se porter
sur ceux dont nous nous occupons........................
.... Le plus grand fonds des idées des hommes est
dans leur commerce réciproque.

CONDILLAC.

A PARIS,

Chez GOUJON fils, Imprimeur-Libraire, rue Taranne,
N°. 737.

VENDÉMIAIRE AN X. (1801).

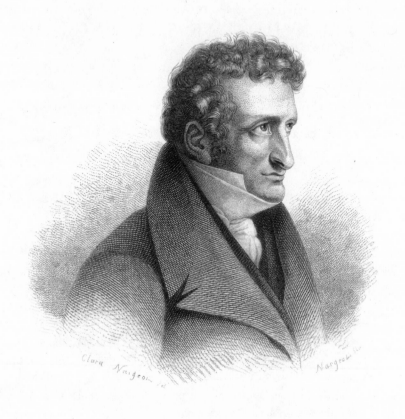

Dr ITARD.

Jean-Marc-Gaspard Itard. Courtesy of the Bibliothèque Interuniversitaire de Médecine (Paris).

intense emotion; 3) to increase his ideas by giving him new needs and multiplying his relations with other people; 4) to lead him to the use of speech by means of imitation and "the urgent law of need"; 5) to exercise simple mental operations upon the objects of his physical needs and then apply them to objects of instruction. In the course of his work Itard formulated new pedagogical principles and invented instructional devices that would win him the admiration of future generations of experts and practitioners. By the time he wrote the report Itard was confident that his hunch had been right. His task was far from complete, but the progress detectable so far suggested that the boy "is not, as is generally believed, a hopeless imbecile but an interesting being, who merits, in every respect, the attention of observers and the particular care being devoted to him by an enlightened and philanthropic administration."[40]

Itard's insistence on his pupil's progress and prospects is understandable, since his intention in writing this report was to impress the Observers of Man and convince Chaptal that his (and Mme Guérin's) task was worth funding. But Itard's portrayal of the wild boy had more troubling underpinnings and effects. While he disagreed with Pinel's assessment of the cause of and prognosis for the boy's idiocy, Itard maintained Pinel's description of the state of the boy's physical and intellectual faculties. According to Itard, an enormous distance separated Victor (after a few months of treatment, "an *almost ordinary* child who does not speak") from "the savage of Aveyron." By retaining Pinel's negative and unsympathetic characterization of the "savage," Itard was able to reinforce Victor's progress – and his own medico-pedagogical achievement. Even if Itard's often-repeated representation of the boy as "a disgustingly filthy child, affected with spasmodic and often convulsive movements, rocking ceaselessly like certain animals in the menagerie, biting and scratching those who crossed him, not showing any affection for those who attended him; in short, indifferent to everything, and paying attention to nothing" was, in context, not devoid of irony and hyperbole (after all, Itard was indicting the curious Parisians who flocked to see the boy upon his arrival), later commentators took it literally and reproduced it word for word. As a consequence of the popularity of Itard's report, Pinel's description of the boy (which it enthroned) eclipsed all prior ones, and his earlier history of encounters and relations (which it made light of) vanished from view. Itard's confidence was only slightly tempered by his concern regarding Victor's lingering speechlessness and budding sexuality. His incomplete observations nonetheless provided "material proof of the most important truths" at which Locke and Condillac had arrived speculatively through sheer genius: a) in the state of nature man is inferior to animals; b) the moral superiority of man results from civilization, his special sensibility, and his faculty of imitation; c) the faculty of imitation weakens with age and isolation, hindering the late learning of speech; d) the dependence of ideas on needs is a constant; e) education must be guided by medicine, "which, of all the natural sciences, can cooperate most powerfully in the improvement [*perfectionnement*] of the human species, by appreciating the organic and intellectual anomalies of each individual and determining therefrom what education must do for him, what society may expect from him."[41]

It is important not to underestimate the complexity of Itard's first report. Although it was rooted in eighteenth-century concerns, it simultaneously initiated a new view of knowledge as intervention (and, we shall see, a new view of the child). Likewise, although it constituted and espoused the *medico-pedagogical* relation between child and adult, it contained telling traces of a different type of relation. Its most arresting passages are indeed those in which the adult evinced careful regard for the child's unclassifiable strangeness: "One morning when there was a heavy snowfall while he was still in bed, on awakening he uttered a cry of joy, left the bed, ran to the window, then to the door, impatiently coming and going from one to the other, escaped half-dressed, and gained the garden. There, giving vent to his joy by the most piercing cries, he ran, rolled in the snow, and gathering it by handfuls, feasted on it with incredible avidity." On these occasions Itard perceived a wider range of emotions in the child, including regret and nostalgia for his lost freedom and a special, *aesthetic* connection to nature: "When the rigour of the weather drove everybody from the garden, that was the moment he chose to go there. He went round it several times, and finished by sitting on the edge of the pond. I have often stopped for whole hours and with inexpressible pleasure, to examine him in this situation; to see how all his spasmodic movements and the continual rocking of his whole body diminished, subsided by degrees, replaced by a calmer attitude." Victor could not be interested in ordinary children's toys and games, yet he derived intense pleasure from simple things: "If sometimes, despite the keen interest this young orphan inspired in me, I took upon myself to excite his anger, I let no occasion pass of procuring him joy; and certainly no difficult or costly means were necessary to succeed in this. A ray of sun, caught on a mirror, reflected in his room and turning about on the ceiling; a glass of water let fall drop by drop and from a certain height upon his finger tips, while he was in the bath; a little milk contained in a wooden porringer that one placed at one end of the tub, and that the oscillations of the water made drift, little by little, amid cries of joy, into his grasp: this is nearly all that was needed to amuse and delight this child of nature, often to the point of ecstasy." In a revealing passage, Itard registered Victor's lack of appreciation of his medico-pedagogical care and his affection for Mme Guérin:

The friendship he has for me is much weaker, and this is how it should be. The care Madame Guérin takes of him is of a kind which is immediately appreciated, and what I give him is of no sensible use to him. This difference is so obviously due to the cause I indicate, that there are times when I am welcomed: those which I never employ for his instruction. If, for instance, I go to his room, in the evening, just after he has gone to bed, his first movement is to sit up for me to kiss him, then to draw me to him by seizing my arm and making me sit on his bed. Then he usually takes my hand, carries it to his eyes, his forehead, the back of his head, and holds it with his upon these parts for a very long time. Sometimes he gets up with bursts of laughter, and comes beside me to caress my knees in his own way, which consists of feeling them, rubbing them firmly in all directions and for many minutes, and then in some cases laying his lips to them two or three times. Say what you will, I confess that I lend myself without fuss to all this childishness.

Scattered throughout the report, this and similar passages help us distinguish Itard's medical pedagogy from the *personal* relation he was sometimes able, and willing, to establish with Victor.[42]

Itard's report achieved its purposes. The philosopher and Observer of Man Joseph-Marie Degérando (1772–1842), reviewing it for the Class of Moral and Political Sciences of the National Institute, of which he was a member, supported Itard's notion of "moral idiocy" caused by extreme circumstances. Having himself observed and studied the boy, Degérando verified that Itard's successes were almost miraculous and foretold even greater progress in the future. Through Itard's efforts, "the hopes of the philosophers are beginning to be realized and the zeal of the friends of humanity to obtain its reward."[43] But after a few calm months Chaptal resumed his threats to cut the expenditures associated with the boy's training, thus eliciting a series of letters and progress reports to justify its continuation. In 1802 Sicard transmitted the results of an examination conducted by himself, Pinel (who was an old friend of Chaptal's), and another eminent physician, Jean-Noël Hallé (1754–1822). Led by Itard, Victor had performed many tasks and exercises that demonstrated the development of his senses of sight, touch, and hearing, and of his imitative faculty. To accentuate Victor's progress, Sicard once again devalued his earlier condition. Compared to ordinary children, who enjoyed so many resources from which he had been deprived, the progress made by this poor creature under Itard's care seemed minimal. But if one compared the Victor of the present with "that young savage who had nothing of the human species except the mechanical structure," then the magnitude of his progress was made visible. The examining authorities recommended that the treatment/training be continued until the boy stopped making progress, since only then could the true extent of his capacities and perfectibility be estimated: "This is the experiment whose success or lack of success will establish the nature of this intelligence, which one could not at present declare null without temerity, and perhaps without a kind of barbarity." Sicard's report indicated that Victor's training was proceeding along the lines set out in Itard's published work, testified to the approval which by this time Itard had garnered from Sicard and Pinel, and made clear that Itard's superiors backed his contention that the boy's true condition could only be known in the future, at the end of the medico-pedagogical intervention.[44]

In an undated and incomplete manuscript on mental illness, Itard defined idiocy as a lesion affecting both the intellectual and the affective functions, either inherited or acquired "by moral ineptitude or by a long isolation." Apathy and indifference were common symptoms: "We may communicate with [idiots], but they never communicate with us (this reciprocity being a characteristic of perfectible beings) unless regarding the objects of their first needs." If, as Condillac believed, the greatest source of men's ideas is their dealings with each other, it was "incontestable" that a man deprived from infancy of all society would find himself "reduced, like most idiots, to purely animal functions." What Itard claimed was that there were *two* kinds of idiocy – caused by natural functional inaptitude or absolute lack of education – and that only the first one was untreatable. Furthermore, natural idiocy could only be identified as such *a posteriori*, after education, guided by medicine, had exhausted all possible means to instruct/cure an individual. Appearance and symptom did not determine a person's potential or perfectibility. Itard was thus able to explain his decision to care for the wild boy, despite his miserable state and Pinel's negative prognosis, without giving up the idea of idiocy: "I dared believe that this kind of idiocy could be cured, because this state only seemed to be a natural consequence of his long isolation, because I had had occasion to observe that this being, so limited, so stupid relative to our customs and the new objects around him, seemed to rise above himself every time his own needs were at stake, and then his attention, his memory, his judgements, became evident and prodigiously extended." Victor was beginning "to trace all the letters of the alphabet reasonably well, to copy many more complex figures, to sew"; from the progress of his faculty of imitation, Itard augured that he would "at least be able to become a good draughtsman or copyist." Victor was displaying intense curiosity, of a type never found in cases of natural idiocy, which for Itard was "an extremely favourable circumstance." While at first it was impossible to attract his notice, at present he watched "with the greatest attention" whatever one did in his room. Victor was being taught numbers and sign language: "He has got some ideas of the first numbers indicated by the fingers. Reciprocal relations have greatly improved. By means of the signs of the deaf-mutes, one may make him present all the objects in his room, demand *an action* and determine the visible qualities of objects and even their number, provided that they do not go beyond the first numerical additions. As speech is not progressing, we have taken another road to determine his progress."[45] Because both Itard's 1801 and Sicard's 1802 reports were written to ensure the continuation of the treatment, it would be fair to suspect that they might have overrated Victor's progress, however unwittingly. The assessment contained in this unfinished text is therefore especially important in that it not only does not conflict with those reports but hints at even greater advances.

In mid-1804 Chaptal decided to cease funding Itard's and Mme Guérin's work with Victor and refused to hear any entreaties. Still, the minister accepted that by then it would not have been right to confine the wild boy in a hospice, as he had acquired certain rights owing to the attention he had received, and asked the Institute's administration for advice as to what was to be done with him. On 21 July the administrators of the Institute drafted a reply. They confirmed that Victor's case merited special attention, "whether because of his bizarre fate or because of the hopes aroused by his first education," and informed Chaptal that Itard had expressed the wish to take care of him for three more years, "undertaking to provide him with the care and supervision he needs" without demanding "any salary for his efforts." What they suggested as a just and humane arrangement was that Itard be remitted a sum equivalent to what the government would spend on Victor if he were registered as an imbecile in a hospice.[46] But this desperate and moving letter was not sent because around that same time Napoleon asked for Chaptal's resignation. The new minister, Champagny (whose general secretary was Degérando), never again questioned Victor's presence at the Institute or begrudged its cost.

Two years later Champagny urged Itard to write another report on his work with the wild boy: "I know, Monsieur, that you have attended both generously and diligently to the education of the young Victor, entrusted to you five years ago. It is important for humanity and for science to know the results." Itard promptly complied with the minister's request but noted that he would rather have "condemned to an eternal oblivion" work "whose result offers much less the story of the pupil's progress than that of the teacher's lack of success."[47] Itard did not say it in the report, but Victor's education had already ended. It is strange and baffling that whereas in July 1804 Itard seemed ready to commit himself to Victor's care exclusively out of interest and affection, not long afterward he terminated the treatment on his own. What happened between 1804 (when Itard most firmly voiced his commitment to Victor) and 1806? The second report presented the development of Victor's sensory, intellectual, and affective functions. Itard underlined the many areas in which Victor had made great strides, yet he did not conceal that he was increasingly frustrated by his pupil's slow and limited intellectual attainment and disappointed by his failure to learn spoken language. Itard's efforts met with two other sources of resistance: Victor's lack of motivation and frequent disruption of the lessons, and his awakening sexuality, with whose intense and intensely confused manifestations Itard was unable to deal successfully: "I saw this eagerly awaited puberty arrive, or rather explode, and our young Savage consumed by desires of an extreme violence and startling continuity, without sensing what was their aim, and without experiencing the slightest feeling of preference for any woman."[48] Did Itard lose interest in Victor once the opposition to his work subsided? Did Victor undergo a change for the worse that wiped out his earlier progress? Was Itard simply ready to move on? In the closing words of the report, Itard reiterated his plea for the wild boy's case: "Regardless of the point of view we use to envisage this long experiment, whether we consider it as the methodical education of a savage [homme sauvage], or we only see it as the physical and moral treatment of one of those creatures ill-favoured by nature, rejected by society, and abandoned by medicine, the care that we have taken of him and that we still owe him, the changes he has undergone, those that can be hoped for, the voice of humanity, the interest inspired by such an absolute abandonment and such a bizarre destiny, everything recommends this extraordinary young man to the savants' attention, to our administrators' solicitude, and to the Government's protection." Itard was no longer willing to devote his own time to Victor, but he never completely gave up his sense of duty and responsibility towards him.[49]

The ambivalent tone of the second report fed later suspicions that Itard came to view his work as a total failure and his former pupil as an incurable idiot. In fact, Itard himself included in the report hints as to how he wanted it to be read and judged. He insisted that Victor, "to be judged soundly, must be compared only with himself," and enhanced the comparison by further depreciating his earlier state: "I will not retrace for you, Sir, the hideous picture of this man-animal as he was when he came out of his forests." Itard was not present when the boy came out of "his forests" and the people who were did not describe him in those terms. Still, by denigrating the boy's condition before the medico-pedagogical experiment Itard magnified the transformation he effected in him and thus his own scientific and peda-gogical contribution: "Such was the state of this child's physical and moral faculties, that he was placed not only in the lowest rank of his species, but also at the last rung of the animals, and one could say that in some mea-sure he differed from a plant only in that he had the faculty of moving and uttering cries." Regardless of his personal feelings in connection with the outcome of his work, Itard must have been very pleased with the evalua-tion of his report by the third class of the National Institute, which officially underwrote the interpretation he had suggested. First, the class marvelled at "the distance that separates the point of departure from that which he has reached" (Victor must be compared only to "himself" – the filthy, dis-gusting, dull, hideous, and animal-like, even plant-like, savage of Aveyron). Second, the class "recognized that it was impossible for the teacher to put into his lessons, his exercises, and his experiments more intelligence, dis-cernment, patience and courage, and that if he has not obtained a greater success, this must be attributed not to a defect in zeal or talent, but to the imperfection of the organs of the subject on whom he worked" (Victor's remarkable changes were due to Itard's efforts and talent – and his unremit-ting deficiencies to his own imperfection). Third, the class recommended that the report be published, as it comprised many interesting observations the knowledge of which would prove extremely useful "to all persons who are involved in the education of young people." The observations, techniques and conclusions arrived at by Itard during his work with Victor would contribute to the improvement of the education of all children. On 26 November Champagny, who had ordered the evaluation, let Itard know that his report would be printed at government expense and at the imperial printers because in it "men involved in the education of childhood will find new and useful views."[50]

Let us pause for a moment to reflect on what has happened. Itard's experiment – the observation *and training* of a wild child – has made visible general (medico-pedagogical) methods and principles useful to everyone engaged in the education of (*both* normal and abnormal) children. The meaning of the wild child, Itard's experimental subject, has shifted from potential representative of man in the state of nature to potential stand-in for *the child*. This emerging understanding of Itard's work rested on the erasure of the accounts and descriptions of the wild boy made before his first miserable months at the Institute for Deaf-Mutes and on Itard's own construal (which was indebted to Pinel's) of his original state.[51]

After Itard's desertion, the authorities of the now Imperial Institute for Deaf-Mutes had second thoughts with respect to Victor's presence there. In July 1810, in a letter to the new minister of the interior, Montalivet, they put forward several reasons why Victor should be removed. The wild boy (then a young man) was not deaf, and since despite Itard's efforts "his intelligence has not developed but very slightly about certain material objects," Sicard was of the opinion that he suffered from "complete idiocy" and would not progress any further. Victor was "unsociable" and could not live with other children: "It is impossible to subject him to any rule; he cannot therefore stay in an Institution where the maintenance of order and discipline are crucial." To complicate matters, Victor required special arrangements that were "a source of abuse and inconvenience." The authorities objected to the continuous presence of a woman, who moreover received frequent visits from her daughters, in an institution devoted to the education of boys. Yet for so many years "an object of the Government's charity," Victor seemed to have "acquired rights not to be deprived of it, and even to continue to enjoy it according to the habits he has been led to contract." The authorities made a proposal that reconciled "the interests of the Government, of the Institute for Deaf-Mutes and of the young savage, with the duties of humanity": Mme Guérin would seek accommodation for herself and Victor outside but very near the Institute (so that both could remain under institutional supervision) and the government, through the Institute, would continue to pay Victor's expenses and Mme Guérin's salary. The proposal was approved, and in mid-1811 Victor and Mme Guérin moved to 4 impasse des Feuillantines.[52] At precisely the same time Montalivet asked the Institute's authorities to admit a young deaf-mute who had been found in January roaming the fields around Loriol, near Valence, in the department of Drôme. While the young man seemed to have passed the age when he could be admitted for free, the minister requested that an exception be made due to his extreme destitution: "He is more or less in the same situation as Victor of Aveyron." The administrators wrote back immediately, politely rejecting the minister's proposal. The boy's age and the habits he must have undoubtedly contracted in his wandering life would make him "incapable of profiting from the lessons and the care that would be given him." As the young savage might bring with him "the contagious example of depraved habits," his stay at the Institute would be "fruitless for him and dangerous for the others." The same authorities that eleven years earlier had been so intent on bringing the savage of Aveyron to Paris now proclaimed that the newly found savage should stay right where he was, at the Drôme hospice, to prevent the repetition of experiences "about which Victor of Aveyron has only too well shown us the difficulties as well as the uselessness."[53]

Victor's later years were spent in obscurity. Three brief accounts illustrate the scope of views and attitudes prevalent in those years. Claude-Henri de Saint-Simon (1760–1825) appropriated Victor for his progressive conception of human intelligence. Since the state of the boy's intelligence before his return to society must have been "very near that of the first generations of the human species," by observing him we were directly observing the intelligence of the "first men." For Monboddo, Peter had typified the first stage in human progress; by the same token, Saint-Simon used Victor as a living example of the first term in the "series of different nuances observed in the development of human intelligence." Resuming old debates, he argued that the Savage of Aveyron proved that the idea of God was not innate and conventional signs were indispensable to form and combine ideas.[54] In contrast, Franz Josef Gall (1758–1828) and Johann Gaspar Spurzheim (1776–1832) treated Victor not as a savage but as a true idiot. Whereas other observers had repeatedly stated that in appearance the wild boy did not differ from other children, Gall and Spurzheim saw in him the physical stigmata of idiocy: "He is an imbecile to a high degree. His forehead is very little extended on the sides, and very compressed on top, his eyes are small and very sunken, his cerebellum is little developed." The expectations awakened by the wild boy were unwarranted: "That is the outcome of all the hopes aroused by him, the numerous efforts made, and the patience and kindness manifested in her conduct towards him by a beneficent woman." Like Pinel, Gall and Spurzheim framed Victor within the domain of mental pathology, but unlike Pinel they added visible deformities to support their diagnosis. Victor and the other savages found in forests were not examples of natural man but "miserable creatures of an imperfect organization" who were abandoned because of their idiocy and "cannot receive any instruction or education." Their condition proves that education and circumstances can only modify and improve man insofar as he possesses the necessary physiological dispositions.[55] Finally, Virey, who had studied the boy in 1800, had little to say about his present condition in 1817: "Today, he understands many things, but without articulating any words ... [He] remains frightened, half-savage, and has been unable to learn to speak, despite the efforts made to teach him."[56]

Since his "discovery" until the moment when he stopped being interesting, a string of observers captured the wild boy in writing, proffering descriptions, diagnoses, conjectures, and prescriptions. But we do not know what the two people who actually took care of him, Clair Saussol and Mme Guérin, thought of him. How did they see Victor, and how did they understand their relation to him? Actions sometimes speak louder than words. Several documents refer to the close relation between the boy and Clair, but the accounts diverge as to the boy's feelings for him, some claiming that he was indifferent and others that he loved the "poor and respectable old man" very much. There is no question that Clair must have learned to care deeply for the boy in the few months they lived together, since before leaving Paris to return to Rodez he "promised to come and take him again and act as a father to him, if Society ever abandoned him."[57] Mme Guérin, who lived with Victor and looked after him from the outset of the medico-pedagogical experiment until his death, was undeniably the most significant person in his life, much surpassing Itard. The available evidence does not tell us what her original status at the Institute was. In his reports Itard gave her credit for her invaluable assistance, her competent performance of her duties, and her sincere attachment to Victor, which, we know, was fully reciprocated. Mme Guérin had a husband, whose death is recorded in Itard's second report, and daughters who visited her (and, we assume, Victor) at the Institute. One of them, Julie, eleven or twelve years old in 1801, may have inspired one of the few words Victor uttered spontaneously. After the girl's weekly visits to her mother, he was "often heard to repeat *lli lli* with an inflection of voice not without sweetness."[58] When on 5 April 1811 the authorities officially notified Mme Guérin of the new arrangements touching her and Victor, they appealed to her affection for him to make her comply: "The particular care you have devoted to him until now assures us that you will not want to expose him to further miseries."[59]

Did Itard play any role in Victor's later life? In their 1810 letter to Montalivet, the Institute's authorities had vowed that Itard would not lose sight of him and would act if any sign that further improvements in his ideas or development of his faculties might be expected. Itard looked back on his work with Victor in 1825 in a report to the administration of the now Royal Institute for Deaf-Mutes. He had sacrificed most of his time during six years to the experiment, hoping to take advantage of the wild boy's extraordinary condition to observe "the late development of the instinct of imitation, the influence of imitation on the development of speech and of speech on the formation and association of ideas." Although his diligent care did not produce in the Savage of Aveyron the results Itard expected, he was later able to apply the observations and techniques "suggested by the inflexibility of his organs" to other mute children with happier results.[60] All of Victor's biographers suppose that Itard never saw him again; yet even if there is no evidence that he ever did, there is no evidence to the contrary either. I would like to believe that Itard continued to care for the boy who had launched his career and that he was at least partly responsible for the proposal that allowed him to spend the rest of his life with Mme Guérin – an anonymous and most likely simple life, but neither lonely nor destitute.

FROM HIS DEFINITIVE capture in 1800 until his death in 1828 the shape of Victor's life was determined by other people's decisions. The first (and most drastic) decision was to force him to leave the forest, thus putting an end to his freedom. Was it right to capture the wild boy, to make of him, as Shattuck put it, "a prisoner of culture and society," when he seemed to have passed "the first fundamental test: survival"? Shattuck thinks so, because had he stayed in the forest he would forever have lacked "the benefits of social exchange and a place in a collective life." Truffaut was more emphatic: "For me, Victor's life in the forest was wholly abject. And everything that happened to him in society constituted progress." In the wild, the boy had to endure brutal winters and constant dangers, to which the many scars in his body attested: "Contrary to the wild children of legend who were helped by the animals of the forest, Victor lived in *spite* of them."[61] On the whole,

I believe that the wild boy's captors, while to a large extent following their intellectual curiosity, were also sincere in their conviction that they were doing what was best *for him*. But the boy's voluntary appearance at the tanner Vidal's need not be interpreted as an indication of his *desire* to be captured. He may have sought some human contact that day, as, it seems, he was wont to do in the last few months of his free existence, but he never expected, much less wanted, to be kept there by force and stopped from leaving again.

Even if we concur with the decision to capture the boy as perhaps the only means to ensure his full return to human society and protection from the dangers of life in the forest, it is still necessary to appraise the kind of life allotted him within society. A dramatic passage in Itard's second report outlines the alternatives available at the time: "I went and sat at the end of the room, and considering with bitterness this unfortunate creature, reduced by the strangeness of his fate to the sad alternative of either being relegated, as a true idiot, to one of our hospices, or purchasing, through unheard-of effort, a little instruction that was still useless for his happiness, 'Unhappy creature,' I told him, as if he could hear me, and with real anguish of heart, 'since my labours are wasted, and your efforts fruitless, take again the road to your forests, the taste for your primitive life; or, if your new needs make you dependent on society, you must expiate the misfortune of being useless to it, and go die in Bicêtre of misery and boredom.'"[62] The alternatives were successful reintegration (through education) into society, return to the forest, or confinement in a hospice. The problem was that, after the end of Itard's treatment, none of them appeared viable. The boy had not been thoroughly reintegrated or re-educated, but the political, scientific, and institutional authorities, Itard included, were aware that they were accountable for his new state of dependency. The sense of obligation they continued to feel towards the wild boy until the end of his life, which demanded from them a happier solution than the misery of Bicêtre, stemmed from their understanding that they had replaced his earlier freedom and self-sufficiency with a host of artificial (social) needs.

Victor's benefactors were most likely right in their view that after his Parisian experience he was no longer capable of resuming a free and independent life and required indefinite assistance. Still, there was another alternative, which they failed to consider. Victor could have been returned to Tarn or Aveyron, his region of origin, and placed with a peasant family (as Peter had been) or entrusted to Clair, who had offered to act as his father if society ever abandoned him. What made this alternative unthinkable at the time? The available options, whether enacted or only formulated, were circumscribed by a hierarchy of peoples and places – Paris and the provinces, the city and the country, the authorities (decision makers and knowledge makers) and the people – themselves framed within a project of national unification that in part proceeded through the devaluation and elimination of specific cultural and linguistic elements within the nation. In this setting, it was perhaps to be expected that the Parisian administrators, intellectuals, and professionals involved in the wild boy's case, many of whom, like Itard, had been born and grown up in the provinces and moved to Paris before or during the Revolution to advance their careers, did not see the peasants (equated with savages, when not directly idiots) and rural life (confused with the savage state) as valid alternatives for the boy. In his unpublished manuscript on mental illnesses Itard asserted that a kind of apparent idiocy could be caused not only by lack of verbal communication (as with deaf-mutes before their education) but also by the isolated and rudimentary life led by some populations. As illustration, he referred to the people of a marshy region of France. If an individual from that region were placed beside an inhabitant of the enlightened cities, the former, in relation to the latter, would be "a true imbecile." The Parisian authorities revealed their arrogance in their blindness to the wild boy's proximity to the peasants (which Constans had obliquely honoured by calling him St Sernin) and presumption that their simple and often difficult life was uncivilized and had little value.[63]

In his foreword to the catalogue of the exhibition on the wild boy organized by the Mission Départementale de la Culture of Rodez in May 1992, the president of the mission, Jean Monteillet, noted that for a long time the people of Aveyron felt somewhat embarrassed by their association with the boy, afraid that it might give them a bad image. This is no longer the case, as attested by the exhibition itself, the statue of the boy, by Rémy Coudrain, which stands in Saint-Sernin-sur-Rance since 1987, and the now routine references to the wild boy in local histories and promotional material on the region.[64] For the first time the testimony of the local people (the descendants of the peasants who sighted, captured, and fed the wild boy) has appeared in their own words. Vague details about an episode not registered in the known documents were preserved in the oral tradition. Some farmers of Rougéty, north of Roquecezière, captured the boy and brought him to Amans Foulquier-Lavernhe, a rich landowner who kept him for a few days and tried to tame him through gentleness and mollify him with kindness, but without success. "They said that he was captured here in Rougéti," Alphonse Cambon related:

It must have been at night, poor thing, because it was a lost child raised by the wolves. It was the wolves, I think.

And the doctor who lived at my daughter-in-law's house, here, treated him ... When people tried to capture him he always ran away. Otherwise, he must always be in the same place. They said he had been in the woods of Lacaune ... but they also said he had been in the woods above Sent-Sarnin.

The oral tradition also preserved rumours about the boy's origin. Mme Malaterre of Claparède told René-Charles Plancke that the young daughter of a castle gave birth to an illegitimate child and ordered a servant to make him disappear. The servant hid the baby in the bushes and fed him in secret until one day he found that a she-wolf had taken his place. Mme Malaterre's Lacaune aunt, from whom she had the story, claimed that the family still existed. Adultery, illegitimacy, attempted murder, and remorse recur in the version reported by Henri Calmels of La Bastida (as heard by his brother-in-law from his own parents): this wild child was the bastard of a Parisian queen, "I don't know which one it was, if it was Louis XIV, or Louis XV or Louis XVI, I can't tell you that." A man from Lacaune, charged with the gruesome task of killing the baby, took him to the forest and wounded him: "And he thought the child was dead. But there were leaves, which fell over him, it was the time when the leaves fall it seems, one leaf fell where he was bleeding and the blood clotted, he healed and he lived." The wild boy had a lingering impact on some local communities. All through the nineteenth century, every time the people of Roquecezière gathered for a meal or festival, they remembered his visits to la Vayssière, Tougnetou, la Frégère, and other places. In Madame Gély's family the story of the savage was used to scare the children: "My grandmother, who was born in 1862, often talked to her children about the wild child. She scared them, telling them that if they ran away, the wolves would bring them up, they would make them walk on all fours." But the inhabitants of Saint-Sernin, unlike their counterparts in the surrounding villages and farms, had forgotten everything about the wild boy until quite recently, when they were reminded of him by foreign tourists and visitors.[65]

CHAPTER SIX Victor's Afterlife

> Given the time in history, an almost nonexistent knowledge base
> with regard to educational practice, and total ignorance of "Victor's"
> origins, Itard's work is nothing short of remarkable and profound.
> In its entirety it is a statement for all special educators for all time.
> Its timelessness removes it from the realm of historical curiosity and
> will forever project it toward contemporary brilliance.
>
> L.M. Lieberman, "Itard: The Great Problem Solver"[1]

THE FINDINGS AND PROCEDURES Itard derived from Victor's training were in time to affect not only the subsequent encounters with wild children but also the treatment and care of increasingly larger groups of children. This chapter examines Victor's afterlife, that is, the many ways in which his story was appropriated, interpreted, and reinterpreted within the disciplines and professions dealing with childhood and children during the past two centuries. The numerous textual incarnations and uses of Victor's life and Itard's account of his education expose the changing relations of opposition and identity between wild children and children in general. They underscore the movement from the *wild child* (as exception, monster, or aberration) through the *abnormal child* (object of psychiatry and special education) to the *normal child* (object of developmental psychology, progressive pedagogy, and compulsory education) and reveal how each of these instances contaminates and complicates the other two. The last section of the chapter explores some historical, pedagogical, and ethical issues arising from the discontinuities between Victor's story and his afterlife and points out some tensions inherent in the medico-pedagogical model of the child-adult relation promoted by Itard and institutionalized in the sciences of childhood influenced by him. As it follows the thread of scientific and professional engagement with Victor, the chapter stresses the fact that what underlay the progress of scientific knowledge and the educational feats of intelligent adults was the puzzling presence and haunting memory of a silent child who came out of the forest.

In his article "Idiotisme" (1818), the prominent Parisian alienist Jean-Etienne-Dominique Esquirol (1772–1840) – a friend of Itard's and like him a student of Pinel's – thus epitomized the stories of wild children:

A guilty mother, a wretched family abandon their idiot or imbecile son; an imbecile escapes from the paternal home and gets lost in the woods, not knowing how to find his way back; favourable circumstances protect his existence; he grows nimble to avoid danger; he climbs trees to save himself from peril; pressed by hunger he eats whatever he finds; he is fearful because he has been frightened; he is stubborn because his intelligence is weak. This unhappy child is encountered by hunters, brought to a village, taken to a capital, placed in a national school, entrusted to the most renowned instructors; the court, the city take an interest in his fate and his education; scholars write books to prove that he is a savage, that he will become a Leibniz, a Buffon. The observing and modest physician asserts that he is an idiot. This judgment is appealed; new accounts are written; everyone wants to take advantage of this event; the best methods, the most enlightened care are brought to bear for the education of the so-called savage. But what is the outcome of all these claims, all these efforts, all these promises, all these hopes? That the observing physician had judged rightly. The savage was nothing but an idiot.

Esquirol's general conclusion was that "these men deprived of intelligence, isolated, found in the mountains, in the forests, are imbeciles, idiots, lost or abandoned." Esquirol sided with Pinel (the "observing and modest physician") against Itard. He made this explicit in 1838, the year of Itard's death, when he revisited the topic of idiocy in his treatise on mental illnesses: "This was Pinel's judgment on the *Savage* of Aveyron." But Esquirol also praised the methods Itard applied in the education of the savage: "It is impossible to read anything more interesting than Dr. Itard's two reports on the admirable care our colleague lavished on this idiot to develop his intelligence." And this is how Jean-Baptiste Bousquet (1794–1872), secretary of the Royal Academy of Medicine, summarized Itard's contribution: "to bring up an idiot, to turn an unsociable and disgusting creature into an obedient, bearable boy, is a victory over nature, almost a new creation!"[2] Almost thirty years later, another Parisian psychiatrist, Louis-Jean-François Delasiauve (1804–1893), enunciated a similar reading of Victor's condition before proceeding to praise Itard's work: "It is hard to understand how, with such poor faculties, he was able to secure, by himself, his subsistence and survival for so many years. The logic of hunger has its genius ... The savage of Aveyron was what he had to be, according to his crippled nature. Certain potentials did not exist ... His level was marked by the mediocrity of his judgment and inductive discernment ... His selfishness was no less a natural consequence of his incomplete organization."[3] This then is the first appropriation of the story, insinuated by Itard himself in his second report: the outcome of Itard's rash experiment demonstrated that Victor was not a savage but an idiot or imbecile, as Pinel had claimed, but precisely for that reason it was remarkable that the young doctor had been able to effect such an extraordinary transformation in him. The more the wild boy was believed to have been an idiot – and the more his initial condition was disparaged – the more Itard's accomplishment stood out as both admirable and exemplary.

This rendering of the story received a more positive and practical turn in the writings of Édouard Séguin (1812–1880), widely recognized as the founder of what is now known as special education. Séguin recounted that when in 1837 Itard was asked to treat a young idiot, he declined the commission because of his poor health but agreed to supervise Séguin in this task. During their brief collaboration Séguin learned the medico-pedagogical principles discovered by "his illustrious teacher" and used them as the starting point for his own pioneering work in the education of idiots, to which he devoted the rest of his life, first in Paris and then in the United States (a Saint-Simonian socialist, Séguin left France after the defeat of the 1848 revolution). According to Séguin, while Itard had failed to cure or fully rehabilitate Victor – and even if his diagnosis, "based upon a metaphysical error," had been wrong and Pinel's right – he had succeeded in proving what until then was unthinkable: that idiots were *educable*, and he had laid down the bases upon which their education should be conducted.[4] Through Séguin's widespread influence, the wild boy's memory was kept alive – and the reduced interpretation of his condition (founded on Pinel's and Itard's accounts) was entrenched. Late nineteenth- and early twentieth-century textbooks and overviews of idiocy, mental retardation, or mental deficiency routinely inserted references to Itard and Victor. In these texts, the history of mental retardation is construed as the move from mistreatment and neglect to enlightened concern, treatment, and education, a battle between obscurantism and progress in which doctors and philanthropists play the starring roles while the "idiots," like Victor, are filthy and disgusting examples of flawed humanity that must be reformed or hidden away. Just as praise of Itard is invariably accompanied by certainty about and depreciation of Victor, in the triumphalist history of mental retardation the objects of study and treatment are devalued and the (medical and philanthropic) transformation imposed on them is magnified.[5]

Here are some examples of how Itard and Victor are represented in these works. For William Ireland, while Itard's pamphlet was "plainly the work of a superior mind" he "overestimated the mental capabilities of his pupil" and the result of his venture "proved the correctness of Pinel's diagnosis"; still, Itard's method of education "has been of use in the training of idiots." Martin Barr specified that Itard's work was "the first successful demonstration of the possibility of educating an idiot by physiologic means with a philosophic aim." Even if "unwittingly," Itard was "the discoverer of a reflective power in idiots that once awakened might be trained." Likewise, Pierre Pichot first pointed out that Itard's "starting point was not quite correct" since the boy was feeble-minded "and no educational method could make up for that." The theoretical foundation of Itard's pedagogical method, "the sensual philosophy of Condillac," was "much too fragile." Yet Itard must be commended both for his courageous attempt to educate "a subject who was looked upon by all as a mere curiosity" and for the "educational technique" he invented.[6] Although the overblown exaltation of his work was tinged with slight condescension (his discovery of the educability of idiots was momentous but unintentional; he adhered to outdated and inadequate theories that misled or blinded him), from the late nineteenth century until roughly the 1960s Itard was approached mainly as a predecessor or precursor, a groundbreaking historical figure who had to be given due credit in the brief historical reviews that introduced textbooks and handbooks of mental retardation and deficiency. In this vein, the tenth edition (1963) of *Tredgold's Textbook of Mental Deficiency (Subnormality)* stated that it was Itard who "first described attempts to train a subnormal child," anticipating "by a century and a half some part of modern theory and practice in connection with the teaching of young or slow learning children."[7] Two side effects of the link between Victor and idiocy were that he was sometimes included, together with other wild children, in classifications of idiocy, and that his case could serve as an example of the condition in general.[8]

By the 1960s, professionals in the field of mental retardation had no doubts concerning Victor's diagnosis. But as the field grew and broke down into subfields, researchers and practitioners started to perceive Itard differently, as not just a revered forerunner but also a model or inspiration for present theory and practice. They claimed his legacy (medico-pedagogical principles and instructional techniques) for particular methods and approaches within the field and interpreted his goals and strategies in light of their own. More detailed analyses of Itard's reports led to revaluations of Victor's condition and progress. For instance, John F. Gaynor reinstated Itard's view that the cause of Victor's retardation was the long period he had spent in isolation in the wild while rejecting Itard's estimate of the boy's progress: "He is in danger of being remembered as the man who considered his efforts to educate Victor a failure, rather than as the author of specialized training for the mentally retarded."[9] Itard's technique was revaluated as well. While certainly innovative for its time, had it been good enough to elicit the best possible outcome? Would Victor have made further progress had Itard employed a more sophisticated technique – such as the one propounded by the author(s) of the article or book in question? Many modern professionals manifest a strong personal identification with Itard, that is, they see *themselves* in him. As they appropriate Itard and profess to recognize their own commitments and methods in his, professionals consistently position Victor as the consummate object of knowledge and intervention – or *child*.

In Thomas S. Ball's *Itard, Seguin and Kephart* (1971) we find one of the most conspicuous cases of massive identification with and appropriation of Itard. Ball's aim was to develop an approach to sensory education that would integrate the Skinnerians' behaviourism and Kephart's cognitivism. Itard and Séguin must be included in this discussion, he explained, because they were the "true pioneers and innovators of sensory education" and because "the assumptions upon which the whole field was based might best be understood by returning to their original sources." The book opens with a lyrical account of Ball's own relation to Itard. Ball (of Pacific State Hospital) first read Itard's "classic" reports on the wild boy of Aveyron some years after completing his doctorate:

It was a beautiful, deeply moving experience, timed at precisely the right moment in my life and career ... As I have read and reread Itard, the hiatus of years that separates our lives has slowly disappeared. Each time, he becomes more of the teacher-physician-scientist-humanitarian and sensitively responsive human being. Although I do not view this in a mystical sense, my mind has become the scene of a dialogue involving three parties: great men of my contemporary experience,

Itard, and myself. As I know these contemporaries better, I know Itard better. With enhanced understanding of Itard, I understand more deeply my own reactions to what I have personally experienced. Out of the chemistry of these interactions I begin to come in contact with what I would like to call *wisdom*. It is with whatever wisdom I can bring to bear upon this topic that is so close to my heart that I proceed with the dialogue.

The subjective and emotional tone of this passage starkly contrasts with the behaviourist terminology and unmitigated scientism that pervade the rest of the book. Ball got carried away again when depicting the link he sensed between (his) Itard and his contemporary hero, Kephart:

In many respects I understand Kephart better through Itard than I do through Kephart himself. This is because I see in Itard's work with Victor a brilliant and penetrating, yet exhaustive, clinical documentation of sensory education carried from its most rudimentary level on to the development of abstract functioning. In part, the limitations of this material lie in the fact that it is based on a single case. But what it lacks in this respect is more than compensated by the breadth and scope of what can be truly described as a monumental effort – a work of genius. And it turns out that Itard's presentation does, in fact, have great generality. I can find in many of his experiences and observations exact counterparts to my own and those of others.

Since Itard was "the point of departure, the fountainhead of the field of sensory education," it was imperative that his work be understood "as clearly as possible within a modern framework." And this is what Ball did: he recast Itard's work with Victor in terms of "the theoretical framework of operant conditioning" and "the concepts and methodology stemming from Pavlov's original formulation of the orientation reaction." Ball maintained that Victor's progress was greater than many, including Itard, were inclined to admit, but he also believed that the boy would have benefited from a better technique. As to Victor, Ball (predictably) equated him with a rat: "Like a rat pushing a lever which leads to the presentation of a food pellet, for Victor, presenting the word cards led to the presentation of a reinforcing object."[10]

Even as the behaviourists saw Itard as a proto-Skinnerian, professionals of a different bent, who focused on other elements of his work and described and labelled it differently, saw in it an anticipation or reflection of their own concerns and practices. In the final chapter on "Psychotherapy" of *Psycho-*

logical Problems in Mental Deficiency (1949), Seymour B. Sarason, professor of psychology at Yale, emphasized, as the central factors of Itard's success with Victor, the individualized attention Itard bestowed on his pupil-patient, his open attitude towards Victor's prospects, and the intersubjective relation established between them. Itard's experiment illustrated "the degree of behavioral change which can be effected by efforts which are planned, intensive, personalized, and therapeutically oriented." In Sarason's opinion, Itard's feat showed the validity of psychotherapy as a method for treating defective children: "Had the boy been treated in accord with the diagnosis made by the authorities of the day there probably would have been no change in his behavior, a finding which then would have been utilized as proof of the validity of the diagnosis of incurable idiocy. The hopeless attitude which is expressed today regarding the defective individual's amenability to psychotherapy seems also to be a result of diagnostic labels." A decade later, Sarason and Tomas Gladwin indicated that the "most important conclusion" to be drawn from Itard's work was that "even in severely defective individuals the quantity and quality of interpersonal relationships is an important variable in determining the level of complexity and efficiency of psychological functioning." Victor was still grasped as "severely defective," but the accent shifted from intelligence and language to personality structure and emotional expression. Sarason and Gladwin measured the "phenomenal" progress Victor made under Itard's care not in words uttered or read but in "the development of various ego functions, the capacity to delay responsiveness ... [and] the development of a surprisingly complex personality."[11]

Two somewhat unusual textual uses of Itard and Victor in the journal *Mental Retardation* expose how, by the mid-1970s, both of them were firmly ensconced in the field. First, Victor was declared "the most eminent retardate" based on the relative amounts of space granted various individual cases in well-known texts and reference books on mental retardation from 1908 through 1974.[12] Second, in 1977 S.A. Warren, the journal's editor, printed a fictive "letter from an editor" to Itard, dated 1 April 1809, as an April Fools' Day joke. In it, Itard was notified that the reviewers were "impressed" with his "five years of diligence in study of the wild boy, Victor," but his manuscript was rejected (as, the fictional editor guessed, it had already been by other editors) because the study was "marred by major flaws in experimental design." Itard was advised to redo it: "select a larger sample (e.g., 60) of wild boys of the same C.A. [chronological age] and number of years in the woods, assign them randomly to experimental and control groups, apply the treatments again, perform appropriate statistical tests, and re-submit. You could provide better support for your thesis if you employed on each subject several standardized measures such as the WPPSI, Binet, Porteus Mazes, Lincoln-Oseretsky, ITPA, McCarthy, VRT, AAMD ABS, Reading Free Interest, Purdue Pegboard, TROCA, Bialer-Cromwell Locus of Control, and some anxiety, self-concept, and academic tests." The "editor" sympathized with Itard's plight ("We understand that publication may be necessary to you if you are in a struggle for University tenure") but reminded him that tenure was granted "on demonstration of a national reputation, preferably a good one. With work of this calibre, you surely cannot expect to attain any kind of reputation." To crown the joke, Warren had the fictional editor counsel Itard to "consult one of the vanity presses" for "someone may be interested in what appears from your excellent (if pre-scientific) descriptions to be clear indication that a profoundly retarded, asocial child can be changed to one with relatively good self help and occupational skills. The document may be of passing interest as the first of its kind to demonstrate the possibility of 'educating intelligence.'" Warren's tongue-in-cheek letter poked fun at and amiably criticized the field, pointing out the many ways in which Itard's reports deviated from current standards for acceptable (and publishable) research and implying that contemporary works of comparable worth could face unfair rejections to the profession's detriment.[13]

The success of Warren's joke hung upon the very fact that by then both Itard's reputation and the standard version of the story (Victor was retarded, Itard proved the educability of idiots) went unchallenged. Changing attitudes, labels, and treatment options have shaken the field of mental deficiency and retardation (now more likely to be called developmental or learning disability) in the last few decades; however, no change has shaken Itard's position as pioneer and model. In Lawrence M. Lieberman's words, "the Wild Boy of Aveyron is not a model of diagnostic teaching. It is the model ... It is a tribute to Itard's genius that he discovered and implemented perhaps the most important truth of all: Education must be in harmony with the dynamic nature of life." Lieberman furnished "modern translations" of Itard's medico-pedagogical aims because, as a special education curriculum, they have been "occasionally equalled but seldom surpassed."[14]

We need to consider the two major alternative explanations for Victor's condition. The first one is the old eighteenth-century notion, taken up by Itard himself, that prolonged isolation could cause an *acquired* type of idiocy in an originally "normal" child. As Harlan Lane put it, "the obvious explanation for the differences between Victor and almost any other rural French adolescent of the same era lies in Victor's experiences during his years of isolation in the wild." Lane pointed to his survival in the wild as evidence of the boy's initial normality: Victor's "deviant behavior in society" was simply the obverse of his "adaptive behavior in the forest." Octave Mannoni (philosopher, anthropologist, and Lacanian psychoanalyst) detected in the boy's adaptation to forest life a sign of *exceptional* (rather than defective) qualities.[15] Although this view accounted for Victor's wild life, it appeared to flounder before his limited recovery after his return to society. As Itard had already surmised, two possible beginnings of answers to these questions could be that the known and unknown vicissitudes of Victor's childhood – abandonment, abuse, murder attempt, social isolation, capture, and further neglect *within* society – might have had long-term effects (what we now call trauma) and that certain skills may only be learned in early childhood (what we now know as critical periods).

The second alternative explanation, which fully returned Victor to the domain of pathology and professional expertise, is infantile autism. The concretion of the link between Victor and autism had some interesting twists. First, the link can be traced back to the 1959 publication of Bruno Bettelheim's "Feral Children and Autistic Children." Bettelheim advanced the theory that wild children were "severely autistic," but perhaps bowing to the then prevailing opinion, he made an exception of Victor: "Most of the so-called feral children were actually children suffering from the severest form of infantile autism, while some of them were feeble-minded, as was possibly the Wild Boy of Aveyron."[16] Second, the "discoverer" of autism, Leo Kanner, who dedicated many pages to Victor's (and Itard's) role in the history of mental retardation, never associated the wild boy with autism.[17] Third, Bettelheim's contention that parents, especially mothers, were responsible for the onset of autism provoked an intense critical reaction on the part of other experts. But the suggestion that wild children might indeed be autistic proved so attractive to professionals embarking on the establishment of a new field of practice and expertise that they adopted it even as they rejected its first proponent. Finally, in his major work on autism, *The Empty Fortress* (1967), Bettelheim seemed to have changed his mind with respect to Victor's condition: "Unlike Pinel, who thought the boy feeble-minded, I tend to agree with Itard's original opinion: that this boy was not feeble-minded but, likely as not, was reacting to the conditions of his life with what we now would call infantile autism."[18]

The late discovery of autism raised a problem: why had it not been identified and described before? Experts willing to dispel the notion that autism is a disorder of our time and to demonstrate that, even if unrecognized as such, it affected all kinds of children in all times and places, welcomed the opportunity to latch onto Victor and Itard. Seven years after Bettelheim's seminal article, John K. Wing and Lorna Wing noted that "the clinical syndrome has only relatively recently been adequately delineated by Kanner so that past insights, such as those of Itard in 1799 and Witmer in 1920, were not recognized as more generally applicable to a substantial group of similar children." The fact that we now recognize autism and distinguish it from other disorders like mental retardation is read as a signal of *our* enlightened regard for children. In the same child whom the specialists in mental retardation conceived as palpably retarded, the autism experts spotted autism one hundred and fifty years before Kanner first described and named it: "To the modern reader there can be no doubt that the wild boy of Aveyron showed most of the diagnostic features of autism – whatever the original cause. The details of his behaviour are uncannily familiar."[19] The experts were so stricken by the uncanny familiarity of these telltale details that they did not see the need to attend to the context in which they were registered and their concrete place in the overall story, even though Lane cautioned that a conscientious assessment of *all* the available evidence afforded a more intricate picture. For Lane, "the similarities between Victor and autistic children seem to be exaggerated" – Victor's rapid mood changes were provoked by specific events, usually his transactions with people; he was not emotionally withdrawn and displayed affection for others and the desire to please them; he was not obsessed with order and excelled at practical manipulation; he used a gestural language and communicated his needs, desires, and feelings very effectively.[20]

Lane's argument, backed by extensive acquaintance with the historical evidence, did not persuade the experts. In the most extended and famous discussion of Victor as an autistic child, the chapter "Lessons from the Wild Boy" in *Autism: Explaining the Enigma* (1989), Uta Frith dealt with Lane's objections summarily "in the light of current knowledge." Lane's observations did not rule out autism because they "fit older autistic children very well." Frith cited selected passages from the accounts contained in Lane's own book as evidence of Victor's "serious impairment in reciprocal social interactions," "specific intellectual impairment," "characteristic impairment of sensory attention," "lack of imaginative play," and "stereotypies." She contended that the major diagnostic feature of autism, "autistic aloneness," was evident in numerous scattered incidents of his life, in particular his visit to Mme Récamier: "It is as if, for Victor, minds did not exist. It follows that he is unconcerned about the effect his behaviour has on other people's opinion of him." In a stunning reversal, Frith argued that Victor's survival in the wild, which Lane had wielded as solid indication that he could not have been retarded or psychotic, was downright facilitated by his autism: "autistic individuals seem to be peculiarly qualified – better than normal children are – to lead the rugged, solitary life that Victor lived when roaming the forests. In the case of a normal child it would be more difficult to explain why he did not seek refuge with people. Villagers, by all accounts, were often nearby and ready to help him. If he was autistic this may not have occurred to him. Perhaps he found it impossible to differentiate well-meaning people from creatures of the wild."[21] Frith used Victor not just to substantiate autism's long lineage ("Autism is not a modern phenomenon, even though it has only been recognized in modern times") but to buttress her stand in the controversy about its cause. In opposition to Bettelheim's psychoanalytic view of autism as the child's response to a pernicious kind of parenting and an extreme environment, Frith defined autism as a congenital cognitive and developmental impairment best understood as the inability to mentalize, or lack of a "theory of mind." Autistic children, like Frith's Victor, are unable to "recognize the existence of other people's minds," lack empathy, and have great difficulty communicating with others. Frith avoided a sweeping argument like Bettelheim's (all wild children were autistic) and called into play the *contrast* between two wild children, (autistic) Victor and (non-autistic) Kaspar, to bring out the essential features of autism and prove that it could not be caused by prolonged deprivation of human contact. In her singleminded search for symptoms, however, Frith passed over the many details and anecdotes in the accounts of Victor's life that exhibit a boy profoundly involved with others and attuned to their feelings and states of mind, such as his reaction to Mme Guérin's sorrow on the death of her husband and the multiple frustrations, conflicts, and joys he visibly experienced in his dealings with Itard.[22]

The appropriation of Victor for autism had several side effects as well, with regard to the theory of mind, child psychiatry and child psychosis, and professionalization. In connection with theory of mind, the association worked both ways. At first the lack of a theory of mind was proposed as the underlying malfunction uniting all of Victor's "symptoms"; subsequently,

Victor's condition was itself probed as a means to obtain insights into the theory of mind supposedly applicable to all children. As Peter Mitchell (for whom "Viktor" [sic] was "an archetypically autistic boy") maintained in *Introduction to Theory of Mind* (1997), since autism "practically amounts to either a deficient or a deviant theory of mind," its study is "particularly relevant to investigations into the development of a conception of mind."[23] More generally, child psychiatrists saw in Victor the prototype of the psychotic or emotionally disturbed child and correspondingly awarded Itard, for his work with him, "the distinction of being the first modern child psychiatrist."[24] In 1969 Françoise Brauner and Alfred Brauner proclaimed that, inasmuch as Victor adapted very well to stable material situations and only remained weak in social and affective predicaments, the proper diagnosis for him was not mental deficiency but child psychosis (deep problems of the personality, whose real cause is unknown and which may result in severe obstacles to intellectual development). Almost twenty years later the Brauners reserved a special place for Victor and Itard in *L'enfant déréel*, a history of "autisms" in literature and clinical practice.[25] Moreover, as the subdisciplines and professions ministering to "exceptional children" multiplied, more of them laid claim to Itard as *their own* predecessor. Dennis E. McDermott was looking for the "real founder of child and youth work"; while searching for early references to "any form of humane treatment of disturbed, delinquent, or otherwise troubled kids," he came upon Itard. In him, McDermott found "a person I could easily relate to": "He worked intensely in a residential setting. His 'client' was so unsocialized that he had been given the name 'The Wild Boy.' His methods were such models of good child care work that they are, or could be, used today." The "insightful" and "caring" Itard stands as "a credible model of professionalism for our own times." Interestingly, McDermott remembered Mme Guérin's contribution: "Perhaps future historians will be able to tell us more about Guerin, and we will be able to talk more accurately about the 'co-founders' of child and youth work."[26]

The interpretations and appropriations of Victor and Itard do not bear only upon "abnormal" children. One troublesome property of the concept of normality is that the boundary between normal and abnormal is never fixed and exceedingly permeable. Already in the first decade of the nineteenth century, the evaluators of Itard's second report tied together his work with Victor and the much more comprehensive project of childhood and youth education in general. In Itard's individualized effort to train an extraordinary child they sensed the point of departure for attempts to bring forth the right approach to all children. Half a century later, and after having adapted Itard's program of medical education for use with large numbers of retarded children, Séguin claimed that, with further adaptations, Itard's methods and principles could be fit for "the training of mankind."[27] While Séguin himself did not undertake this mission, in the early twentieth century the education of the wild boy of Aveyron was made relevant to all children by Maria Montessori, who modelled her scientific pedagogy on it. By insisting on the centrality of his work as an inspiration for her own, Montessori installed Itard as a harbinger of progressive and "child-centred" education. Like the other appropriations, Montessori's operated by fastening on selected elements of Itard's account of his work. Montessori applauded Itard's minute observation of his charge: "A student of Pinel, Itard, was the first educator to practise *the observation* of the pupil in the way in which the sick are observed in the hospitals." She hailed the experimental character of Itard's endeavours, which she saw as "practically the first attempts at experimental psychology." In Itard's writings, Montessori discerned the origin of the conjunction of medicine and pedagogy and the first intimations of the kind of early childhood education anchored in science that she would elaborate in her "Montessori Method."[28] To comprehend Montessori's pedagogical innovations, her followers and commentators also scrutinized Itard's reports, hence reinforcing the belief that they prefigured the tenets of contemporary child-centredness. Itard "anticipated the principles and practice of twentieth century education," wrote Robert John Fynne, because he realized "the great educational role of the child's organic needs" (mental, moral, social, aesthetic, and physical); conceived the idea "of creating new needs and of making them permanent and operative for further development"; encouraged and utilized "the feeble spontaneity of his pupil," and found a place for "pleasure, interest, and imitation" in his training.[29]

For Montessori, the task of scientific pedagogy was to facilitate the individual child's development. But whereas in Itard's program for Victor's education "development" was meant in an active sense, as *making* the child's faculties develop in a certain way through direct intervention, the creation of specific needs, and the manipulation of his environment, in Montessori's pedagogy "development" functioned equivocally. In practice her goal was the same (active) type of development underscored by Itard, yet in theory she misleadingly declared that the child's development is *naturally* programmed and best takes place spontaneously under conditions of "freedom" – the very conditions scientifically made possible by her method. Montessori's work relied on, and most vividly disclosed, the conceptual and practical shift from the wild child, through the retarded child, to "the child." Thus she observed: "If a parallel between the deficient and the normal child is possible, this will be during the period of early infancy *when the child who has not the force to develop* and *he who is not yet developed* are in some ways alike." If development was natural and followed a single pattern in all children, it was legitimate to formulate analogies between Victor and young children: "In the education of little children Itard's educative drama is repeated."[30]

Montessori conceived of Victor as mentally retarded, but to her mind there was no qualitative difference between normal and retarded children. The slippery concept of development, which authorizes analogies between young "normal" children and older "abnormal" (retarded or backward) children, and therefore between the "wild child" (as one form of the retarded child) and "the child," supports not only contemporary child-centred pedagogy but also most fields of research and practice involving children. It made sense to psycholinguist Roger Brown to begin *Words and Things* (1958) with the story of Victor because, he believed, it sheds light on language acquisition *in general*: "The doctor's methods of instruction were founded on an analysis of the basic psychology of language which is the same as the analysis on which the present book is founded." Itard's instruction and Victor's learning provided Brown with paradigmatic examples of the psychology of language. Because he construed the relation between Itard and Victor as the prototypical teacher-pupil or adult-child relation, Brown was able to characterize the "Original Word Game" as "the game of linguistic reference that Victor played with Itard and all children play with their parents."[31]

Victor and Itard have been assigned foundational and paradigmatic roles in the fields of mental retardation, autism, and pedagogy; consequently, *critical and alternative positions* have also proceeded by revisiting and reinterpreting their story and its implications. Within the field of mental retardation, but from a psychoanalytic perspective, Maud Mannoni reread Itard in the course of her articulation of a psychoanalytic approach to the treatment of mentally retarded children (she was dissatisfied both with the educationalist's faith in the power of education to remake the other in the self's image and with the psychoanalyst's refusal to engage with children deemed uninteresting on account of their speechlessness). What Mannoni found "touching" about Itard's experiment with the (retarded) wild

boy was precisely that Itard strove "to bring him into the world of speech";
still, his "preconceived ideas about the nature of language" obstructed "his
pupil's path toward his possibilities." The main lesson Mannoni derived
from Itard's "mistake" was that professionals working with retarded children, be they psychoanalysts, physicians, or educators, must "start first
with themselves," that is, by questioning their own attitude to the different
child: "What was the trap into which Itard fell at the very outset? Are not his
reactions still a determining factor in our own relationship with a retarded
child?" Mannoni, while praising Itard for having at least attempted to reach
Victor, concluded that in the end the relation established between them was
not "a proper human relationship" – one in which self and other, professional and patient, adult and child, *communicate* – but rather a relation of
submission, a form of "subjection of the child to the Other."[32]

In reference to autism, we have seen that experts who espoused a biological or organic explanation for the syndrome cared much less about Itard's
medico-pedagogical intervention than about Victor's symptoms as genuine indicators of autism. For them, Itard's role was that of an observer and
recorder, and the success or failure of his experiment was secondary relative
to whether he did or did not comprehend that Victor's diagnostic features
were different from those of a mentally defective child. From the periphery
of the field, Douglas Biklen, a proponent of "facilitated communication" and
defender of an unorthodox view of autism, returned to Victor and Itard in
his book *Communication Unbound* (1993), in the section "What Is Required
in Order to See the Person?" Facilitated communication assumes that what
causes the autistic child's mutism or unusual speech is not a cognitive disorder but "apraxia," namely, the inability to have the body do what one wants
without help from others. Biklen did not challenge the view that Victor was
autistic or disabled, yet he did not dwell on the question of diagnosis or the
boy's symptoms. On the contrary, he was interested in pinpointing what
exactly permitted Itard to "observe, educate, and understand Victor with
optimism" even though the boy's appearance and behaviour seemed to por-
tend lack of ability. Biklen cast Itard as someone who faced two hundred
years ago the same quandary that facilitators confront today: what is the
proper attitude to be adopted before a child who appears strange, uncom-
municative, disabled? According to Biklen, Itard was not daunted by Victor's
strangeness because he believed in "educability" and was willing to entertain "multiple possible explanations for what he observed." While performing his educational task, Itard seized upon "evidence of competence" as a

sign that "other abilities of a similar nature could and would follow" and took Victor's responses to be "as much a reflection on Itard the teacher as on Victor's innate or learned qualities." Biklen's generous reading extended to the boy too. Through Itard's efforts and Mme Guérin's "warm, persistent spirit," Victor became "a caring, expressive, competent person in their eyes and possibly in his own as well." In Biklen's opinion, the facilitator must bring to the relation with autistic and other seriously disabled children the same personal traits that allowed Itard to relate to and communicate with Victor despite his odd appearance and distressing behaviour.[33]

From the point of view of pedagogy, some critics reviewed Itard's reports for clues as to the ambiguities and misunderstandings inscribed at the very heart of modern education. For Octave Mannoni, the problem with Itard (and his followers in special and early childhood education) was that his arbitrary preconceptions prevented him from seeing the real child before him. Itard failed to realize that Victor was not "a blank screen" but an individual with a history and a great deal of accumulated knowledge, however unconventional. To stress the unidirectional character of the pedagogical relation instituted by Itard, Mannoni imagined a reversal of roles: "send Itard into the woods at La Caune with the savage, to see what he would learn there that would be really new to him." By clinging to his *a priori* notions and glossing over "all that his pupil had not learned from him," Itard lost the chance of being himself re-educated by his savage. Still, Mannoni warned contemporary educators and psychoanalysts that even if the advances in knowledge and theory made since Itard's time may enable them to make out the inadequacies that provoked *his* failure, "they can tell us nothing about our own." In "Un admirable echec" (1995) Sophie Ernct re-examined Itard's reports as founding texts of modern education. Since Itard was a precursor of modern pedagogy, it is necessary to delve into his reports to see if they make visible the essential risks of pedagogical thinking; since Itard's reporting was detailed and careful, it is possible to make our own judgments on the success or failure of his aims, procedures, and medico-philosophical principles. Ernct even-handedly analyzed the pedagogical relation between Itard and Victor and unravelled Itard's "failure" within the terms of that relation, without having to resort to temporally or conceptually prior deficiencies in the boy. Like Octave Mannoni, Ernct admitted that our superiority over Itard – our ability to benefit from the progress of knowledge and our position of exteriority in the fact of reading – only means that we may stay clear of his mistakes but does not protect us from committing those peculiar to our own time, of which we are unaware.

Itard's reports raise questions (about the emergence of humanity, the relation between humanity and language, the foundations of education) that
are still our own. But their value, Ernct insisted, lies not in the answers they
may offer (they offer none) but in their power to foster thoughtfulness in
contemporary readers.[34]

The story of Victor and Itard has thus been appropriated by experts and
practitioners in the fields of mental retardation, autism, and child-centred
pedagogy and reinterpreted by critics within and at the margins of each of
these fields. There is one more way in which the story was rewritten, and
that is through further research into and reassessment of Itard's life and
work. Historians of medicine long supposed that Itard's medical contribution was restricted to his discoveries and inventions in the area of ear,
nose, and throat diseases; however, since the late 1970s Thierry Gineste, a
French historian of psychiatry and a psychiatrist himself, endeavoured to
reconstruct Itard's psychiatric contribution. Whereas the other psychiatric or psychotherapeutic renderings of the story rested on selective or sim-
plified readings of Itard's reports and (less often) other accounts, Gineste
engaged in a painstaking reconstruction of the surviving documentary evidence. Even though Gineste's research undoubtedly revolutionized the state
of knowledge about Victor and Itard, the interpretation he imposed on the
evidence was a new appropriation, a myth of origins, a dogmatic epic of
"great men" in pursuit of the truth through the very elision of the *child*. The
title of Gineste's 1992 article, "Jean Marc Gaspard Itard: Psychotherapist of
the Wild Child," gives away his viewpoint. The entire story of the wild boy
is fixed with reference to a single domain: "In this climate, and according
to Itard's own acknowledgement, his care of the wild child was nothing but
a long psychotherapy." Gineste argued that, while Pinel and Esquirol very
quickly "perverted" moral treatment (or psychotherapy) by turning it into
"institutionalized policing," Itard alone, in his treatment of the wild boy,
confronted its "impossible pain." Through moral treatment of a child who
"would never speak, regardless of the care he was given, and who, after a
relative improvement, would finish by sinking again into autism and cata-
tonia," Itard experienced a painful encounter with *himself* that originated
a "new understanding of man" and allowed him to grasp the true nature
of madness. Thus Itard must be recognized not just as the founder of child
psychiatry but as one of the founding pillars of modern psychiatry.[35]

But Gineste trod on dangerous ground, because his interpretation is contingent on Itard's *silence*. After ending his involvement with Victor, Itard
turned away from "mental alienation" and devoted himself to the treatment

and education of deaf-mutes; according to Gineste, this was a "renuncia-tion" prompted by the very fact that what Itard had learned in his moral treatment of Victor (about himself, about "man") was "unspeakable": "it is by what is audaciously hidden in his work, rather than what is noisily explicit in it, that [Itard] remains a monument of medicine. In spite of a tradition that keeps him in the turbulent role of adolescent rebelling against the father, in fact he compels us not to be blinded by a cosmogony in which the myth of the founding father hides the truth, that which is pierced by the eyes of children, who are, as you well know, eager to know."[36] Just as he rejected one myth (Itard as the rebellious adolescent taking on Pinel, the founding father of psychiatry) Gineste inaugurated a new one, grounded on the unspoken (and unspeakable), in which the child, "eager to know," is Itard himself – while Victor, the real child in the story, has completely vanished. In the final analysis, for Gineste the wild boy was merely the "occasion" for Itard's momentous discovery. The paradox is that Gineste both maintained (rightly) that to understand the story of *Victor* "everything must be taken into account" and propounded a reductive view of *Itard*'s historical signifi-cance that relied on the unsaid and unwritten.[37]

How can we account for the enduring and seemingly inexhaustible appeal of the story of Victor and Itard? How can we explain its hold on resolute adherents of diverse and opposed schools of thought about, and practical approaches to, the care, education, and treatment of children, all of whom in some measure identify *themselves* with it, perceive in Victor's condition that of the children with whom they are concerned, and recognize in Itard's principles, goals, and procedures an anticipation of their own? What is it that makes of this story such an invitation for ongoing and unrestricted identification and appropriation? One reason is that, unlike other accounts of "wild children," Itard's reports bear unimpeachable scientific credentials and their authenticity cannot be questioned. But there is more: the story of Victor and Itard has become a legend, the perfect embodiment of one kind of child-adult relation. It is thus incredibly easy for adults (teachers, doctors, parents) to identify with Itard as the boy's rescuer, saviour, maker. The medico-pedagogical legend encircling Victor and Itard is so irresistible that it overshadows all other elements of Victor's life. Ultimately, with few exceptions, the appropriations and rereadings of the story presuppose and reproduce the glorification of Itard, at the cost of devaluing, debasing, or simply forgetting the wild boy: "Whether Victor was normal or retarded, Itard won ... If normal, then it is thanks to Itard that we have an extensive

and perceptive account of bringing the 'savage' part way back to civilization. Compared to him, the lowliest Australian bushman or African Pygmy
is highly civilized and surrounded by a thick sheath of cultural and social
behavior. On the other hand if Victor was organically (or ever functionally) retarded, then Itard performed an almost uncanny feat of redeeming
the unredeemable, of finding a place for a stone the builder rejected. Either
way he was the miracle worker of his era."[38] And in an age of mass media,
it would be unwise to ignore (and hard to exaggerate) the impact in the story's reception and endurance of François Truffaut's *L'enfant sauvage* (1969),
singly responsible for making many people fall in love with it. Truffaut's
explanation of his decision to play the role of Itard is both powerful and
instructive:

I feel that if I had given the role of Itard to an actor, this would have been of all my
films the one that would have satisfied me the least, because I would have done only
technical work. All day I would have been telling some man "Now take the child,
make him do this, take him there" and that is what I wished to do myself ... From
the day I decided to play Itard, the film took for me a complete and definitive meaning ... I felt that the role was more important than that of director, because Doctor
Itard manipulated this child and I wanted to do it myself; but it is likely that there
were also deeper meanings. Up until *The Wild Child*, when there were children in
my films, I identified with them, while here for the first time I identified with the
adult, the father.[39]

TO CLARIFY MY ARGUMENT that the story of Victor, the wild boy of Aveyron, is inextricable from the emergence of the child as an object of knowledge and intervention and to show how he embodied the shift from the earlier perception of wild children as *savages* to the new realization that the
wild child is *a child*, I must return to the Society of Observers of Man. In
a paper read at the Observers' public meeting on 7 July 1801, Jauffret summarized the society's interests and projects. Since the science of man, the
most noble of all, was also the most neglected, the Observers of Man were
determined to rectify the situation by undertaking an ambitious research
program embracing the differences between man and the animals, the varieties of the human species and variations between individuals, the origin
of languages and ideas, and the faculties of the soul. What is more, the Observers, Jauffret explained, attached enormous importance to the collection

of well-made observations on the first developments of the human faculties: "This task, as new as it is interesting, indicated by the Society to the true friends of philosophy, is no doubt surrounded by numerous difficulties. But these difficulties are not insurmountable; and why, besides, would one not find a certain appeal in the pleasure and the honour of overcoming them? Why would one not find the same charm in considering with an attentive eye the first glimmer of the developing mind, in keeping a detailed journal of the progress of intelligence in a child, in seeing the birth of his faculties one from the other, than one finds in watching closely the habits and industry of an insect, in observing the blooming of some foreign plant?" In an age in which the scientific study of children does not need any justification, we may be taken aback by the lengths to which Jauffret had to go to entice his listeners to apply themselves to the new task. As added enticement, the Observers offered a prize, announced almost a year earlier but to be given in the eleventh year of the Republic (1802–03), for the best essay that would "determine, by daily observation of one or several newborn children, the order in which the physical, intellectual, and moral faculties develop, and to what extent this development is assisted or opposed by the influence of the objects surrounding the child, and by the influence, even greater, of the persons who communicate with him." The prize had been announced at the public meeting held on the very day of the wild boy's arrival in Paris: 6 August 1800.[40]

Although the Observers initially approached the wild boy as a savage, his import was later reframed in accordance with the new problematization of the child. Jauffret's injunction to study children included a recognition that children (unlike insects or plants) were not then seen as particularly attractive objects and that the study of children was beset with practical and epistemological difficulties. Itard's medico-pedagogical approach, which fused knowledge and intervention, "solved" the problem of how to study the child. Whereas the forbidden experiment assumed that the means to study children was to prevent them from receiving any education (understood as corruption of an original nature), Itard demonstrated that children could be studied in and through the process of education. And it was in the course of Itard's experimental education that Victor was divested of one set of meanings and relocated in the new conceptual universe. Some historians of eighteenth-century human science have noticed weighty points of contact between Itard's concerns and those of Lord Monboddo. For Antonio Verri, this is because Monboddo's entire work "indirectly" addressed the problem of human formation and therefore of education.[41] I agree with Verri's claim to a certain extent, but I want to suggest that a world of difference lies in that word *indirectly*. The contrast between Monboddo and Itard – between their responses to the wild children they encountered, marked by the different questions they posed and the practical forms the encounters took – allows us to gauge the change I am trying to highlight.

The emerging interest in the child, like most intellectual mutations, entailed continuity and rupture at the same time. In part, it must be related to the ongoing interrogation of the savage. The child was conceived of as another figure of the uncivilized; in that sense child was close to wild child. But the child was more familiar and more available for scrutiny than the rare wild children; after all, all human beings are uncivilized (or yet to be civilized) at the beginning of their lives. But the new interest in children also arose from a transmutation of perfectibility (as the distinctive mark of humanity, as man's potential to become something other than what he is, as the boundary separating man from animal and signalling the progress from savage to civilized) into the idea of *educability*. Educability, like perfectibility, denotes becoming and potential, yet by placing children's capacity to learn in the foreground, it also calls attention to adults' duty to shape children, to guide the development of their physical, intellectual, and moral faculties, to mould their environment to facilitate this development, to secure normal development by correcting individual abnormalities. This then is the crucial difference between Monboddo and Itard: the former functioned within the framework of perfectibility as indefinite potential; the latter made possible the rise of educability as a demand for concrete intervention. Monboddo was interested in the *historical* origin of man; Itard (through Victor, the wild *child*) zeroed in on his *biographical* starting point – the child.[42]

Moreover, "the child" would become intelligible within a normality/ abnormality continuum. Hacking has claimed that during the nineteenth century the old way of thinking about people, or "Human-Nature-Thinking," was displaced by the new idea of "normal people." To illustrate this displacement he pointed to the many research grants that focus on questions of normality or abnormality: "How many are about a contrast between normal and somehow abnormal children, be they gifted or hindered? Lots, I am told ... How many, in their grant proposals, state that they are about to investigate the nature of children?" In fact, in the eighteenth century (during the heyday of "Human Nature") the "nature of children" was not a major concern of scientists and philosophers either. The child emerged as an object of scientific knowledge concurrently with the displacement from "human nature" to "normal people." And it was through the idea of normality (or normal development) that the difference between the extraordinary (the wild child) and the ordinary (the child) could be erased: it became one of degree, not kind. First assimilated to the abnormal child – retarded, deficient, insane, deviant, disturbed, disabled – the wild child came to function as an adequate representative of children in general because the boundary between normal and abnormal is singularly fragile. Normality is not an inherent quality with which the child is born but the product of a particular kind of intervention. This is another way of saying that all children are (and all development is) potentially abnormal, that knowledge about children is indistinguishable from intervention, and that the dominant form of this intervention is *normalization*. Every child, like the wild child, is subjected to normalizing intervention. In *The Taming of Chance* Hacking analyzed the "coming into being" of laws about people, which are "statistical in nature" and obtain their power from the idea of the normal: "People are normal if they conform to the central tendency of such laws, while those at the extremes are pathological. Few of us fancy being pathological, so 'most of us' try to make ourselves normal, which in turn affects what is normal." Victor transcended his own time and place in large part because his life coincided with the first adumbrations of the idea of the normal; since, unlike most of us, he did not try to *make himself normal*, he also uncovers the limits of this idea. Never fully "tamed," the wild child resists normality as a concept and a principle for the intervention of adults in the lives of children.[43]

Just as Victor was identified with "the child," Itard's medical pedagogy came to be the prototype of all knowledge/intervention involving children. In 1802, in a little-known text, Itard elaborated his view of the relation between medicine and pedagogy: "If the physical and moral education of children were enlightened by the insights of philosophical medicine, its course would become more certain, and its results happier." The "main defect" marring the education practised in Itard's time was that "it is essentially the same for all children" instead of being adapted to "the innumerable variations that the state of the intellectual faculties presents in each individual." Medicine, "considerably ennobled" by its recent attainments in the moral treatment of insanity, could "acquire yet another lustre by shedding light on the course of education," because to it belonged the study of individual differences not only in man's physical constitution but also in the "moral" (psychological) realm. The shortcomings of current education were most patent "in the case of those it has left so far behind ordinary people; the idiots, for instance, or those individuals whom we commonly call slow-witted." If one were to judge by the progress made by the wild boy of Aveyron, Itard concluded, the future of medically informed education looked promising. In this text, even more than in his classic reports on Victor, Itard foreshadowed the bases of modern education and the conditions of possibility for its universalization: education must, firstly, observe and respond to children's individual differences and, secondly, take the most-deprived and less-gifted children as its standard.[44]

Itard's medical or experimental pedagogy operated through direct intervention in Victor's life – by shaping his environment, creating needs, eliciting behaviours, thoughts, sounds, feelings – because it presupposed an *active* view of development. The doctor-teacher's task was to *make* the child's faculties (not the child him- or herself) develop. Yet Itard's pedagogy has come to us under a different guise, as the origin of *child-centredness*, in which development is assumed to be a natural and spontaneous process and education is understood as the facilitation of the child's own development by responding to the child's own needs. This is how Montessori reinterpreted (and absorbed) Itard's work, and how it is presented in recent appraisals. "It is to Itard's credit that he did not view the pupil as a little adult but as a developing child," writes Lane. "The format of the instruction is not determined then by some logical progression in the subject matter to be taught but rather by a genetic progression tailored to the individual – his history, physiology, affective needs, intellectual and social maturity." Alain Hirt asserts that Itard "had the intelligence not to consider his pupil as an adult to be moulded but as a child the way he is; to be accompanied, to be stimulated taking his affective needs into account and helping him keep in his memory all the traces of his learning." For Itard (according to Hirt), as for modern educators, the child was not "a small-size adult" but rather "a different being that must be helped in his development according to stages of development that must be respected."[45] In the interests of historical truth and conceptual clarity, it is important to underline the fact that child-centredness and natural/spontaneous development, far from being the principles grounding Itard's pedagogical practice, are the central tenets of the contemporary pedagogical myth. If there is one thing about Victor concerning which Itard's reports leave no doubt is that he *did not develop* in the modern sense of the term. On the contrary, he *learned* only as a consequence of the tenacious efforts and conscious choices made by Itard while engaged in a close personal relationship with him. Itard conceived pedagogy as intervention and engagement, and I see this as a good thing. The problem is not intervention but the denial of intervention. The rhetoric of child-centredness and the "developing child" obscures, and ultimately debases, pedagogical action (the adult's intervention in the child's life) and naturalizes the adult's decisions and values. If, as adults, we acknowledge our multiple direct and indirect interventions in the lives of children, then we can discuss the hows and the whys of those interventions – and perhaps we may even care to ask children's opinions on the matter. But if adult intervention is disguised as a mere response to children's own needs, then all serious discussion is foreclosed, and only the experts *on children* have the right to speak.[46]

While I am not troubled by the interventionism of Itard's pedagogy, I believe it is open to criticism in other ways. Itard's "failure" to meet his own educational expectations in relation to Victor is sometimes contrasted with Sicard's astounding success with his most famous student, the deaf-mute Jean Massieu (1772–1846), whose education Sicard described in *Cours d'instruction d'un sourd-muet de naissance* (1800). This is how Sicard portrayed the young Massieu before he entered the school for deaf-mutes in Bordeaux: "He had never seen any other people besides his family, who never took the trouble to communicate even simple physical ideas to him ... Massieu was the man of the woods, not yet knowing but purely animal habits, startled and frightened by everything. Coming to Bordeaux, he believed he was just changing residence, and imagined that he would be placed in charge of another flock ... How far was this simple child from realizing that he was coming to be instructed and to learn how to become human, when he regarded himself as the equal of the animals he tended!" Sicard's portrayal of the uneducated Massieu bears an interesting resemblance to Itard's depiction of the wild boy of Aveyron. Sicard generalized this characterization to all congenitally deaf people. The uneducated deaf person is "a kind of walking machine whose organization, in its effects, is inferior to that of animals"; if we compare him to a savage "we are still overrating his miserable condition," because he is inferior to the savage both from the point of view of "the moral" and in ability to communicate with others. The deaf person "in his natural state" lacks ideas and morality, is apathetic and incapable of affection. "We must soften this beast," Sicard proclaimed, "humanize this savage, teach him that he is not alone in nature; that not everything refers to him."[47]

But there is an alternative account of the deaf person "in his natural state." On 6 August 1800, the day when the wild boy arrived in Paris and the Observers of Man announced their prize for observations of children, Massieu himself presented to the Observers, in sign language, the account of his life and his education he had prepared two years earlier at Jauffret's request. This is how Massieu told his story:

Until the age of thirteen years and nine months, I remained in my village, without ever receiving any education ... I expressed my ideas by manual signs or gestures. The signs I used then to express my ideas to my parents and to my brothers and sisters were quite different from those of the educated Deaf-mutes. Strangers never understood us when we expressed our ideas with signs; but the neighbours understood us ... Before my education, when I was a child, I did not know how to read or write; I wanted to read and write. I often saw young boys and girls going to school; I wanted to follow them, and I was very envious of them.

I asked my father, with tears in my eyes, for permission to go to school.

When Massieu was invited to enter the Bordeaux school for the deaf, his father told him that he was going there "to learn to read and write." Like Itard, Sicard diminished the condition of the child before education to stress the changes brought about by education and thus magnify his achievement. Yet in his own account Massieu claimed that before he met Sicard he had not lacked ideas, interests, feelings, or means of expression. It was Massieu's *eagerness to learn* that led to his being brought to Sicard's attention in the first place. For Sicard, as for Itard, education was a process of humanization or civilization, in which an incomplete or defective child must be transformed into a full (civilized) human being. They viewed education as the process through which human beings are *made* rather than as a relation of teaching and learning in which human beings engage *as human beings*. Sicard himself offered a different, possibly more honest, picture of his relation with Massieu: "Not a day passed in which he did not learn more than fifty names, nor any day in which he did not in turn teach me the signs for the same objects whose designations I had made him write. Thus, in a happy exchange, while I taught him the written signs of our language, Massieu taught me the *mimic* signs of his." The pedagogical relation between Itard and Victor arguably could never have accommodated such symmetry, but it was a relation of teaching and learning between human beings nonetheless.[48]

Sicard's fame fed on his public presentations of his pupils, who were the living proof of his success: "A school for Deaf-Mutes exists right in your midst. Suspend your judgment; silence your doubts for a moment; go there and propose your problems; ask questions to my pupils; their answers will solve your uncertainties." One would like to sympathize with Itard's disappointment when he realized that Victor would never be able to participate in the Institute's public presentations nor, like Massieu, relate his story to the Observers of Man. But throughout the many hours Itard spent with Victor, patiently and obstinately devoted to his instruction, he was unable to prevail over the one decisive difference between his pupil and Sicard's: Massieu's eagerness to learn. Unlike Massieu, Victor did not enter into the pedagogical relationship willingly, and in the circumstances this could not be blamed on Itard. Still, Itard failed to instil any eagerness in the boy or communicate to him the purpose and meaning of what he was trying to accomplish. Itard enforced a strict separation between everyday life and education; he thus paid scant attention to the many things Victor did do and like in everyday life – when he was alone, with Mme Guérin, or with Itard outside the classroom – and did not take advantage of them to make the boy's education meaningful *for him*. Itard himself was painfully aware that the ingenious exercises he devised for Victor, the same ones that won him the admiration of later generations of educators, had no meaning whatsoever for the boy. Victor became tired and impatient because Itard presented him with increasingly difficult tasks "of which, in truth, he could not conceive the end, and of which it was quite natural that he should weary." In this context, the tantrums with which Victor frequently interrupted the lessons may be seen as expressions of resistance to exercises that he had every right to experience as imposed and artificial.[49]

A comparable dynamic unfolded in the domain of communication and language. Itard acknowledged that the boy was able to express all his needs by signs and gestures: "Each of his wishes is manifested by the most expressive signs, which have in some measure, as have ours, their gradations and their synonymy ... He is no less expressive in his way of showing the affections of his soul, above all impatience and boredom." For Itard, Victor's gestural facility corresponded to Condillac's "language of action": the "primitive language of the human species, originally employed in the childhood of the first societies before the work of many centuries coordinated the system of speech." Itard was nevertheless dissatisfied with the fact that the boy's communicative achievement was, and remained, non-verbal. Indeed, he saw Victor's facility with non-verbal communication as the main obstacle to his acquisition of *true* language: speech. Itard undervalued both the only type of communication in which Victor showed some kind of mastery and the few words he did learn to articulate. After inordinate efforts, Itard succeeded in having Victor utter the word *lait* – but only *after* the milk had been poured into his cup, and not before (as a request), which is what Itard wanted: "One can see why this kind of result was far from fulfilling my intentions; the word pronounced, instead of being the sign of need, was, relative to the time when it had been articulated, merely a futile exclamation of joy. If this word had left his mouth before the thing he desired was granted, that would have been it; the true use of speech would have been seized by *Victor*; a point of communication would have been established between him and me, and the most rapid progress would have sprung from this first success. Instead of all this, I had just obtained a mere expression, insignificant to him and useless to us, of the pleasure he felt." Itard dismissed, and did not encourage, Victor's words – not only *lait* but also his other words, *lli lli* and *oh Dieu!* – because the boy did not use them to make his needs known (the "true use of speech") but to express his joy and his pleasure. It is perhaps because he could not appreciate the role of pleasure in language or, for that matter, in education that Itard failed to make Victor's learning pleasurable. As Octave Mannoni observed, Itard was "incapable of seeing what was happening before his eyes," that is, that he was continually communicating with Victor.[50]

Itard is often praised for his willingness to engage (as a doctor, a teacher, and a person) in a relationship with a child whose appearance and behaviour bespoke total lack of ability in most other people's eyes. As Itard argued in "Vésanies," a firm pronouncement on a child's innate ability or inability to benefit from education (perfectibility or educability) cannot be made until all possible educational and medical means have been tried. This is what Itard did: he engaged with the child to the best of *his own* ability, knowledge, and principles. This is his lesson. But the medico-pedagogical relation between adult and child reached a limit: the child could not progress any more, and the adult lost his patience and his interest in the child. Because the wild boy failed to meet all his expectations, the doctor-teacher was disappointed and severed not only the medico-pedagogical relation but also the *personal* relation between them. At this point – that is to say, at the other end of the medico-pedagogical relationship – we should heed the silent lesson of Mme Guérin, who did not subordinate her involvement with Victor to the latter's demonstration of ability or competence.

PART FOUR Variations on a Theme: Brutalization, Abuse, and Freedom

CHAPTER SEVEN

Wolf Children

> To an almost superhuman degree [Kamala] survived psychologically and achieved human estate. In this Frankenstein paradox of feral and human lies the riddle of her existence. The fates spun a tangled skein and we shall not succeed in fully unraveling it. Some of the threads of the skein will prove to have a forbiddingly subhuman aspect. There will be a reluctance to find such apparent degradation in a human being.
>
> A. Gesell, *Wolf Child and Human Child*[1]

MY ACCOUNT OF THE STORY OF Victor of Aveyron and its reception in the sciences and professions concerned with children showed how the link between wild children and children in general was forged and elaborated. Through the diverse interpretations and appropriations of his story, Victor was transformed into (and made to represent) a generic child. In the last two chapters I turn to the wild children discovered in the past two hundred years. In the second half of the nineteenth century, and primarily throughout the twentieth century, the wild child existed – in discourse, in adults' imaginations, and perhaps in reality too – in three distinct incarnations: the *wolf child*, the *confined child*, and the *free wild child*. What these chapters explore is how these different forms of the wild child offered vehicles for fantasy, projection, and identification. The children reputedly reared by wolves and other wild animals in remote colonial or postcolonial locations stand at maximum spatial, cultural, and conceptual distance from the "civilized" adult and, in their likeness to animals, appear to be most estranged from the human condition. The confined children are not found "far away" or "out there," in some exotic wilderness but right here in our midst, in a human-made environment (dungeon, attic, locked room), and to this minimum spatial distance (from us) corresponds a maximum of possibilities for psychological investment and identification. The wild child who remains free is conceived of as a figure of pure and perfect harmony with nature and attests to the civilized adult's desire for another kind of life, even though, I claim, advanced civilization in fact makes possible the articulation of that desire.

In my retelling of the recent stories of wild children, scientists and professionals of childhood once more play prominent roles. We see them manifest interest in the children; strive to authenticate or dismiss their stories; endeavour, directly or indirectly, to extract knowledge from them, and interpret their cases in light of various theories and frameworks. Still, my contention is that from the outcome of the modern scientist's engagement with wild children we learn more about her or his dreams and aspirations than about either the individual wild child in question or "the child." I attend as well to non-scientific meanings and uses of the wild child, suggesting that our (civilized adults') shifting sense of distance from or proximity to them largely reflects our self-understanding and present position in the world, and I consider how our inordinate preoccupation with the wild child – which, I argue, is in many ways a preoccupation with *ourselves* – may impinge on our relations with real children.

The modern wolf children (and other children associated with wild animals) must be distinguished from the animal-raised children of ancient myth and legend and from the early modern European wild children. Many ancient myths contain the narrative motif of a (generally male) child, exposed or lost, who is nursed and protected by an animal, then saved by shepherds or hunters, and who eventually grows up to be a hero or a ruler. The child's bond with the animal signals the hero's special destiny and *superhuman* character, that is, his possession of both human and animal traits: intelligence, strength, fearlessness, ferocity, cunning, resilience, and so on. The mythical and literary heroes have consistently provided a set of references against which the "real" animal-raised children were perceived, written about, and explained, and in turn some scholars see in the latter evidence that the former might have had a basis in reality; however, the two kinds of story are not to be confused one with the other.[2] In the same way, virtually all the wild children found in Europe before the nineteenth century were believed to have been nurtured by or lived in the company of wild beasts, wolves and bears in particular. While strikingly resembling the earlier stories with regard to the children's strangeness and fate, the more recent accounts of animal-raised children stand out in two respects: first, they are not located in Europe but in "exotic" places (India, South Africa,

Burundi, the Syrian Desert, the Sahara Desert, Uganda, Sumatra); second, they gave rise to new questions and distinctive debates. The earlier stories of wild children were obviously recorded because they were deemed curious and extraordinary, but before the mid-nineteenth century what puzzled and unsettled observers and readers were the children's appearance and behaviour. How could a visibly human child so completely lack attributes and skills held to be essential to humanity? In contrast, from the mid-nineteenth century on the children's condition, while still unpleasant, was no longer unsettling, for the diagnostic categories designating various forms of mental and developmental pathology could more or less account for it. The source of intense puzzlement and insurmountable controversy was now the purported animal association itself. The crucial question became simply whether the stories of wolf and animal-raised children are (and could ever be) true. Is the animal-nursed child within the realm of physical, biological, and psychological possibility? Was a human child ever raised by a wolf or another wild animal?[3]

The first cluster of texts on wolf children – Sleeman's account of seven cases, all of them boys, from the Indian region of Oude (or Oudh, now Uttar Pradesh) and the British and North American articles that took them up, disseminated them, and examined them critically – inaugurated the pattern that characterizes the modern discourse on wolf children. Sir William Henry Sleeman (1788–1856) heard the stories of the wolf boys during his stay in Sultanpoor, by the Goomtee (Gomati) River, in the course of his official investigation of the political situation in Oude.[4] Many children were carried off every year by the numerous wolves living in the neighbourhood of the town and along the banks of the river, and on very rare occasions, it would appear, the wolves did not immediately kill them. All of Sleeman's stories shared similar elements: the first sighting and capture (the boy is sighted by a trooper or soldier in the company of a female wolf and some cubs; the capture takes place after a difficult pursuit during which the boy is often dug or smoked out of the den and subdued by force while the wolves may be killed or taken captive as well), the description of the boy's condition (he does not speak, walks or runs on all fours, and abhors clothes; he has calluses on knees and elbows and odd food habits, including a ravenous appetite for raw meat, and may smell offensively; he is afraid of or indifferent to human beings and attached to other animals; he constantly seeks to escape but is not violent), and the incidents following the capture (the boy is taken to a village or town where a series of local and British authorities take charge of him; he changes hands several times; he may be recognized and temporarily reclaimed by his parents; he does not recover and either dies soon or escapes[5]).

As a rule, stories of animal-raised children are not given singly but juxtaposed to similar ones. While Sleeman did not relate his wolf boys to other wild children (and we do not know if he was familiar with any of them), his account, itself made up of several stories that support and reinforce one another, constitutes a list of cases in its own right. How did Sleeman acquire so much information about so many cases? He did not state how, but it is likely that, his curiosity having been aroused by one or maybe two of the stories, he inquired about more instances of the same phenomenon. Nor did he say whether he himself encountered the wolf boys either but cited testimonies from direct and indirect witnesses. At times Sleeman's account reads like the record of an interrogation; for example, Boodhoo, a Brahmin cultivator, took care of the fifth boy for three months, and then his father claimed him: "What became of him afterwards [Boodhoo] never heard. The lad had no hair upon his body, nor had he any dislike to wear clothes, while he saw him. This statement was confirmed by the people of the village." The first stories Sleeman heard determined the questions he put to his subsequent informers and thus influenced the shape of the later stories. To a certain extent the parallels resulted from Sleeman's method of finding out information. He also inserted some intricate anecdotes, like this one, told of the sixth boy:

One night while the boy was lying under the tree, near Janoo [the man who looked after him], Janoo saw two wolves come up stealthily, and smell at the boy. They then touched him, and he got up; and, instead of being frightened, the boy put his hands upon their heads, and they began to play with him. They capered around him, and he threw straw and leaves at them. Janoo tried to drive them off but he could not, and became much alarmed; and he called out to the sentry over the guns, Meer Akbur Alee, and told him that the wolves were going to eat the boy. He replied, "Come away and leave him, or they will eat you also;" but when he saw them begin to play together, his fears subsided and he kept quiet. Gaining confidence by degrees, he drove them away; but, after going a little distance, they returned, and began to play again with the boy. At last he succeeded in driving them off altogether. The night after three wolves came, and the boy and they played together. A few nights after four wolves came, but at no time did more than four come. They came four or five times, and Janoo had no longer any fear of them; and he thinks that the first two that came must have been the two cubs with which the boy was first found, and that they were prevented from seizing him by recognising the smell. They licked his face with their tongues as he put his hands on their heads.

The clearly legendary motif of the former foster siblings returning at night to play with the captive wolf child resurfaced in some of the later stories.[6]

The context in which Sleeman's account was produced and received prefigured that of future stories of Indian wolf children. Against the political background of British imperialism (and its aftermath), the stories were collected and recorded by colonial officials and administrators with a taste for the jungle and some scientific pretensions (defined in opposition to the natives' superstition and unreliability); the recorders of the stories were several times removed from the original witnesses (usually natives) of the children's association with wolves; the wolf children were surrounded by an assorted mixture of native villagers and aboriginals, soldiers, local rulers, servants and merchants, Anglo-Indians, Indian Army officers, and missionaries; at the receiving end, the stories were retold in meetings of British, Indian, and North American scientific societies, reprinted or summarized in scholarly journals, popular magazines, newspapers, and books and consumed and debated by naturalists and humanists who demanded authentic evidence and objective truth but were also deeply imbued with the ancient myths and legends (in the late nineteenth century the stories of Indian wolf children appealed mainly to zoologists, physical and cultural anthropologists, philologists, and mythologists; from the beginning of the twentieth century, they attracted the interest of child psychiatrists and psychologists, sociologists, social psychologists, and other experts on children, development, and socialization).

Likewise, the controversies provoked by Sleeman's account set the terms for all future treatments of wolf and animal-raised children. Some of the issues were raised by Sleeman himself. Although in his view the evidence was satisfactory and the authenticity of at least some of the cases established beyond doubt, he brought to the fore the question of evidence in stories of animal-raised children and introduced the distinction between a more legitimate or credible form of wild child (without animals) and a more suspicious form (with animals). "That he was found as a wild boy in the forest there can be no doubt," Sleeman affirmed of his seventh case, the old man of Lucknow; "but I do not feel at all sure that he ever lived with wolves." Furthermore, he stressed the pernicious long-term alterations produced in the children by their life with animals (through both adoption of animal traits and deprivation of human contact): "From what I have seen and heard I should doubt whether any boy who had been many years with wolves, up to the age of eight or ten, could ever attain the average intellect of man." The ostensible and seemingly irreversible brutalization of Sleeman's wolf boys was so extreme that the initial state and limited recovery of other known wild children paled in comparison. No observer, reader, or reviewer ever mistook a wolf child for "natural man." Sleeman noticed as well that all his cases involved *children*. Since no human adult had been found living with wolves, he concluded "that after a time they either die from living exclusively on animal food, before they attain the age of manhood, or are destroyed by the wolves themselves, or other beasts of prey."[7]

Once they reached the metropolis, the stories created great ferment and were integrated into the growing list of wild children. They also lost much of their plausibility. For some readers, Sleeman's authority and his familiarity with the Indian situation sufficed to make them "unimpeachable,"[8] but others had qualms about the nature and quality of the evidence. Professor Owen, of the British Association for the Advancement of Science, who read some of the stories with "much interest," did not see "very great improbability" in them but could not accept them at the Zoological Section "because the facts are related at second-hand."[9] At a meeting of the Cambrian Archaeological Society, Gilbert N. Smith read a letter from Sleeman himself on the subject of the wolf boys, which, "though backed by such good authority," was received "with considerable incredulity." Smith was disinclined to pronounce a definitive opinion, hoping that further information "from Indian experience" would corroborate or disprove the stories. More resolute, "L." declared that Sleeman's name and reputation alone could not confer authenticity upon such "strange and improbable" stories and that written testimonies of witnesses and medical examinations were in order. "As the question stands upon the facts related in this pamphlet," "L." asserted, "there is no satisfactory proof of any boy having been found in the care of wolves, or in their company." And Tylor, whose "Wild Men and Beast-Children" was the first extended scholarly discussion of wolf children, did not challenge the boys' "brutal condition" but dismissed their link with wolves, for which "we have no other evidence than that of natives, and it is pretty well known what Oriental evidence is worth as to such matters." Tylor did not rule out the wolf child phenomenon in principle – "It would be, perhaps, imprudent to assert that it is *impossible* that children might be suckled by wild beasts, though the fact that the she-wolf drives her cubs away to shift for themselves before they are a year old is not very compatible with the notion of a child being an inmate of the family for several years; we can only say that it is very improbable and not to be believed but on the best of evidence" – but ended on an uncertain note (with a very current ring to it): "I cannot see that the whole evidence on the subject proves anything whatever, except the existence of the stories, and the fact that there have been and still are people who believe in them."[10]

The stories also spurred speculation, of two kinds. The event itself was probed. Why would the child be spared by the wolves? How exactly would wolves rear a human child? What would drive them to feed the child for many years, when this is "an office which wolves are not in the habit of performing for their own young"? How could the child "avoid falling a prey to other wolves and wild beasts"? And were the structure and physiology of the growing human body consistent with the kind of locomotion, habits, and nourishment presumed in the stories?[11] The wolf children's condition also inspired generalizations about "man":

But what, then, is man, whom mere accidental association for a few years can strip of the faculties inherent in his race and convert into a wolf? The lower animals retain their instincts in all circumstances ... Man alone is the creature of imitation in good or in bad. His faculties and instincts, although containing the *germ* of everything noble, are not independent and self-existing like those of the brutes. This fact accounts for the difference observable, in an almost stereotyped form, in the different classes of society; it affords a hint to legislators touching their obligation to use the power they possess in elevating, by means of education, the character of the more degraded portions of the community; and it brings home to us all the great lesson of sympathy for the bad as well as the afflicted – both victims alike of *circumstances*, over which they in many cases have nearly as little control as the wild children of the desert.[12]

For this author, the wolf children carried a serious message that philanthropists and politicians could ignore only at a heavy social price.

The second brood of cases (which spawned the second cluster of texts and debates) was publicized by Valentin Ball in *Jungle Life in India* (1880), a combination of report and journal describing his travels and experiences in the Indian jungle. This time, all the children converged at a single place, the orphanage run by the Church Missionary Society in Sekandra (or Secundra), near Agra, also in what is now Uttar Pradesh. Towards the end of 1872, the Indian newspapers informed readers that a wolf boy had been brought to the orphanage, where he had joined another one who had been living there for some time: "A boy of about ten *was burned out of a den in the company of wolves*. How long he had been with them it is impossible to say, but it must have been for rather a long period, from the facility he has for going on all fours, and his liking for raw meat. As yet he is very much like a wild animal; his very whine reminds one of a young dog or some such creature. Some years ago we had a similar child; he has picked up wonderfully, and though he has not learned to speak, can fully express his joys and grief. We trust the new 'unfortunate' may soon improve too." Intrigued, Ball wrote to the orphanage, and received a letter from the superintendent, Rev. Mr Erhardt, furnishing details on the two children and letting him know that the boy found in 1872 had died only a few months later. In 1873 Ball presented the cases in a paper he read to the Asiatic Society of Bengal, and in August 1874 he visited the orphanage to examine the surviving boy, who "presented an appearance not uncommonly seen in ordinary idiots": "His forehead was low, his teeth somewhat prominent, and his manner restless and fidgety. From time to time he grinned in a manner that was more simian than human, the effect of which was intensified by a nervous twitching of the lower jaw. After taking a sort of survey of the room and the people in it, he squatted on the ground, and, constantly placing the palms of his hands on the floor, stretched forward in different directions, picking up small objects such as fragments of paper, crumbs, &c., and smelling them as a monkey would do." Ball noticed his remarkable sense of smell, on which he depended to identify objects, and "the shortness of his arms," which may have resulted from "his having gone on all-fours in early life, as all these wolf-boys are reported to have done when first captured." Ball's approach to the stories was cautious, because "this subject is one which the majority of people seem unable to discuss without prejudice." Until a thorough investigation could be carried out and conclusive proof obtained, Ball urged readers to "recognise the justice of suspending judgment." In the meantime, he imagined what might have caused the wolves' unusual behaviour: "Firstly, it may be that while one of a pair of wolves has brought back a live child to the den, the other may have contributed a sheep or goat to the day's provision, and that this latter proving sufficient for immediate wants, the child has been permitted to lie in the den, and possibly to be suckled by the female, and has so come to be recognised as a member of the family. Secondly, and, perhaps, more probably, it may be that the wolf's cubs having been stolen, the children have been carried off to fill their places, and have been fondled and suckled."[13]

The enormous interest excited by the Sekandra wolf children can be attributed both to the memory of Sleeman's account, which had whetted people's appetite for such stories, and to clever "marketing" by the orphanage authorities, ever eager to comply with requests for information and to expose the surviving boy to the curiosity of the many visitors who stopped at Sekandra to have a look at him. The wolf children at the Sekandra orphanage had a singular property: they multiplied. When in 1885 W.F. Prideaux wrote asking for precise facts about the two boys (after Lysart notified readers of *Notes and Queries* that two Anglo-Indian friends of his had visited the orphanage and heard the stories of two wolf boys), the then superintendent, Rev. H. Lewis, wrote back indicating that there had already been *three* wolf boys at the orphanage, two of whom had died. In 1887, when Jivanji Jamshedji Modi visited Sekandra, Lewis told him that besides the surviving boy, called Sanichar, the orphanage had been the home of *two other wolf boys* and *one wolf girl*. As Mr Theobald of the Geographical Survey of India aptly remarked, at the Sekandra orphanage the arrival of wolf children "appears to have created no more surprise than the delivery of the daily supply of butcher's meat."[14]

The stories of the Sekandra wolf children conformed to the standard pattern, and the many first-hand accounts of Sanichar concurred in the depiction and appraisal of his strangeness. The Indian wolf children were beginning to constitute a class: "The facility with which *they* get along on four feet (hands and feet) is surprising," wrote Erhardt to Ball. "Before *they* eat or taste any food *they* smell it, and when *they* don't like the smell *they* throw it away." In this case too, however, the key incident, the child's discovery in the company of wolves, was only known indirectly. In support of the theory that the children had lived with and been nurtured by wolves, there was hearsay evidence and the testimony of natives (which counted for little in the eyes of "educated Europeans") and the children's "animal" traits (which could be interpreted as signs of association with wolves but also as symptoms of mental pathology).[15] Thus Prideaux was not persuaded by Lewis's letter: "The only tangible fact is that there have been idiot children in the Secundra Orphanage, but whether those children were in their earliest years nurtured by wolves there is no satisfactory evidence to show."[16] Still, the stories and the children's strange presence were too suggestive and intriguing to be discarded outright, and scientifically informed Europeans were torn between a guarded scepticism and the desire to believe. A compromise position was reached: the existing evidence was too weak to prove the reality of any of the known stories, yet the *possibility* that a human child could be nurtured by wolves (or other wild animals) should not be categorically rejected. The onus was cast on the future. As Ball put it, "According to the law of averages, the next few years ought to produce a case, and it is to be hoped that should one occur, it may be made the subject of the very strictest enquiry by a joint committee of judicial and medical officers."[17] The hope was that the necessary evidence would be collected – by alert scientists, administrators, and medical men – when the *next* wolf child was discovered. Then, if a single case was proved beyond doubt, the others could be retroactively rehabilitated.

By the end of the century there were enough accounts of, and accumulated evidence on, wolf children to warrant the production of survey articles; by the first decade of the twentieth century, wolf children were installed as a fact (or fiction) of Indian life and as such merited an entry in *Things Indian: Being Discursive Notes on Various Subjects Connected with India* (1906), by William Crooke of the Bengal Civil Service (retired). Also by the end of the nineteenth century the "exotic" animal-raised child entered literature and popular culture with striking and lasting power, first in Britain, in Rudyard Kipling's *The Jungle Book* (1894), and almost two decades later in the United States, in Edgar Rice Burroughs's "Tarzan of the Apes" (1912). The stories of wolf-child Mowgli and ape-boy Tarzan, though prompted by the spate of "real" cases and incorporating elements from them, reinscribed the ancient myths. Far from the pitiful, brutish examples of inhumanity depicted in the "real" accounts, Mowgli and Tarzan stood out and excelled among both animals and humans and thus became appealing heroes for readers stirred by imperialist dreams and hungry for vicarious adventure.[18] The third cluster of cases and texts, which would last from 1926 to the early 1940s, was more diverse and diffuse and centred on three cases: Amala and Kamala of Midnapore (Bengal); the boy found with wolves in Miawana (near Allahabad, Uttar Pradesh), and Lucas, the South African "baboon boy." All of them were featured in the most reputable English-language newspapers and incited vehement reactions from the reading public on both sides of the Atlantic.

The story of Amala and Kamala reached the West in October 1926. Bishop Pakenham-Walsh of Calcutta had learned the story from the man who rescued the girls, the Reverend J.A.L. Singh of Midnapore, during a visit to the latter's orphanage in August. Alerted by some villagers in a remote part of his district to the presence of "demons" in the jungle, Singh had discovered instead the two little girls in a den with several wolf cubs. The girls, aged about two and eight years old, were "exceedingly fierce, running on all fours, uttering guttural barks and living like wolves." The younger had died soon after the rescue, but the elder was still living in Singh's orphanage. At first, the surviving girl exhibited "savage ways," fought against wearing clothes "and tore them off even after they were sewn on her," refused to be washed, and ate "with her mouth in a dish." She had learned to say a few words, but was still "weak mentally and neither cries nor laughs," and continued to prefer "the company of dogs to children."[19] Like the other wolf children, the two girls touched the popular imagination and conjured up personal and collective memories. In a "well-known London club," an argument over whether the story was to be believed ended in a fist fight. A few months later, a writer regretted that the wolf girls' return to civilization had been "tragically unlike that of fortunate Mowgli, who throve alike among wolves and men."[20]

In April 1927 a new spurt of flashy headlines on yet another Indian wolf boy temporarily eclipsed Amala and Kamala.[21] A string of letters to the editor (printed in the London *Times* throughout April and the *New York Times* on 17 July) followed the news of the boy's capture. Readers expressed their belief in or rejection of the stories, listed other cases from little-known publications or their personal (or some friend's) experience in India, proffered theories as to how the phenomenon was (or was not) possible, and drew general conclusions about human nature or development. Whereas those with "Indian experience" – ordinary men and women but also high-ranking colonial authorities, Indian Army officers, civil servants, clergymen, and Sleeman's grandson, Lieutenant-Colonel James L. Sleeman – tended to accept the story (and some of them averred that they had met a wolf child in person), medical men were much more reluctant to believe it. For Dr Donald C. Norris (22 April), all such cases could be explained "on the theory that the child had wandered, or been carried, away from home within a day or two of its being rescued," and for Herman B. Sheffield, MD (17 July), alleged wolf children were "nothing but microcephalic idiots." Writing off the stories as mere fables that "emanate from India, that land of rhetorical conceptions and of mental imagery," Sir Robert Armstrong-Jones, MD (25 April), proclaimed that "it is physiologically impossible that man who has taken, perhaps, millions of years to evolve should in less than a decade regress to the brute level solely from a changed environment." In stating what, in his view, was missing from the evidence, Dr Norris insinuated that the wolf children must be left with the wolves, at least for a while, for the sake of scientific observation and truth: "Has anyone ever found a child living in an animal's lair, and left it there, returning from time to time to observe how it was getting on, and to find out how it was fed?" Another reader, Jacqueline Nollet (17 July), repudiated the boy's capture for a different reason: "Have men for 'humanity's sake' the right to take this Miawana boy away from his mother-wolf and from his brotherly playmates, from the jungle's new and enthralling life, and to condemn him instead to an existence devoid of companionship and a life of utter misery just because he was a man and should remain a man?" Nollet's discordant voice raised doubts about the value of enforced civilization and introduced the question of the boy's own rights. Since it had already been proved that wolf children kept in captivity did not live long and remained mentally deficient, she called for the Society for the Prevention of Cruelty to Animals "to have a law voted to the effect that a child saved from starvation, loved and protected by the wolves against ferocious beasts, might be left to live with his wolf family."[22] Twelve years later, and in the face of imminent war, the imagination of the *Times* readers was again awakened by news stories regarding an animal-raised boy. This time, the story originated in South Africa, and the animals in question were baboons. Readers' letters on the "African Mowgli" appeared almost daily from 27 June to 26 July 1939. The correspondents' social and professional profile, the arguments advanced for and against the story's authenticity, and the range of themes that were addressed uncannily repeated the earlier debates on Indian wolf children (Sleeman's grandson, now a colonel, also took part in this debate).[23]

As nothing else was ever known about the Miawana boy, he soon sank into oblivion. Lucas, the South African "baboon boy," at first seemed more promising. But further investigation of his story, conducted by Raymond A. Dart of Witwatersrand University, Johannesburg – upon request by the Anglo-American scientists who were already mobilized around the case of Amala and Kamala – unearthed more evidence showing that Lucas had been institutionalized for most of his life and never lived with baboons.[24] Thus only Amala and Kamala managed to hold the attention of Western readers (especially scientists) past the initial commotion. It is ironic that even though it was long believed that all Indian wolf children were boys, the wolf *girls* of Midnapore ended up as the most famous and documented case.[25] In many respects the girls' story fitted the already established pattern; in others, it was unique. In Zingg's opinion, what set it apart was that "only in this case do we have the record of nine years in human association after the rescue by the man who, in company with several others, saw the children brought again into human society." Not only was the man who rescued (or captured) the wolf girls, the Reverend Singh, known but he had written a diary account of the girls' life in his orphanage. The scientists took Singh's account to be the crucial evidence they had been looking for.[26]

Yet things were not that simple. If, as Singh maintained, the girls had been rescued on 17 October 1920, why had the scientists only heard about them six years later, when one of them was already dead (Amala died on 21 September 1921) and all material traces of their life with wolves had most likely disappeared? Singh later said that the reasons why he and his wife did not reveal the discovery were the children's gender ("If the rescue story became public, it would be difficult for us to settle them in their life by marriage, when they attained that age") and fear that publicity "would lead to innumerable visits and queries, which would be a great drain on our time." The wolf girls' existence was divulged by accident when a letter from Singh's old friend Bishop Pakenham-Walsh inadvertently fell into the hands of a British reporter in 1926. This leak was "a providential boon" for the scientists, many of whom contacted Singh directly to check the facts and request more details.[27] In the end Singh reconciled himself to the limelight, acknowledged the wolf girls' scientific significance, and submitted to the scientists' scrutiny. When the Lecture Bureau of the Psychological Society of New York invited him to tour the United States to show "Kamala, the wolf child" to the American people, he declined only because by then the girl's health had badly deteriorated. After Kamala's death on 14 November 1929, the scientists and the bishop persuaded him that he had the duty to make the full story and his first-hand observations available. But Singh's materials on the wolf girls were less weighty than the scientists had hoped. He had never cared to collect written statements from the men who had been with him during the rescue expedition (to confirm that the girls had been found in a wolf's den) nor allowed doctors or specialists to examine Amala and Kamala (to corroborate the notable physical changes that, Singh claimed, life with wolves had effected in them). To complicate matters, when the controversy was at its peak a different version of the rescue story came to light: in the early 1920s Singh had told Indian reporters that not he but the villagers had found the girls in the wolf's den.[28]

By the late 1930s, when Zingg, then an anthropologist at the University of Denver, was entrusted with Singh's manuscript and granted all publication rights – provided that the profits be sent to the orphanage – scientific opinion on the wolf girls of Midnapore was irreparably divided. For some scientists, like Zingg, the case was "well-authenticated" and the publication of Singh's diary would raise "the subject of feral man" to legitimate scientific status, but for others the case and the diary were less appealing than they had first appeared. Specifically, some scientists were loath to admit as evidence of the reality of a particularly improbable phenomenon a muddled account written by a priest – and a non-white one to boot. The scientists' objections were coloured by the white Anglo-American's prejudice towards the "native" and the secular man's feeling of enlightened superiority before religious faith (or "fanaticism"). What could an obscure, untrained Indian missionary who could not even write good English know about scientific evidence, observation, and objectivity?[29]

Wolf-Children and Feral Man, published in 1942, is a curious, exaggeratedly eager book, an odd assortment of interesting material and protestations that the material (and book) should be taken seriously. Zingg had wished the publication to be a collaborative, almost collective, work and to this purpose he invited the scientists who had evinced interest in the wolf girls to inspect the diary and contribute prefatory comments and explanatory footnotes wherever they thought appropriate. Besides "The Diary of the Wolf-Children of Midnapore (India)," by the Reverend J.A.L. Singh, and "Feral Man and Cases of Extreme Isolation of Individuals," by Robert M. Zingg, PhD, *Wolf-Children and Feral Man* comprised a preface and an appendix ("Chronology of the Wolf-Children") by the Right Reverend H. Pakenham-Walsh (Bishop); an affidavit by E. Waight, District and Sessions Judge of Midnapore, declaring that he did not know the wolf girls personally but there was not "the least doubt in my mind that Mr. Singh's truthfulness is absolutely to be relied on"; four forewords, by Professor R. Ruggles Gates, PhD, DSC, LLD, FRS, Professor Arnold Gesell, MD, Professor Francis N. Maxfield, PhD, Professor Kingsley Davis, PhD; nineteen questions from Dr Wilton R. Krogman of the University of Chicago, given in footnotes followed by Singh's answers; about twenty photographs of the wolf girls and

the Singhs, and a full reprint of the 1833 translation of Anselm von Feuerbach's *Caspar Hauser*. In spite of the editor's and collaborators' high hopes,
the book did not fulfill its stated aim. The recurrent efforts to establish the
authenticity of the wolf girls' story once and for all collapsed under the very
weight of the titles and honours it invoked. The sceptics remained sceptical,
and the scientific defenders of wolf children were back at square one. M.F.
Ashley Montagu noted that, much as he would like to believe the story, "no
scientist can accept as true any statement of a fellow-scientist or the statement of anyone else until it has been independently confirmed by others."
David G. Mandelbaum observed that all that could be asserted from the
evidence at hand was "that there was a child by the name of Kamala at the
orphanage whose behavior was peculiar." Singh was a direct witness, yes,
but the only one; his testimony was first-hand and detailed, yes, but his reliability was open to question (why had he kept the girls' rescue a secret, told
conflicting versions of the story, and lied, or at least withheld part of the
truth?). Ultimately, belief in the story of Amala and Kamala could not be
grounded on indisputable, objective evidence but depended on the subject's
decision to believe. The evidence was there, but rather than command-
ing acceptance it had to be (willingly) accepted, together with the reasons
adduced by Singh for its shortcomings.[30]

After the end of the war, interest in the story of the wolf girls subsided,
but the desire to authenticate or disprove it was rekindled every now and
then. In 1951 William F. Ogburn, a sociologist at Florida State University,
carried out an on-site inquiry with the object of securing additional first-
hand testimonies to either buttress or refute Singh's. "On the Trail of the
Wolf-Children," coauthored by Ogburn and his collaborator Nirmal K.
Bose, anthropologist at the University of Calcutta, shows how their efforts,
far from unravelling a single, progressively more clear and authentic story,
called forth a proliferation of accounts, versions, stories: "A miscellaneous
observation from our interviews and correspondence was that not all persons have as high regard for facts in some sectors of their lives as do statisti-
cians in their laboratories. Story telling, devotion to principles, and even
the love of money may take precedence. Then there was the usual observation that successive retellings of a story produce great departures from
the original version." Every attempt to confirm a single fact or detail from
Singh's diary resulted in many more facts and details in need of confirmation. Every interviewee had a story to tell, but no story perfectly matched

the others – or Singh's. The only conclusion Ogburn and Bose could safely draw was that two girls named Amala and Kamala had lived at the orphanage and that "Kamala at least was an exceptional child in that she talked very little" – that is, no conclusion at all.[31] In 1975, almost fifty years after Kamala's death, Charles Maclean, convinced that it was still possible "to produce enough evidence to satisfy myself and others whether or not a human being had ever been fostered by wild animals," travelled to India to conduct another on-site investigation. Maclean believed that he found what he was looking for. He heard references, in the villages near the presumed site of the girls' rescue, to the sighting, around 1916, of a strange creature in the company of wolves, and he met an old man who remembered having participated in the rescue; but he conceded that the version of events he put forward in *The Wolf Children* rested mainly on his interpretation of Singh's character and motivations. One more time, belief depends not on the objective existence of irrefutable evidence but on the subject's decision to accept the available evidence and interpret it in a particular way.[32]

The failure of every attempt to authenticate or disprove the stories of wolf and animal-raised children once and for all is one of the main reasons why such stories remain poignantly haunting. But, I suggest, the failure is inextricable from, on the one hand, the absence of agreed-upon criteria for *what would count* as conclusive evidence in this situation (what is missing is not only the evidence but also the conceptual framework in which the evidence might make sense) and on the other, a historical process of *distancing*, one of whose consequences is that certain types of life and experience are increasingly out of reach of civilized, and more concretely of Western, adults.[33]

Why were Western scientists interested in the stories of wolf and animal-raised children? As Ogburn pointed out, science is "greatly interested in children reared by wolves, for the light the study of them may throw on the new formulation of the old problem of heredity versus environment, which is concerned with the role of culture and of the learning process in shaping personality": would such children "show any human traits" or "behave like a wolf? Would the heredity of *Homo sapiens* mean that a child so reared would walk erect, talk, invent? Would he have a sense of modesty? Of shame? Would he have a soul? Or would he have no other habits than those of wolves as regards locomotion, hunting, howling, sleeping, and dwelling? Or would he do these things better than wolves?" The most salient implication of the stories seemed to be the primacy of environment in human development. For most scientists, what the wolf child's brutalized condition made visible was that without a human environment human children do not become fully human. G.M. Stratton encapsulated the standard environmentalist rendering: "Lack of association with adults during a certain critical period of early childhood, it seems likely, produces in some or all normal children marks like those of congenital defect. The evidence seems against the romantic view that a civilized community is a chief obstacle to the development of personality. On the contrary, the higher forms of personality become possible only in and through such a community ... We become human only by active intercourse in a society of those who already have become human." A minority of scientists, like Wayne Dennis and Eric Lenneberg, cautioned that the stories of animal-raised children should not be used as evidence of *any* social or psychological theory. Nothing certain could be learned from these cases, first, because the accumulated evidence was inadequate, and second, because even if they were authentic, the many unknown factors in the children's early history made it impossible to ascertain why some of them recovered and others did not. For Lenneberg, "the only safe conclusions to be drawn from the multitude of reports is [*sic*] that life in dark closets, wolves' dens, forests, or sadistic parents' backyards is not conducive to good health and normal development." But the attraction of wolf and animal-raised children was so enduring and relentless that even scientists who dismissed the evidence seemed incapable of reining in their generalizing instinct. M.F. Ashley Montagu did not accept the story of Amala and Kamala, but this did not stop him from advancing general conclusions on the matter: "Given all the necessary normal potentialities, an individual does not become a human being simply in virtue of being born into the species *Homo sapiens*; indeed, he cannot become a human being unless he is exposed to the socializing influences of other human beings."[34]

The most fascinating scientific use of wolf children is a book by Arnold Lucius Gesell (1880–1961) on Kamala, *Wolf Child and Human Child: Being a Narrative Interpretation of the Life History of Kamala, the Wolf Girl* (1941). Gesell's account stood out in three ways: a) he did not explicitly engage with the question of evidence (he did not argue that Kamala's story was authentic but *assumed* it from the start); b) he rendered the story in *maturational* rather than environmentalist terms; and c) he did not expect Kamala to shed light on something he did not know (the answer to some crucial question or the revelation of a secret) but deployed his previous knowledge to explain *her*, and in so doing to confirm and extend his theory of development. "Few men in history have influenced the rearing of children as profoundly as has Dr. Arnold Gesell," said Jack Harrison Pollack in an article appropriately titled "Meet Dr. Gesell – The Man Who Knows Children" (1954). Pollack continued: "During the past half-century his pioneer studies have opened new horizons for millions of parents and helped shape the thinking of countless pediatricians, educators and others working with children." In his long career, Gesell endeavoured to describe as accurately as possible the growth of infants and children, map the lawlike unfolding of behaviour patterns, and determine the developmental norms for each age and stage. He designed elaborate and exhaustive testing procedures and filmed more than twelve thousand children. Gesell was among the first scientists to contact Singh when the story of the wolf girls broke in the West and one of the staunchest sponsors of Singh's diary. Louise Bates Ames, Gesell's former collaborator at the Yale Clinic of Child Development and one of the founders (and later co-director) of the Gesell Institute of Child Development, remarked that "no other publication of Dr. Gesell's attracted such stingingly negative reviews" as his book on Kamala. Why would such a respected and productive scientist stake his reputation as a rigorous investigator by getting involved in this sensational and flimsy story? How did the wolf girl relate to Gesell's "normal child"?[35]

Gesell's interest in Kamala amounted to an obsession. In a letter to Zingg, he justified his intention to publish *Wolf Child and Human Child* thus: "I wrote this exposition from an insistent inner compulsion ... I was so haunted by Kamala and Amala that I could not exorcize them until I had written out a story which would satisfy my own questionings. In so doing I hope I have also written something which will help others, particularly lay readers, for there is a profound, unfathomed resistance to the acceptance of Feral Man. And I should be pleased if my step by step interpretation will break down prejudices of antipathy and scepticism." In the book, he gave a similar explanation: "This book, if the author may begin with a confession, was written from inner compulsion. I have always been intrigued (and who has not?) by the weird stories of feral children."[36] For Gesell, the story of Kamala was "the most singular and perhaps the most remarkable which has ever been told of any human child." *Wolf Child and Human Child* was his attempt to reconstruct it and bring out its "psychological significance." This was not an easy task, for the available information was "far from complete." Gesell admitted that he had been forced "to summon imagination and even invent a few conjectures to fill the gaps of actual knowledge," yet he insisted that his objective was "truth rather than fiction" (3–4). Gesell believed that his account of Kamala's life was truthful because to "fill the gaps" he purposely and overtly relied on his previous knowledge of child development – which he clearly believed to be true. On the basis of his knowledge of "the child" Gesell was able to produce a surprisingly detailed account of Kamala's life. But that was not all. Despite his protestations to the contrary, he resorted to the emotional and evocative power of fiction to lend cohesion to the whole. His recurring references to Kipling's Mowgli implicitly afforded another narrative framework, a romantic alternative to his scientific exposition of the normal child's growth, against which the story of Kamala might be read. Kipling's influence was especially noticeable in two aspects of Gesell's account: the anthropomorphic portrayal of the wolves, the "Mother Wolf" in particular, and the narrative teleology, hinting that, like her fictional counterpart, Kamala managed a triumphant return to the human community.[37] The various discourses activated by Gesell were not fully translatable, though, and a series of unrecognized transpositions must be noted – from Kamala's experience to Singh's diary, from Singh's diary to Gesell's psychological biography, from Singh's wolf girl to Gesell's normal child, from Mowgli to Kamala – each move pushing and testing the limits of representation and translation.

The chapter titles spell out the directionality Gesell conferred on Kamala's life. After the introductory chapter, "The Story of Kamala," the account begins in chapter 2 when "Kamala is Born (Spring of 1912)" and takes her in chapter 3 through her adventure "With the Wolves (1912–1920)," only to return her to her rightful place "With Humankind (1920–1929)" in chapter 4. Chapters 5 to 7 show that at first Kamala retained most of her "Wolf Ways (1920–1922)" but was gradually "Weaned from Wolf Ways (1922–1926)" and in due course recovered her "Human Ways (1926–1929)." In chapters 8 and 9 Gesell tackled the controversy on "Heredity and Culture" and formulated a comprehensive view of "Kamala's Life Cycle." The narrative is structured around what Gesell saw as three great crises in Kamala's life: the loss of human care as a baby when she was carried to the wolves' den; the loss of her wolf life and foster-mother wolf when she was "rescued" by Singh; and the loss of "her younger wolf-child sister Amala" (5). Gesell also stressed the importance of three female figures (the birth mother, the wolf, and Mrs Singh) who successively played the role of mother and facilitated Kamala's transitions and adaptations. Kamala's birth mother had an ambiguous status in Gesell's account. He intimated that the baby was initially cared for and loved ("She experienced the deepest satisfaction when she felt the snug pressure of adult hands, which held her in secure grasp and which rubbed her smooth swarthy skin with sweet-smelling ointment") but could not evade the possibility that she might have been deliberately abandoned by her mother (11–12). No ambiguity taints Gesell's depiction of the wolf; on her first appearance, with gorged teats and eyes "preternaturally mild," the wolf steals the baby – but gently: "a she-wolf whose whole being is warmed by the chemistry of maternal hormones can be as deft and gentle as a woman" (13). Back in the wolf's den, Gesell's she-wolf would not fall short when compared with the best examples of American motherhood: "She licked and cleansed her cubs; she kept the floor tidy; she warmed them when necessary with her shaggy hide. For weeks she filled her breasts for them; and weaned them to flesh by chewing it for them and by preparing tidbits from the kill. She permitted them to leave the den when they were about two months old, but not until they were ten to twelve months old and had shed their milk teeth did she permit them to shift for themselves" (18–19). (Gesell did not explain why the she-wolf might have kept Kamala for so many years when her own cubs had to "shift for themselves" after only one year.) To complete the happy family, when Kamala was about seven years old, "of all unpredictable wonders, what should happen? Kamala's wolf mother adopted another human cub" (23). Who could doubt that, had she been able to speak, Gesell's she-wolf would not have said, with Kipling's, "child of man, I loved thee more than ever I loved my cubs."[38] Kamala's second transition, from jungle to orphanage, constituted a major trauma, "a succession of shocks, privations, and dangers" (45). Having lived with the wolves for so many years, Kamala was bound to acquire "wolf ways," and she could not be expected to shed them "at once, even under the benign humanizing influences of her new-found home" (37). The third mother-figure, Mrs Singh, helped Kamala through this harrowing transition and comforted her after the loss of Amala, around whom "clustered a host of associations, tracing back to the ruined den, now so sorely missed" (49).

Around the story of Kamala's life and growth Gesell wove a general argument concerning the distinction between normality and abnormality and the spontaneous nature of growth. On his authority as an expert in development, he declared Kamala to be "a potentially normal child, who in spite of extremely abnormal isolation retained to the end distinguishing marks of normality" (4). Kamala fell outside the scope of Gesell's definition of feeble-mindedness as "inborn or acquired defectiveness of intelligence" preventing the individual from making "an adequate adjustment to the culture into which he is born": to Gesell, "the available evidence strongly denotes that Kamala was born a normal infant and that she suffered no inflammatory illness or physical injury which destroyed the normal potentialities of her brain development. She presented no sensory defects" (73). (Gesell overlooked the fact that the available evidence said nothing about Kamala's infancy, and that, as no tests had been performed, it could not be known whether she had suffered illnesses or injuries or had sensory defects.) Kamala's normality was demonstrated by her successful adjustments first to the wolf's den and then to the complex demands of human culture. Her story exemplified "the reactions of normal human potentialities under extremely abnormal stress" (xii); that is, what was abnormal in Gesell's view was not Kamala but her circumstances.

Once he had established that Kamala was normal, Gesell could easily insert elements of what he knew to be true of the normal child's development into his narrative account of her early life, of which he knew nothing. Baby Kamala *is* the Gesellian infant: "In her own birthright she was already an active infant bent on creating experience rather than passively receiving it. She almost demanded to be propped up in a sitting position, so that she might survey the universe at eye level, for did not Nature intend that someday she was to stand erect and walk upright?" (12). In the wolf's den Gesell's Kamala continued to grow spontaneously according to his developmental schedules: "She already had good control of the movements and postures of her head. She was learning by alternate flexion and extension of her arms to pivot on her stomach, so she could swing through the arc of a circle. A week or two later she flexed her arms simultaneously and pulled her body weight forward; that is to say, she crawled on her stomach ... All of this came about as we say naturally, which means that it came largely from inborn impulse" (19). Gesell affirmed that Kamala's readjustment to "human ways" was spontaneous as well. Where other social and behavioural scientists had seen incontestable manifestations of environmental influence (e.g., Kamala went on all fours when living with wolves and stood and walked on her knees after two years of life with humans), Gesell found strong confirmation that heredity determines development. To emphasize the developmental/maturational interpretation of Kamala's life, Gesell's last chapter outlined her "life cycle" by means of brief sketches of her "daily life" at "four successive stages of her maturity, namely at five months of age, at five years, at nine years, and at fifteen years" (89). He concluded: "*From the standpoint of genetic and of clinical psychology the most significant phenomenon in the life career of Kamala is the slow but orderly and sequential recovery of obstructed mental growth"* (76).[39]

Unlike most other students of wild children, Gesell granted that the wolf girl was human throughout her ordeal. She acquired "wolf ways," but "by no stretch of the imagination can we say that she became a wolf creature. She must be envisaged as a human infant who was confronted with a monstrously exceptional situation, and who solved it within her capacities as a human being" (21).[40] Gesell's narrative and interpretive effort to "rescue" Kamala for normalcy and humanity is not only refreshing but very moving and definitely commendable. Yet it must also be said that Gesell could confidently champion Kamala's normality and humanity because his Kamala was in great measure a creature of his imagination, his knowledge of "the child," and his desire to make the wolf girl intelligible.

Gesell's overall understanding of Kamala's life was grounded on an overly optimistic assessment of her progress. It is true that Singh's account is often vague and at times contradictory, but Gesell unfailingly "filled the gaps" with the most cheerful interpretation possible, the one that matched his view of Kamala's "whole life cycle." Gesell could assert that Kamala's recovery of "human ways" marked a resumption of spontaneous development because he disregarded the deliberate, patient, and persistent intervention of Singh and his wife and the great pains they took to elicit each new response. Describing how, in August 1922, Kamala began to take her food from a specially made table rather than the floor or ground, Gesell quickly added that "this significant behavior pattern was *not* taught. Kamala was in effect teaching her tutors, for she was displaying to them a new ability which she herself had matured" (41).[41] Gesell downplayed the permanence of some of the most troubling sides of Kamala's behaviour while transforming punctual actions, which Singh mentioned once or twice, into routine behaviour patterns. Each of Kamala's new behaviours was construed as a milestone of development, a skill that would be indefinitely repeated from then on. And whereas each new behaviour denoted Kamala's spontaneous growth and initial normality, all her reversals bespoke, for Gesell, was the success of her adaptation to life with the wolves. He could thus decree: "There is no insoluble paradox in the fact that Kamala both suffered and survived her fate. The seven years in the den took their toll. But when the life cycle of Kamala is contemplated in full perspective we must marvel at the insurance factors which protected her potentialities. We regain a tithe of further faith in Nature, and by the same token in Man" (98). What I find most disturbing about Gesell's rendering of Kamala's life is that her early death did not weaken his certitude that she *survived* her fate. He conceived the girl's life after her rescue from the wolf's den as an ascending line of development and did not give her death a place *in* that line. Kamala's death was obviously a sad turn of events that curtailed her full growth potential, yet as an *external* event, sad but fortuitous, it did not seem to demand a careful (and painful) rethinking of her "life cycle," nor of the implications Gesell wished to derive from it.[42]

Gesell presented Kamala's story as an enactment of pure growth triumphing over environmental hindrance. According to Gesell, development is the unfolding and structuring of inborn patterns of behaviour through the time of infancy and childhood. Normal childhood is an itinerary to be traversed along a single line and at a regular pace by all children, all departures from the prescribed timeline and basic behaviour patterns indicating either retardation or deviation. Central to his conceptualization was the idea that external circumstances could never permanently alter the outcome – normal, retarded, or deviant – determined by the child's "natural endowment." In *Developmental Diagnosis*, Gesell and Amatruda wrote:

Growth potentials are primarily determined. Their limits are fixed by inheritance and constitution; the growth potentials come to realization in experience. The character of the environment, of course, has considerable effect upon the character of the experience. But experience does not create new potentials, nor does it destroy the original potentials ... An ament cannot be lifted to normal mental efficiency by the most favorable environment. An environmentally retarded child responds in a significant way to a more favorable milieu ... [A] normal child is normal and remains, in a developmental sense, potentially normal under environmental adversities. An ament is and remains an ament regardless of alterations of environment.

What this passage proffers is but a technical formulation of the very explanation Gesell read into, or imposed on, Kamala's life. Wolf children were generally seen as a test case in the heredity/environment controversy – in fact, as telling evidence *for* environmentalism. This perfunctory affinity between wolf children and the environmentalists animated Gesell's obsession with Kamala: to counter the prevalent environmentalist interpretation it was necessary to advance and defend an alternative interpretation in maturational terms. Gesell's claim that Kamala was born normal and remained normal despite adversity and extreme experiences was *a demand of his theory*.[43]

Kamala performed yet another function for Gesell. As Esther Thelen and Karen E. Adolph assert, even if Gesell's developmental norms had been arrived at by examining thousands of infants and children, these children had been "carefully sampled from the New Haven community to provide a homogeneous, white, middle-class group of British or German extraction from intact two-parent families." Gesell's "normal child," the basis of his descriptions of normal behaviour and prescriptions for parents, child workers, and paediatricians, originated in a far from representative sample but was "meant to generalize to any infant, regardless of upbringing, environmental opportunities, and racial heritage." Thelen and Adolph are right when they argue that Gesell's "typical child living his typical day" was "clearly male, white, native-born, middle-class, and in an intact family, with a virtually invisible father and a devoted but strangely passive mother who acted without agency in an intermittently compliant culture."[44] Interestingly, these qualities were exactly *what Kamala was not*: she was female, non-white, born in an unidentified Indian village, a social outcast, with a most unusual family (or famil*ies*). In this sense, the attention Gesell paid Kamala becomes meaningful: she implicitly represents all the *other children* excluded from his observations and studies. Borrowing Freud's powerful imagery, we may say that Gesell's obsession with Kamala signals the return of the repressed.

Gesell's imaginary account of baby Kamala would not have been out of place in any of his books on infant growth and behaviour:

Most of the day as well as night the baby kept her eyes closed; but not because she feared the light. One evening at dusk, while she was basking in her corner in the folds of a villager's wrapper, she caught sight of a lighted taper which the mother was carrying across the room quite slowly lest it blow out. The baby's eyes followed the flame across the void. The movement of the eyes was a significant expedition into the outer world. For weeks the infant had lain with head persistently averted to one side, but soon she was able to shift her head back and forth with increased freedom, exploring the universe which was more and more making its vast presence felt. Her arms likewise became emancipated, she flung them outward and then with infantile effort she brought her hands toward the midline as though she were intent to enfold this universe. And one day she succeeded in measure, for when she was about six months old, her dark-eyed brother dangled a rattling gourd before her: she seized it.

By such timely tokens it was evident that the baby was growing in mental as well as physical stature. (11)

In this extraordinary passage, in which the developmental tasks of the examination routinely conducted at the Yale Clinic are restaged in "one of the mud and thatched huts" of Kamala's native village, what Gesell is striving to establish is not Kamala's normality but the cultural neutrality of his testing apparatus and developmental schedules. What was implied in *Wolf Child and Human Child* was that all the world's children, regardless of cultural, historical, or purely biographical variation, provided they were "normally endowed," were essentially (or had the potential to be) indistinguishable from the cute babies and young children daily paraded through the examination rooms and before the hidden cameras of the Yale Clinic. Only minor changes were necessary (lighted taper for dangling ring, rattling gourd for rattle[45]), but the scene of infant growth was essentially – naturally – the same. By claiming her for his own scientific enterprise, Gesell "tamed" Kamala and reduced the enormity of her difference to another instance of the same, an unusual and singularly fascinating but at heart reassuring illustration of his deeply held views. Gesell used Kamala to validate and universalize his theory of childhood and growth. If such a radically different child could be integrated into his developmental scheme, then *any* other child could be integrated as well. In other words, Gesell's theory must be able to explain Kamala in order to prove its claim to be a universal account of development.

Gesell never met Kamala, but as a specialist in children he *knew* her in advance, as it were. But Gesell's approach to Kamala was an exception. In a later encounter between two Western scientists, psycholinguist Harlan Lane of Northeastern University and psychiatrist Richard Pillard of Boston University, and an exotic, animal-raised, brutalized wild child, the scientists once again understood their task as a search for new (and crucial) knowledge. Lane had just published his book on Victor of Aveyron when his former thesis director, B.F. Skinner, forwarded him a report that appeared on 11 April 1976 in the *Johannesburg Sunday Times* stating that a wild boy had been found living with monkeys in Burundi. Like many others before him on hearing about the discovery of a wild child, Lane was elated: "I dared not believe my good fortune if the story was true. The last time a child had been found who was unquestionably feral ... was almost two centuries ago, in 1799."[46] The wild boy of Burundi (who had been named John after John the Baptist) reminded him of Victor: "John had so many of Victor's traits that they were practically twins"; indeed, Lane reasoned that the similarities attested to the story's authenticity: "Surely David Barritt, the journalist who'd written the story, hadn't studied the case of the Wild Boy of Aveyron and then attributed to John the hallmarks of Victor's upbringing" (12). We know better: what John reminds us of is not so much Victor but the Indian wolf children and Lucas, the "baboon boy" of South Africa, whose stories Lane passed over and Barritt could have found in numerous newspaper and magazine articles. After thus connecting John and Victor, Lane went on to transpose what in his view had been the consequences of the encounter between Victor and Itard to the potential encounter between John and contemporary researchers. Victor had been found "at the dawn of psychology and psychiatry, when no one knew how to study a deviant child, much less treat one," and yet "mankind had reaped immeasurable benefits from his capture" and treatment: "Modern methods for educating the deaf, the retarded, and the normal preschool child arose directly out of the efforts to train him" (4). If that was then, "how much more could we now learn with the tools of modern psychology and medicine! How much more could we discover about what it means to grow up in society from this terrible experiment of nature, which chance had designed and which science could exploit? And how much more could we contribute to the education of handicapped children everywhere by undertaking the training of this latest, and perhaps last, wild child, raised in the forests utterly cut off from society" (5). Upon his own admission, Lane knew nothing about Burundi, but this did not diminish his certainty that going in search of his own wild child was the right thing to do.[47]

In an outstanding display of energy and enthusiasm, Lane and his friend Pillard organized a trip to Burundi. Like others before him, Lane regretted that the boy's caretakers were teaching him things (to the detriment of his valuable wildness): "All this teaching the boy is well and good, but it is obliterating the traces of life in the wild and is destroying his value as a scientific discovery" (11). While planning the trip, Lane and Pillard considered what they would do "with the jungle boy once we reached him" (18). The strategy they decided on was twofold: first, they would follow Itard's model, that is, they would study John by rehabilitating him, laying emphasis on sensory training (reconceived as behaviour modification); second, they would have John admitted to the Shriver Center of the Fernald School for retarded children in Boston. They would take advantage of everything that had been discovered and invented since Itard's time, in the belief that their greater knowledge and more sophisticated techniques would lead not only to a more successful training of the wild child but also to more valuable knowledge being extracted from him. For Lane and Pillard, John as a wild child was also a generic child, a child that could stand for every child. His cultural context, social and geopolitical position, ethnic and linguistic background, and previous personal experiences did not have to be taken into account except as obstacles to the identification of what was important about him. The two American researchers presumed that, in the name of science, they could turn up in Burundi – a country that a few weeks earlier they had not known existed – obtain unrestricted access to the child and all the resources they needed (vehicles, assistants, translators, medical facilities), quickly ascertain what John really was and, if he proved to be a true wild child and therefore worthy of study (and expenditure), take him to the United States to give him back his language and his full humanity while making him reveal his secrets.

The North American media and the public became interested in the new wild boy, but this time more people voiced the opinion that he was probably better off in the woods and should not have been captured in the first place. Lane received a letter from three students who were "very disturbed to hear about your rehabilitation program for a child who appears to be living in an environment suited to his needs." Science, they wrote, "seems to have no place or understanding for this boy and we feel it is very inhumane to bring him back to a society based on our needs. Is it not possible to observe him in his environment? What are your motives for this 'experiment'?" A university professor was concerned as well: "My concern is why you feel the child, after reportedly living in the jungle for four years, *needs* to be 'rehabilitated.' Why are 'civilized' people always trying to 'civilize' the 'uncivilized'? Why do we feel civilization is so much better?" (42). Lane was "saddened" by these responses: "What a grim commentary on our lives! Is life in the home sweet home so punitive that we prefer life in isolation, scrabbling for food, fleeing predators, neither giving nor receiving love?" (43). Lane may be missing the point. Some people's refusal to share his enthusiasm and hopes did not simply spring from a misguided idealization of the wild child's wild life. In question were precisely the scientists' quest and efforts: their knowledge might not suffice to offer the boy a better life and the knowledge they thought they would extract from him might not be so valuable after all.

Lane and Pillard went to great lengths to appear open, humane, enlightened, and good-humoured, but their words and actions betrayed the overconfidence of the Western scientific researcher (and the white American male) storming into the unsuspecting Third World, which, like the wild child, functions as the underside of civilization and development. On their way to Burundi, Lane and Pillard stopped for a few days in Paris to get visas: "I [Lane] have had a decade-old love affair with Paris and somewhat briefer affairs with a few of its inhabitants. It is the most cultured city in the world, the apogee of what society has to offer in literature, art, architecture, food, dress. The city of Hugo, Toulouse-Lautrec, Escoffier, Cardin – what better point of departure for studying a wild child utterly cut off from society?" (27). Bujumbura, Burundi's capital, seemed to them "more like a giant village than a city, and after Paris, it was hard not to find it decrepit and filthy" (84). Doctors, diplomats, and other Westerners living in Bujumbura warned Lane and Pillard that John might not be what the newspaper report suggested: "What constitutes a good account of events is not the same in Burundi as it is in America" (88). When they met John at the Gitega orphanage, they were not particularly impressed by the "strange-looking child" (99), but they dutifully proceeded to examine him and subject him to many tests, first at the orphanage, then at the Bujumbura hospital, and finally in Nairobi, Kenya.[48] In parallel, Lane and Pillard made inquiries about the boy's history and found out that John, whose real name was Balthazar Nsanzerugeze, had spent his early years in orphanages and mental institutions, not with monkeys: "It may be difficult to believe, but this discovery left us not crestfallen but exhilarated; the tangle of facts, rumors, people and places was unraveling. The awful possibility that we would never solve the mystery had receded ever so lightly" (147). The testing continued anyway, and after a consultation with all the participating physicians in Nairobi, John/Balthazar was diagnosed: autism and profound retardation, for which there was no treatment.

Pillard pondered "John's future." In a large institution in the United States, like the Fernald School, "where the stress of working is so great that some wards have an almost complete turnover of personnel every few months," nobody would "know John or learn to care about him"; at the Gitega orphanage "he has Sister Nestor and Petronille, who adore him, and a stable environment." Pillard concluded: "Given that there is nothing we can offer in the way of treatment, I feel more than satisfied with the care he will get in his native land" (173). Is it too cynical to think instead that Balthazar, a poor African boy, was valueless to science and thus not worth the effort and expense? That had John's "wildness" been established, the loving care and stable environment his native land could offer him would have had to give way to the technically and scientifically superior options found in the United States, however anonymous and loveless?

Having displayed their efficiency and accomplished their mission, Lane and Pillard left Burundi less than ten days after their arrival. They were sad to leave the new friends they had made in Burundi, but not John/Balthazar: "At that moment he didn't enter our minds. If you think that is strange or hardhearted, you must try to understand the difference between caring for a friend and caring for a patient ... Balthazar was our patient and our puzzle; we had done what we could for and with him; we felt complete" (176–7). They had fun; they would do it all over again, but still the discovery that John was not a feral child was a disappointment: "The opportunity for science would have been magnificent ... it would have been the find of the century" (179, 180). The disappointments multiply, but the dream that science may, one day, succeed in wrenching the wild child's secrets lives on. As for John, he died at the orphanage in 1985.[49]

CHAPTER EIGHT

Confinement and Freedom

Genie was about the richest source of information you can imagine.
... There were kinds of questions that I felt she might shed light on.

Jay Shurley[1]

IT MAY BE THAT "exotic" wild and animal-raised children are just too un-
wieldy. They may be too elusive, too far away from the centres of scientific
knowledge production, too radically other to be studied properly. Their
wildness, taken to be the outcome of a long period spent in isolation or
with animals in the wild (forest, jungle, desert, mountain), is what makes
them valuable and excruciatingly desirable but by its very nature cannot be
controlled or observed. It is not difficult to understand the excitement of
a group of scientists when they discovered a child who appeared to be the
perfect surrogate for the slippery wild child. This was Genie; she was found
right here, in our midst, and her early life held no mysteries, it seemed, since
for more than a decade she had almost never left the confines of a room
in her parents' home in Temple City, California. Tempted by a child who
promised to reveal the secrets associated with the wild child while bearing,
in her being and history, none of the wild child's annoying uncertainty, the
scientists transformed the confined child into a full-fledged wild child.

Susan Wiley, renamed Genie by the scientists, first appeared in the news
in November 1970, when the *Los Angeles Times* reported that her parents,
accused of having kept her "a virtual prisoner since infancy," were arrested.
Although the girl was thirteen years old, she was unable to talk or walk,
wore diapers, and did not know the most basic life skills (like chewing).

Her limbs and muscles were partially atrophied owing to physical restraint and inadequate activity. The Wileys' neighbours, who remembered having seen the girl playing in the yard now and then, thought she was mentally retarded. Genie was admitted to Childrens Hospital, Los Angeles, for malnutrition.[2] She was without question a horribly abused and extremely deprived child, but at first glance there was nothing "wild" or "savage" about her. Her case was undoubtedly a police matter, and various kinds of medical, educational, and welfare professionals would have to exert great ingenuity to find the way to rehabilitate her, heal her physical and psychological wounds, and restore her to a fuller life. But the doctors and researchers who became involved in Genie's life were not satisfied with helping her – they wanted to study her. For people in general, Genie was an object of pity; for the scientists, she was an object of knowledge. The name the scientists gave her, "Genie," indeed marked her transition from an abused child to a more extraordinary object of study. As a matter of fact, this was not the first time that scientists had related confined children and wild children. Still, while earlier cases of confined children – Kaspar Hauser, Anna and Isabelle, Anne and Albert, Yves Cheneau – had been *compared* to wild and animal-raised children to highlight variations in the condition produced by, and long-term effects of, different degrees and kinds of isolation, none of these children was, like Genie, *identified* as a wild child from the start. Because the scientists construed Genie as a wild child, hence as singularly valuable and precious, research was given primacy in her case over all other considerations.[3]

Genie was "rescued" from her parents' home and admitted to Childrens Hospital at the same time that Truffaut's *Wild Child* opened in Los Angeles. When, in May 1971, the professionals and scientists in charge of her case organized a conference to make decisions concerning how she would be treated and the specific type of research that would be carried out on her, they arranged to have a private screening of *The Wild Child*. The film worked its magic, and the scientists identified Genie with Victor. "It was awe-inspiring to us because here was the first case that had been documented in any scientific way," said Howard Hansen, head of the psychiatry division of Childrens Hospital. Jay Shurley, professor of psychiatry and behavioural science at the University of Oklahoma and expert in social isolation, remarked that "the impact on the whole group was stunning ... All of us saw in the movie what we were prepared to see to confirm our biases."[4] The label "wild child," borrowed from Truffaut's film, stuck permanently to

Genie. She was characterized as a wild child in the scientific publications resulting from the research on her and in the more recent critical investigations of her story. What was there in common between Victor and Genie? Both children were unable to speak and had not had the chance to learn many skills deemed essential to humanity and socialization; both had had little contact with other human beings and little exposure to human culture of any kind. But there the commonalities end. In one case isolation took place in the wild, the outdoors, nature; in the other, in a locked room in a house on the outskirts of one of the largest cities of the most developed country in the world. In one case the child lived a rugged and dangerous but eventful existence; in the other, she endured ongoing neglect and abuse at the hands of a small group of people. The child experienced, in one case, maximum autonomy and freedom, unrestricted mobility, and the pressing need to provide for his own subsistence; in the other, total physical restriction, helplessness, and dependence in a bare, human-made environment. Yet both children were considered to be epistemologically equivalent, in the sense that, for the scientists, study of Genie, and what could be learned from her, were equivalent to study of Victor. Susan Curtiss, then a doctoral student in linguistics and later a professor at the University of California at Los Angeles, thus linked Genie to Victor (and, by extension, herself to Itard): "The Wild Boy of Aveyron died over a century ago, but another adolescent who affords us equally rich opportunities for study has been discovered in our own time: Genie."[5] History appeared to be repeating itself, to the scientists' great good fortune. Victor had made Itard famous; what professional and personal rewards would Genie not have in store for whoever was there, ready to grab them?

Genie's newly conferred status as a wild child had several consequences. She was portrayed as other wild children usually are: "Genie was unsocialized, primitive, hardly human." The recent change in her life (from the locked room to the hospital) was couched in the language of discovery. This is how Curtiss closed the heartbreaking narrative of Genie's childhood: "Genie was admitted into the hospital for extreme malnutrition. She had been discovered, at last."[6] Like other wild children, she was interpreted as a guilt-free version of the forbidden experiment. Experimental deprivation "ha[s] not and cannot be carried out for obvious reasons," Curtiss maintained, but "experiments in nature" (which she defined as "tragic alterations of the normal human condition not purposefully induced by the scientific community") offered a valid alternative for scientists wishing to verify various hypotheses about human development. For Curtiss, "Genie is such an experiment in nature."[7] (A simple objection to this claim would be that even if the scientists did not "purposefully induce" Genie's "tragic alterations," neither did *nature*.)

As I suggested earlier, the more the forbidden experiment is seen as a moral evil, the more the study of the wild child (as a natural or accidental instance of the forbidden experiment) finds some justification in the idea that, by forcing the child to reveal her secrets, the scientist is at least giving some meaning to her unspeakable suffering and deprivation. In this way, the study of the wild child, however intense or intrusive, is not seen as exploitation but as a duty, even more so since none of the previous cases known in the literature had been properly and systematically studied: "The case of Genie assumes even more importance, then, because of its unique character, and because, from the time she emerged from isolation, a team of psychologists, psychiatrists, neurologists, and linguists have been working with this amazing child."[8] What exactly did the researchers expect to learn from Genie? Since Genie, like other isolated and wild children, was "in a retarded state of development," they wanted to know "whether a child so deprived can 'catch up' wholly or in part."[9] The research focused on language acquisition. It was determined that Genie had not yet acquired language and "was faced with learning her first language when she was 13 years, 7 months of age." The main question was whether language could be acquired at such a late age. Genie's learning (or not learning) would bear on Lenneberg's critical-age hypothesis and on the relation between language acquisition and brain lateralization: "Is there a critical period for language acquisition? If so, what kind of language development is possible beyond the critical period? Are language acquisition and language lateralization interrelated? Will language be lateralized if acquired after puberty? If so, will it be lateralized to the left hemisphere as it is in normal human brains? What happens to cerebral organization in general when one of the brain's basic functions fails to develop?" Curtiss's questions are certainly important, but one cannot help noticing that they lack the breadth and poignancy of the questions that obsessed eighteenth-century thinkers and attracted *them* to wild children.[10]

Curtiss's *Genie: A Psycholinguistic Study of a Modern-Day "Wild Child"* (1977) presented and analyzed the linguistic data collected between 1971 and 1975 while Genie lived with David Rigler, professor at the University of Southern California and chief psychologist in the psychiatry division of Childrens Hospital, and his wife Marilyn.[11] Itard had described in his reports the educational program he designed for Victor and the vicissitudes of the medico-pedagogical relation established between him and the boy as the program was implemented; in contrast, Curtiss described the tests she designed for and administered to Genie and the girl's performance in them, as well as her linguistic comprehension and spontaneous production in informal situations. Curtiss's account leaves no doubt that Genie was incessantly and exhaustively tested but says little about the concrete educational or therapeutic means that may have been employed with her. This is not a casual omission: the scientists were functioning within a model of "acquisition" associated with spontaneous development ("Since her emergence she has been acquiring her first language primarily by 'exposure' alone"[12]) and could therefore neither design a deliberate intervention to teach Genie language nor discuss openly the teaching interventions that were in all likelihood taking place. Curtiss's stated purpose was to watch the emergence of Genie's innate linguistic structures; her task was not strictly to maximize Genie's learning but to ascertain whether linguistic development could resume after a prolonged period of abnormal deprivation. Testing Genie was "often extremely problematic and difficult," especially at the beginning, because she was inattentive and unpredictable. Yet testing constituted the bulk of the research: "As Genie became more testable, as we became more familiar with testing her, and as her language developed, new tests were constructed and old ones were modified, thereby increasing the range of linguistic elements and structures tested, and making each test a more reliable instrument for assessing Genie's knowledge of a particular linguistic feature or structure at any given time." Testing (which, in Genie's case, overshadowed teaching and treatment) is not mere observation; it is a kind of intervention, but one in which the adult does not take an active part in the child's learning but assesses the extent of the child's own development.[13]

Since the linguistic research carried out on Genie concerned the resumption of suspended but normal development, the scientists had to defend the claim that Genie's retardation had been caused by isolation and deprivation only and discard two other possibilities: that she was congenitally retarded ("On the basis of what is known about the early history, and what has been observed so far, it appears that Genie was normal at the time of birth and that the retardation observed at the time of discovery was due principally to the extreme isolation to which she was subjected, with its accompanying social, perceptual, and sensory deprivation"), and that her early experiences had left lasting psychological scars that affected her general development (Curtiss told Rymer that Genie's "problems with language were not related to any distress or emotion"). The scientists granted that Genie's early experiences had been distressing but they did not view them as *traumatic*, that is, as the root of her present deficiencies.[14] After several years of work with Genie, Curtiss concluded that the girl had been acquiring language: "We must keep in mind that Genie's speech is rule-governed behavior, and that from a finite set of arbitrary linguistic elements she can and does create novel utterances that theoretically know no upper bound. These are the aspects of human language that set it apart from all other animal communication systems. Therefore, abnormalities notwithstanding, in the most fundamental and critical respects, Genie has language."[15] Curtiss took this as demonstration that a first language could be acquired, at least to a certain degree, beyond the critical period. From the comparison between Genie's "far from normal" language and that of normal children, Curtiss drew implications pertinent to the processes of language acquisition and lateralization in general.

All in all, Curtiss's *Genie* – like Truffaut's film, or Itard's first report, or Gesell's book on Kamala for that matter – conveyed an unwarrantedly optimistic sense of Genie's progress: "My work with Genie continues, and Genie continues to change, becoming a fuller person, realizing more of her human potential. By the time this work is read, she may have developed far beyond what is described here. That is my hope – that I will not be able to keep up with her, that she will have the last word."[16] By the time the book was published it was clear that Genie's life had taken a dramatic turn for the worse and that her "development" had suffered in consequence, but for some reason Curtiss chose not to refer to what happened to Genie after 1975. The National Institute of Mental Health, which had been funding the research, rejected David Rigler's application for an extension of the grant, and the Riglers gave Genie up. In the summer of 1975 Genie went to live with her mother (in the same house where she had been confined until the end of 1970), but the latter found life with her daughter too difficult and gave her up as well. From then on Genie lived in a succession of foster homes; she was mistreated and physically abused again; she lost the few skills she had learned at the hospital and at the Riglers', and she stopped speaking altogether. John Miner, a lawyer and since 1972 Genie's legal guardian, saw her some time after she left the Riglers' home: "Her regression was just overwhelming." Then a nasty fight erupted between the scientists and Genie's mother. In October 1979 Genie's mother filed a suit against the scientists and hid Genie away.[17]

In the end, and contrary to Curtiss's hopes, Genie did not realize more of her human potential, nor did she have the last word. The scientists involved in her life proved unable not only to rehabilitate her fully despite their advanced knowledge and techniques but also to provide her with a stable and loving environment in which, even if she never got to be talkative or smart, she could at least be happy and safe from further abuse and neglect. Science could neither save Genie nor justify her earlier suffering. What was learned from or through her was much less, and much less certain, than what the scientists had expected.[18] What makes Genie's story unbearably sad is not just her confined and deprived childhood but what happened to her after her purported discovery. It is however still too close to us, and perhaps more time has to pass before we may be able to understand it, to unravel the conflicts of interest and desire that traverse it, and to judge its protagonists. In the letter he sent Jean Butler in August 1971 (responding to her accusations that the scientists were exploiting Genie), Rigler wrote: "If this child can be assisted to develop in cognitive, linguistic and social, and other areas, this provides useful information regarding the critical role of early experience which is of potential benefit to other deprived children. The research interest inherently rests upon successful achievement of rehabilitative efforts. The research goals thus coincide with [Genie's] own welfare and happiness ... This child is not for sale, but in our view and in the view of funding agencies, knowledge obtained from study of this unique child is important knowledge to be employed for humanitarian purposes."[19] The scientists may have been sincere in their belief that their study of Genie, like Itard's study of Victor, was predicated upon the child's successful recovery. But it is possible to descry two key differences in the way Victor and Genie were handled. To begin with, Genie was never allowed or encouraged to form genuine and lasting relationships with people who cared for her as a person. Besides, even had they wanted to, the scientists in Genie's story, unlike the authorities in Victor's, did not have the power to make binding decisions regarding her life and future. For better or worse, their actions and claims were open to challenge – by other scientists, the funding agencies, Genie's mother, the welfare services. Genie was utterly helpless, but the adults around her, all of whom wanted something from her and had much to say about her, were either powerless or unwilling to give her what she most needed.[20]

Unlike Lane and Pillard, who did not see John of Burundi as a particularly appealing child, the scientists that surrounded Genie emphasized how attractive and special she was. James Kent, psychologist at Childrens Hospital and child abuse expert, declared: "I was captivated by her ... she had a personal quality that seemed to elicit rescue fantasies ... She was very special to me ... I was very attached to her." And David Rigler: "I think everybody who came in contact with her was attracted to her. She had a quality of somehow connecting with people which developed more and more but was present really from the start. She had a way of reaching out without saying anything but just, somehow, by the kind of look in her eyes, and people wanted to do things for her." Curtiss waxed sentimental when reminiscing about Genie: "She was fragile, and beautiful, almost haunting, and so I was pulled, I was very drawn to her, even though I was nervous and had no idea in many respects what to expect ... I could tell as all of us could just looking at her that there was a lot to Genie, and that what we had to do was to make sure we gave her opportunities to express, find a way to take what was latent and express it or somehow then, you know, acquire it, because the potential just seemed so great."[21] Curtiss wrote that Genie "has enriched my life beyond measure"; she announced: "I would pay a lot of money to see her." When read against the reality of Genie's life, such proclamations ring hollow. In court, Miner stated (in defence of the Riglers): "It was a matter of my not being able to understand how people not related to this child could undergo what, in fact, she was subjecting them to in terms of the strain on the household." In the attempt to justify why the Riglers gave Genie up, what Miner conjured up was no longer the beautiful, attractive, and uncannily communicative "genie" but a child so unsocialized and demanding that it was hard to see why anyone not "related" to her would want to put up with her. Miner's words at least sound sincere. Curtiss's too, when for a moment she suspends her effusiveness and simply admits, "I was really at the right place at the right time."[22]

The scientists who studied Genie turned to history to back their view that she was a "wild child" worthy of scientific attention. This being the case, it is curious that they did not relate Genie to Kaspar Hauser, the confined child whose fame matches (if not surpasses) Victor's. Kaspar, like Genie, is said to have spent most of his childhood in a kind of prison, where his most basic needs were met though he could not move and had no contact with other people and almost no sensory stimulation. Kaspar emerged from his isolated and deprived childhood in a state comparable to Genie's, yet unlike Genie he "recovered" almost completely. After a relatively short time he could speak, write, and engage with people in social situations. He gave evidence of an acute sensibility and a lively, if eccentric, intellect. Kaspar's recovery contrasts sharply with the lack of substantial progress shown by most of the other wild children, including Genie. In an article published in 1978, Nicole Simon called attention to this fact: as a "counterexample" to most reports of wild children, Kaspar's case undermines the common view "that early environmental deprivation causes an irreversible disruption of development, especially language development." For this reason, it "cannot properly be ignored in any discussion of the effects of environmental deprivation on later development, especially those that cite the work of Itard with Victor of Aveyron."[23] Simon's warning would seem singularly relevant to the research just then being carried out on Genie, but Simon did not mention Genie. The relation, or rather the absence of any relation, between Genie and Kaspar is a conspicuous departure from the rule that writings on wild children always tend to reinforce or fabricate links between the various stories. In this case we discern the opposite phenomenon: two confined/wild children who are kept apart even though relating and comparing them would seem to be the obvious thing to do. One reason, I suggest, is that both Kaspar and Genie have a tenuous relation to the class "wild child." Being peripheral examples, their status as wild children is strengthened if they are related to a prototypical case like Victor's, but it might be fatally weakened if they were related to one another.

Kaspar Hauser's is one of the best-known and most often revisited stories of the last two hundred years. He mysteriously appeared on 26 May 1828 in Nuremberg. He could say only a few words, whose meaning he did not understand, had trouble walking, and looked frightfully confused. His astonishment at people and things convinced observers that he was seeing them for the first time. Attempts were made to disentangle the mystery of his origin, and baffling details about his imprisoned childhood and rumours about his true identity began to circulate. Kaspar's education was undertaken by Georg Friedrich Daumer (1800–1875), who had studied with Hegel and Schelling; his plight attracted the attention of the respected jurist Anselm von Feuerbach (1775–1833), while Philip Henry, earl of Stanhope (1805–1875), proclaimed his intention to adopt him. Kaspar was wounded on 17 October 1829, while he was living at Daumer's. At the end of 1831 he was moved to Ansbach, where he lived with Johann Georg Meyer, a schoolteacher. On 14 December 1833 Kaspar was stabbed in the chest at the Court Garden in Ansbach, and he died on 17 December.[24]

Kaspar's story brought about controversy and lent itself to many different uses. Already during his lifetime there were two currents of opinion regarding his identity. Was Kaspar the legitimate heir of Baden, kidnapped as a child to change the line of succession to the throne, or was he nothing but a clever liar and impostor as Stanhope and Meyer insinuated? Was he attacked by a stranger in 1829 and murdered by a stranger in 1833, or were his wounds self-inflicted?[25] What concerns me here is not who Kaspar really was but how his story came to intersect with those of wild children. When Kaspar appeared in Nuremberg, the people who first encountered him wondered "whether he should be considered as an idiot or a madman, or as a kind of savage." Dr Preu, the physician who examined Kaspar, referred to him as one of those children who grew up in the wilderness with animals. But Feuerbach expressly dismissed any connection or resemblance between Kaspar and wild children: "By no means an idiot or a madman, he was so mild, so obedient, and so good-natured that no one could be tempted to regard this stranger as a savage, or as a child grown up among the wild beasts of the forest."[26] Kaspar began to be discussed in relation to wild children in the second half of the nineteenth century and was fully integrated into the list in the first half of the twentieth century.

The initial response to Kaspar was analogous to the reaction to the wild girl of Songi. Kaspar, like Marie-Angélique, did not at first understand the meaning of his own words or other people's questions; soon after his "discovery," however, an inexplicably minute story about his early life was afloat. In a proclamation written less than two months after Kaspar's appearance, the mayor of Nuremberg, Jakob Friedrich Binder (1787-1856), indicated that the boy's strange behaviour "provided no reason to assume that it was occasioned by idiocy or dissimulation, but rather led one to believe that this young man, from childhood, had been deprived of all human society and kept prisoner, isolated in an animal-like state in the most inhuman manner." In Kaspar's case, as in the wild girl's, the child's strangeness was immediately ascribed to a cause, but whereas the wild girl's observers perceived her as an exotic savage (imputing her strangeness to life in the wild and lack of contact with civilized people), Kaspar's observers suspected that his condition was the result of a horrible crime. To a degree this explanation was grounded on observable facts, that is, on Kaspar's physical and behavioural peculiarities, which Binder and others read as signs of an isolated, confined, and deprived childhood: the softness of his hands, the simplicity of his food (he would only take bread and water), the sharpness of his senses, his bodily weakness, slow and swaying gait, sensitivity to daylight, aversion to loud sounds and crowds, and especially "his lack of words, ideas, and concepts about all objects, living ones and metaphysical ones, in remarkable contrast to his obvious attempts to make himself understood and to understand, and the manner in which he speaks, in short broken sentences." Kaspar's reported qualities (innocence and gentleness; devotion to those who were kind to him; obedience and submissiveness; love of order and cleanliness; a desire to learn; fondness for music and drawing) were not those of a savage. Or was he truly the *noble* savage, in whom nobility of nature and nobility of blood were joined? For Binder, Kaspar's refined sensibility and "extraordinary mental gifts, which had not been dulled in spite of a long and terrible incarceration," pointed to a high birth: "His limited understanding, although it was in the most obvious contrast to his enormous intellectual curiosity and an extraordinary memory, suggest[s] an excellent hereditary predisposition." Artificially kept in a childlike state, uncorrupted by society, and the unwitting victim of other people's passions, Kaspar radiated innocence and immanent nobility: "The fact that in his prison he was able to speak with his toys, before he had seen the unknown man and had been instructed by him in language, proves that the crime against him goes back to the first years of his childhood, perhaps between his second and fourth year, and therefore had begun in a time when he was able to speak and was perhaps already the object of a noble education, which, like a star in the dark night of his life, shines forth from his entire being."[27]

Binder's proclamation contained the full story of Kaspar's imprisonment and arrival in Nuremberg. Most of this information could not have been read in Kaspar's body and actions nor (rightly or wrongly) inferred from them, and was set out as if it had been recounted by Kaspar himself. How did Binder obtain so many details if the boy indeed could neither speak nor understand others yet? Did Kaspar, and did Marie-Angélique a century earlier, make themselves understood in other ways, or were the stories imagined by their interlocutors? We know that when Marie-Angélique learned French she corroborated the earlier rumours about her past, at the same time noting that she could not be sure whether she was remembering or repeating what she had heard others say. Likewise, when Kaspar learned (or remembered) German he confirmed the story rehearsed by Binder, but the reliability of his memory could not be objectively ratified. As Georg Philipp Schmidt von Lübeck maintained in his essay "Über Kaspar Hauser" (1831), at first Kaspar was "unable to give any explanations due to a lack of words and concepts," but after he learned to speak it was "just as impossible due to a lack of pure and undistorted recollection."[28] Kaspar's interlocutors, like Marie-Angélique's, played an active role in the reconstruction of his memory. They took him to castles and dungeons where he might have spent his early life, entreated him to describe his dreams and make drawings, and introduced him to people who were supposed to have been part of his former life. Kaspar's story, like the wild girl's, raises questions about the relation between memory, language, and self. Memories of the past would guarantee the subject's present identity (lost prince, exotic savage), but in practice memory cannot be reconstructed except in murky, impure, dialogical ways.

Feuerbach called the crime committed against Kaspar Hauser a crime against the life of the soul or "a partial soul murder." According to Leonard Shengold, soul murder is "primarily a crime committed against children." By the same token Jakob Wassermann saw in Kaspar's story "the tragedy of the child, the general tragedy of the child, or, differently stated, the repeated recurrence of an innocent soul, unspotted by the world, and how the world stupidly and uncomprehendingly ignores such a soul."[29] In the past few decades there has been a sweeping reconceptualization of crimes against children, now increasingly included in the broad category of child abuse. As part of this trend, not only was Kaspar's story rendered in terms of child abuse but through it the other stories of wild children were reconsidered as well. To be sure, in all accounts of wild children the underlying implication is that, if the child was not accidentally lost, some crime was committed against him or her – abandonment, neglect, physical harm, attempted murder. Still, in the many readings and uses of the stories since the seventeenth century the central concerns were the children's wild life, strangeness, and transformation; that they were victims of some sort was taken for granted but seldom placed in the foreground. In contrast, in two recent books child abuse was proffered as the key factor in Kaspar's story, and by extension in the stories of wild children in general.[30]

In John Money's *The Kaspar Hauser Syndrome of "Psychosocial Dwarfism"* (1992), abuse is conceived as physical brutality and neglect. In Jeffrey

Moussaieff Masson's *Lost Prince: The Unsolved Mystery of Kaspar Hauser* (1996), abuse is a catchall term that nonetheless has a deep truth: sexual molestation. Money, a medical psychologist, paediatrician, and sexologist at Johns Hopkins University Hospital, argued that deprivation (neglect and abuse) affects children's physical growth. In the historical figure of Kaspar Hauser, after whom the "Kaspar Hauser syndrome" was named, Money found decisive evidence of how "isolation, abuse, and neglect in childhood might induce a syndrome of overall physical and mental growth retardation, following which catchup growth would be at best only partial and incomplete." What Money was interested in were not the psychological consequences (trauma) but the direct physical effects of abuse and neglect (cessation of growth), and not child *sexual* abuse but severe brutality or protracted deprivation and confinement of the kind experienced by Kaspar and Genie. He intimated that, like Kaspar, other wild children (he mentioned Victor, Kamala and Amala) may have had "an extensive history of violent abuse."[31]

Masson offered *Lost Prince* as a groundbreaking, up-to-the-minute scholarly work on Kaspar Hauser, "Europe's most famous wild child"; however, to all intents and purposes the book exists solely as a platform for the reiteration of Masson's favourite ideas. For him, Kaspar's entire story was an extended illustration of "abuse": "Regardless of who he really was, here is somebody who was abused."[32] Since, as Steven Marcus notes, many people before Masson saw Kaspar as the victim of others' crimes, why did Masson affect to be disclosing an explosive secret along the lines of his famous and controversial *Assault on Truth*? And since Kaspar may have been the victim of many crimes, beginning with his kidnapping as a baby and ending with his murder in 1833, what specifically was Masson referring to when he claimed that Kaspar was abused? For Masson, the *real* (deep, momentous) abuse experienced by Kaspar was not his imprisoned childhood, his isolation and deprivation, or his murder but some concealed (repressed) incident of sexual molestation perpetrated by an unidentified abuser. What made Masson think that Kaspar may have been sexually abused was precisely the absence of any record or memory. Although Kaspar did not remember his imprisonment as an unhappy time, especially in relation to the discomforts and pain he endured later, Masson begged to differ: "To speak of his 'happiness' in his dungeon may have only been a device that enabled Kaspar to speak of how unhappy he was made later. He suffered a different series of deprivations once he was discovered, and different kinds of trauma, and it is always difficult to compare traumas. Moreover, we do not know the full extent of what Kaspar Hauser suffered in his dungeon." The implicit meaning of Masson's words is that *Kaspar* did not know the full extent of his suffering in the dungeon and his contemporaries did not *want* to know (nor do *we*), but *Masson* knows: Kaspar was sexually abused.[33]

All the evidence Masson could adduce to back this supposition is indirect. First, he presents the recent data on the "reality and pervasiveness of childhood sexual abuse" and findings relative to the forgetting of memories of this abuse: the "actual data on the forgetting of real events that were traumatic and sexual in nature ... cannot be ignored if we wish to consider the possibility that Kaspar Hauser did not remember everything that had happened to him while he was in prison." (But why would anyone else wish to consider that possibility?) Second, he points to Freud's "omitted" letters, which demonstrate that sexual abuse of children was rampant in his day: "the climate in German-speaking countries" in Freud's time "was no doubt the same as it had been some sixty years earlier at the time of the case of Kaspar Hauser." Third, he reminds us that nobody *asked* Kaspar if he had been sexually abused, and what better indication that a giant conspiracy of silence was in place? Finally, Masson detected an unmistakable sign in the rumours that the relationship between Kaspar and his would-be protector Lord Stanhope was tinged with homosexual undertones: "Children who have been abused are often targeted later in life by older men who recognize the symptoms and take advantage of the vulnerability that is the legacy of sexual abuse." The contemporary debate on recovered/false memories is, in Masson's view, "directly relevant" to Kaspar's story: "It would be pure speculation to suggest what may have happened to him in his dungeon. We have almost no clues, and Kaspar Hauser himself provided few data. He remembered almost nothing. However, he did recover some memories, and might, over the course of a normal lifetime, have recovered many more. He was never given the opportunity." This was then another way in which Kaspar was "abused": uncaring people, like those who now refuse to believe the recovered memories of abuse victims, never gave him "the opportunity" to remember what had *really* happened to him: "There were many who doubted, on no very solid ground, the story of Kaspar Hauser, and claimed that he fabricated his early life of trauma, just as there are people today who believe *no* account of abuse." Or, perhaps, he did remember what he had been through but chose not to talk about it: "Is it not possible that there are no general rules, and that each person will react differently, some forgetting permanently, some repressing, some remembering permanently, and some simply unwilling to talk about it, with anyone? How can we be certain that Kaspar Hauser did not belong to this latter group, and simply elected not to talk about certain things he knew?"[34] How can we, indeed.

Masson construed the "fascination" with Kaspar's story as "a hidden acknowledgment of the reality of child abuse": Kaspar was "abused by his parents or parent when he was abandoned as a newborn infant; abused by whoever kept him for twelve or fourteen or sixteen years locked in a dungeon; abused by Lord Stanhope for political reasons; abused by an unknown assailant who tried to murder him for reasons that could only have been obscure to Kaspar Hauser; and finally abused by the man who stabbed him to death." His reasoning was two-sided. On the one hand, Masson could confidently assert that Kaspar was abused (both in the broadest sense of abuse, exemplified in the passage just cited, and in his own preferred sense, sexual molestation) because he knows that a great majority of children (if not all) are abused. Thus instead of furnishing positive evidence that Kaspar was abused he challenged *us* (the unbelievers, the abusers) to prove otherwise. On the other hand, Masson conceived Kaspar as a figure with whom all abuse victims can identify: "The abuse to which Kaspar Hauser was subjected, while practically unique, is not really so foreign to our own experiences. Therein, I believe, lies the key to the endless fascination." Ultimately, Masson was not drawn to Kaspar as a real person who once lived and suffered in the world but saw in Kaspar a representation of himself: "The modern reader (could it have been any different for readers in the last century), including myself, desperately wants to reconstruct Kaspar Hauser's actual feelings, memories, and experiences while he was in his dungeon. We want to know if this story is true and, if so, what it says about human nature – that is, what does it mean for us?" Masson's appropriation of Kaspar is a consummate instance of the modern assimilation of "the child" to the adult self: "To think about the suffering of Kaspar Hauser and the mysteriousness of it is to think about our own past suffering in an attempt to undo that mystery, recover our past, and emerge scathed but whole." Masson insists: "Something about his perplexity in the face of the world touches a chord deep in everyone: *Kaspar Hauser, c'est moi!*" I am Kaspar Hauser. In Masson's hands, the confined wild child disappears, collapsed into *myself* as a child. Kaspar Hauser, object of maximum identification, allows Masson to feel really sorry for himself.[35]

Go run the ring, run it thin with trespass:
Until we forgive
What we fetter to free ourselves.
O wild child I see you restless in the thorn
And in the burning sky.

Is this my link?
Have I shortened the leash?
Must I lock your eyes onto the mirror
Of my fear, my fear for them. . . .?
Where is the chain I broke,
Are my arms wrapped by death?

J. Fairfax, "The other child?"[36]

IN THE LAST two chapters we have been travelling along a straight line. Moving in one direction, we found the wolf child – the distant, most inhuman and brutalized form of the wild child. Unintelligible, almost unthinkable, the figure of the wolf child is not one with whom we can easily identify, but for that very reason it exerts a special kind of pull: the fascination of the exotic, the obscure, the primitive, the most *radically other*. Moving in the opposite direction, we found the confined child, who, unlike the wolf child, presents us with no mystery, because her or his confined life is one of maximum control and immobility. The confined child sitting alone in a dungeon or locked room, all day, day after day, is an image that troubles us but that we have no trouble imagining. And, we have been told, the confined child is in essence an abused child like most (or all) of us; it is *us*, indeed; it lives *in* us and discloses our truth, our (past) selves, our inner child. Now let us turn in a different direction, away from the straight line and towards what would be the third vertex of a triangle, to find the third modern incarnation of the wild child. The "free" wild child is for the most part a creature of our imagination and desire: the desire to leave the wild child alone, to celebrate and preserve the wild child *as wild child*. To this day, there is only one "real" story of a free wild child: the gazelle boy of the Sahara Desert. This, then, is the last wild child we shall encounter in this study.

In 1960 Jean-Claude Auger (born in 1934), a poet, painter, solitary traveller, and explorer, found a boy living with a herd of gazelles in the Tiris, then part of the Spanish Sahara. Unlike all the other discoverers of wild children, Auger did not capture the boy but rather observed him in his "natural environment" for almost a month. But even though he did not want the boy to be captured or studied, he communicated his find in a series of letters to Théodore Monod, of the Institut Français d'Afrique Noire at Dakar. His curiosity aroused, Professor Monod asked Auger for more precise details, but the latter refused to provide them. Monod insisted; Auger did not budge, at the same time teasing Monod with the fascinating descriptions he did supply and with hints that he was keeping the best to himself. In Auger's reticence Monod recognized an attempt to resist the scientific appropriation or exploitation of the gazelle boy; on 29 May 1962 Monod wrote: "I understand very well that the appetite for precision of 'observers' such as ourselves irritates you a bit, because you would be perfectly satisfied with 'the poetic aura' of things."[37] It may be that Monod eventually managed to persuade Auger that the gazelle boy's existence should be made public, or that Auger changed his mind on his own (the wave of interest in wild children started by the publication of Malson's *Les enfants sauvages* in 1964 and the release of Truffaut's film in 1970 may have had something to do with the change), for Auger wrote a full account of his encounter with the gazelle boy and published it in 1971 under his other name, Armen. Monod contributed a preface, in which he endorsed Auger-Armen's testimony just as he evinced some dissatisfaction with the text itself: Armen should have separated the raw materials (his observations and notes) from his poetico-mystical comments. As it stood, Armen's book was not, for Monod, a serious scientific document but "a very personal testimony of great psychological interest, even if it teaches us as much about the author's inner life as about the details of his adventure." Monod hoped that qualified researchers would search for the gazelle boy to make more systematic observations "while knowing how to respect his freedom, without one more time attempting the lamentable experiment of the wild children captured by force and condemned to a cruel fate in the name of 'Civilization.'" Monod thus upheld the legitimacy of the scientific desire to study the wild child (and repeated his frustration with Armen's imprecisions) while accepting the notion that wild children must not be captured but observed in their "natural environment."[38]

Armen characterized his unexpected encounter as an "extraordinary experience ... the most moving to have befallen me in the course of five years of travelling round the earth." His first sighting of the boy was a "vision" of an "unknown, fabulous creature in a world apart." The thought of capturing him did not cross Armen's mind. He was overwhelmed by the wild boy's presence, resolved to extricate the spiritual meaning of his existence. To this purpose, "the inward attitude of approach to the event" is "of unforeseeable importance." Armen's account contains elements common to most accounts of wild children. First, there is a description of the unnamed boy (if Armen gave him a name, he did not make it public): "The child, now clearly visible, shows his lively, dark, almond-shaped eyes and a pleasant, open expression (not sullen like wolf-children and other children reared by carnivorous animals); he appears to be about ten years old; his ankles are disproportionately thick and obviously powerful, his muscles firm and shivering; a scar, where a piece of flesh must have been torn from the arm, and some deep gashes mingled with light scratches (thorn-bushes or marks of old struggles?) form a strange tattoo – not always a life of paradise!" Second, there are observations on the boy's life and behaviour. Armen considered both the traits that he seemingly adopted from the gazelles and those that set him apart (as human): "Living in closer proximity to the child, even during the deepest hours of the night, I have another surprise: I see him suddenly upright, his neck stretched and chin jutting forward, strangely immobile – he is staring with large, ecstatic eyes at the full moon." Third, there are conjectures about the boy's origin: he may have been lost, perhaps fallen from the basket at the side of the camel where nomad babies are usually placed, when he was seven or eight months old (Armen explained that nomad children, more precocious than middle-class European children, can already stand at this age). He may then have been found by a herd of gazelles in which one of the females had just lost her fawn. Fourth, there is a view of the boy's general condition: Armen did not think that he was deliberately abandoned (as "abnormal"): "His 'response' to his 'milieu' is adequate, a sign of normality in relation to his particular environment (normality in itself does not exist)."[39]

But in crucial ways Armen's response to the boy was unique. He did not cover up the "animal" aspects of the boy's life and behaviour, yet for Armen this "animality" was neither disgusting nor disturbing. In part, he claimed, this was because of the range of his experiences as an explorer of remote lands and non-Western cultures. He was enthralled by what he perceived as the gazelle boy's perfect harmony with the herd, with nature, with the universal order of things. During the weeks he spent with the herd, Armen tried diverse methods to make contact with the boy: first, by means of the gaze ("He catches sight of me, his eyes staring in amazement, perhaps even terror, though I too am hidden behind an isolated cluster of thorn-bushes"); then, by playing a few notes on a simple flute, which after a few days catch the boy's attention ("The child watches from a distance, as if transfixed");

and finally by imitating the gazelle's (and the gazelle boy's) behaviour – their sniffing and licking, which, Armen guessed, was "some kind of code signifying acknowledgment, contact, and almost recognition." Through this last method (in other words, through his own adoption of gazelle behaviour) Armen reached "the transparency and plenitude of a new state, of a rare 'communication'" in "a painful moment of extreme intensity ... an instant of deadlock violence" of the kind that "confers meaning and value on an existence." Armen explored new forms of communication "between myself and the child, between the child and the herd, and between the animals and myself – perhaps exchanges of a kind unforeseen and inconceivable in the present state of the human mind, especially the European mind which, in this technical age, is becoming increasingly alienated from the primary reflexes of communication and primitive 'participation' (in the sense in which the shamans understand the term)." Because in the last few days of his stay with the gazelles Armen detected a code in their sounds and gestures (movements of the head and hoofs), he inferred that the boy's case was one of cultural substitution: "a gazelle 'culture' has almost entirely replaced a human 'culture,' by an imitative process of education." His provisions long gone, and having become "a shadow of myself, surviving only by my passion for the child and his gazelles," Armen reluctantly left "this life which I have been living at the boundaries of unreality." Upon his return to Europe he decided to conceal the boy's precise whereabouts, "for what was at stake was the safety of a creature still too fragile to defend himself against the enterprises of men, well-intentioned or otherwise." Despite Armen's precautions, American officers of the NATO base of Villa Cisneros, in the Rio de Oro, attempted to capture the gazelle boy in 1966 and again in 1970. If they had succeeded, Armen said, "every American in deepest Texas would have seen the child on his little screen, stuffed with tranquilisers and, on his arm, a Hollywood-style native girl darkened with sun-tan, between advertisements for hot dogs and biological washing-powders."[40]

The figure of the free wild child represents a new attitude to the wild child in general. No longer miserable, brutish, and essentially inhuman (deprived of the essential characteristics of human being), the free wild child lives in equilibrium with the environment. The desire to leave the wild child alone marks a change in the evaluation of the wild child's wild life, and this change may be seen as the obverse of the Western civilized adult's dissatisfaction with civilization and yearning for a different kind of life – a fuller, more meaningful existence. The free wild child thus offers a new channel for the expression of the anticivilization sentiments that have been a strong undercurrent in the West since at least the Industrial Revolution. Armen, writing when the 1960s counterculture was still on the rise, remarked that it would be "senseless" to want to transform the gazelle boy into "a candidate for our producer-consumer civilisation, dressing him in a lounge-suit and tie or in dungarees (or condemning him to stagnation in some home for deaf-mutes or idiot children)," precisely at the time "when an increasingly large proportion of the younger generation is rejecting the 'values' of our Western civilisation."[41] The figure of the free wild child is inextricable from the notion that, as Freud warned us, civilization involves constraint, and this constraint is the source of our discontent. The realization that the "uncivilized" may be left to exist as such *without danger to the civilized subject* is tied, on the one hand, to the political and philosophical critiques of imperialism and colonialism (as the project to impose civilization on the other for our own benefit), and on the other hand, to the simple fact that we are no longer *striving* to achieve civilization (and differentiate ourselves from the other on the basis of our advanced civilization) but are for better or worse completely *in it* – whether we want it or not, trapped perhaps.[42] From this position, it becomes easier to identify with the wild child as the embodiment of the self's desire.

Armen argued that knowledge of, and through, the wild child can only be obtained by living with the wild child in his (or her) own environment. Furthermore, he announced that the kind of knowledge held by (or in) the wild child is not of the kind that interests scientists but is instead a spiritual revelation. The free wild child is the civilized adult's guide – away from, or beyond, civilization: "In my innermost self, the wild child whom I discovered by chance has unexpectedly become, as it were, the point of convergence of my long and obscure 'quest' for fulfilment across five continents."[43] Armen not only wanted to relate to the gazelle boy in the latter's own terms but endeavoured to become *like* the wild child. In this reworked form, the encounter with the wild child is a transformative experience *for the subject*. I said before that the gazelle boy of the Sahara Desert is the only free wild child to date, but the last few years have seen a proliferation of free wild children in literature and film. Think for instance of the silent wild boy in David Malouf's novel *An Imaginary Life*, who encounters Ovid in exile, becomes the poet's guide, and eventually allows him to experience his own metamorphosis; or the wild woman played by Jodie Foster in Michael Apted's *Nell*, who pleads in court to remain free and untransformed – and wins. In John Fairfax's poem cycle *Wild Children*, the wild child is the speaker. Captured, the wild child reclaims his (or her) identification with animals:

I found them.

They are mine, I am theirs.

Tamed, trained, civilized, the wild child yearns for freedom:

They come to me with keys

In their voice, with chains

For hands, with thorn in their eyes.

They sound me a name ...

O I cannot recall my forest.[44]

To a great extent the figure of the free wild child emerged in reaction to the appropriation of wild children by the scientific establishment and *for* scientific knowledge – the conviction that scientists should study the wild child, transform the wild child, reveal the wild child's secrets, and in so doing advance our knowledge of the normal child (and our strategies to normalize children). But the free wild child has more troubling connotations as well. Armen claimed that one of the reasons for his opposition to the gazelle boy's capture was the "established fact" that children who have spent several years in the wild are not "readaptable."[45] The desire to leave the wild child alone carries an (implicit or explicit) admission of our own limitations: our attempts to "rescue" the wild child have failed. The fate of most wild children – early deaths, lack of recovery, visible unhappiness – shakes our belief in our individual and collective capacity to respond to the child's needs and in the power of our knowledge to restore and console a lost, abandoned, or suffering child. When I first encountered the stories of wild children, I also believed that the best response to the wild child might be to leave her or him alone, and I questioned the adult's right not only to capture but also to transform, humanize, civilize, educate. But now I am not so sure. The danger is that the recognition that we do not know how to intervene without doing harm may lead us to stop trying and may in this way reinforce the global tendency away from social and ethical obligations towards the vulnerable other (and children in general).[46] Rather than an overdue recognition of the (wild) child's otherness, the desire to leave the (wild) child alone may be a silent confession of the adult's inability or unwillingness to commit fully to the *other child* who demands from the adult not normalizing but meaningful and ethical interventions.

The
Other Child

Silence is possible only in the human world (and only for a person).

Mikhail Bakhtin[1]

IN *Centuries of Childhood*, his groundbreaking study of childhood in history, Philippe Ariès put forward the provocative claim that the idea of childhood did not exist in the Middle Ages and the Renaissance and was "discovered" in Western societies during the sixteenth and seventeenth centuries. Ariès's argument inspired a heated and protracted controversy among historians of childhood. As an antidote to more extreme responses (uncritical acceptance or wholesale rejection), some historians have proposed a moderate interpretation of Ariès's claim: what pre-modern societies lacked was not *the* idea of childhood but *our* idea of childhood, for childhood is always historically and culturally specific. Even though in many respects this position appears convincing, Ariès's original formulation retains a mysterious force and defies attempts to dismiss or rewrite it. Ariès did not say that childhood changed but rather that it was discovered – like the native Americans and the wild children. He observed that modernity brought about the discovery of the *idea* of childhood, corresponding to "an awareness of the particular nature of childhood ... which distinguishes the child from the adult."[2] The concept of discovery is a peculiar one. It positions an object in relation to a subject in such a way that a change in the status of the object is effected merely through a change in its position relative to the subject. We say that something is discovered when it appears or is revealed to *our* eyes, when we come across it or become aware of it; or we say that something is discovered when it becomes part of what we know, of the sum of our accumulated knowledge. Thus for Susan Curtiss, Genie was discovered when she was admitted into Childrens Hospital ("She had been discovered, at last").[3] To elucidate Ariès's claim we may think of a change affecting not the object discovered (the child) but the subject (the adult). In other words, the "discovery of childhood" may indicate a change in our (adults') perception of the child in relation to us.

A transformation of this sort was detected by psychohistorian Lloyd deMause, whose characterization of the history of childhood as "a nightmare from which we have only recently begun to awaken" has proved as controversial, and to a degree as foundational, to the field of history of childhood as Ariès's argument. According to deMause, an adult (by which he means a parent) who is "face to face with a child who needs something" may have one of three reactions: projective (the child becomes an instrument for the projection of the parent's unconscious), reactive (the child is used as a substitute for the parent's own parental figures), or empathic (the parent responds to the child's own needs). In the course of history, relations between parents and children "evolved" in the direction of increasing empathy, passing through six "parental modes": infanticidal, abandonment, ambivalent, intrusive, socialization, and helping. In deMause's version of the history of adult-child (or parent-child) relations, the most crucial occurrence is thus the gradual increase in the adult's capacity to empathize with the child, to "regress to the level of a child's need and correctly identify it without an admixture of the adult's own projections." The "discovery" of childhood would then refer to the adult's recognition of an essential similarity or affinity between the adult and the child facing her or him.[4]

Like deMause, sociologist Norbert Elias was interested in the broad historical transformation in feelings and behaviours that led adults to "discover" childhood, but he construed this transformation as an increase in distance. Elias argued that the contemporary standard of "civilized" behaviour, encompassing the individual's relation to food, elimination, sex, and other bodily functions, is the outcome of a "civilizing process" that took place in Western societies since the Middle Ages. As social differentiation became more pronounced, people were compelled to attune their behaviour to one another, to be more conscious of their own and others' conduct and bodily functions. The civilizing process follows a pattern, beginning with lack of restraint (a certain form of behaviour is acceptable or goes unnoticed), passing through external restraint (a new standard is imposed through advice and education and enforced by the group through fear of social disapproval), and ending in self-restraint (the standard is internalized, the civilized behaviour becomes automatic, and the existence of the restraint itself goes unnoticed). As the bodily restraints increased, the thresholds of shame and disgust were lowered. Elias's account of the changing standard of behaviour in the civilizing process sheds light on the intense reactions of observers to the utter strangeness of wild children and the minute attention they paid to their habits and ways of making physical contact with others. As Western adults were themselves experiencing (and enduring) a civilizing process, they were both fascinated and revolted by these telling cases of uncivilization. In the wild child, adult observers could ascertain, at the same time (but in different ways and to different degrees depending on the time period and their particular social position), the measure of their own civilization and the fragility and artificiality of their behavioural restraints. And once civilization became thoroughly ingrained – the civilized standard of behaviour is now "imprinted on the individual from early childhood as a kind of second nature and kept alert in him by a powerful and increasingly strictly organized social control"[5] – the wild child's meaning shifted. No longer a threat to the adult's still-to-be-achieved civilization, the wild child came to embody a lost instinctual "freedom."

Elias maintained that the civilizing process altered the relation between adults and children. As he put it, "the distance in behavior and whole psychical structure between children and adults increases in the course of the civilizing process." Since "even in civilized society no human being comes into the world civilized," each child must be compulsorily and automatically subjected to an individual civilizing process through which he or she is made to "catch up," "to a greater or lesser degree and with greater or lesser success," with the standard reached by the society over many centuries.[6] For Elias, the "discovery" of the child was a by-product of the historical production of civilized adults (that is, of a standard of civilized adulthood). The civilizing process gave a new content to the universal difference between adult and child. Under normal circumstances, the child's uncivilized state does not last long; when the circumstances are "abnormal" and the child's uncivilized state is prolonged beyond what society deems acceptable, a wild child may be born.[7] Many years before Ariès, Elias suggested that discovery and civilization are inseparable from childhood in modernity, both literally and metaphorically. The child is associated with the "savage" as the other of civilization – its starting point and beyond. The wild child, that fascinating, elusive figure in which "child" and "savage" meet in a single body, highlights the transformation (in the adult subject) and the increasing distance (between civilized adult and yet-to-be-civilized child).

The adults who encountered the wild children were faced with a moral challenge: what to do with them? How to respond? This challenge may indeed be generalized to any relation between an adult and a child. How can the adult reconcile the conflicting demands, on the one hand, to approach the child as *another subject* whose integrity, separateness, and freedom ought to be maintained, and on the other, to *care for* the child, intervene, interfere, educate, mould, change? In "The Crisis in Education," Hannah Arendt affirmed that the existence of children in the world imposes an obligation on all adults. According to Arendt, adults' responsibility towards children – who are "newcomers by birth" and people "in process of becoming" – is double: they must not only provide what is necessary for children's well-being and growth but also introduce children into an old world that existed before their birth. The adult encounters the child as a representative of the world into which the child is born a stranger. Only by fully assuming this responsibility can the adult create the conditions for the child's "becoming," for the manifestation of "the uniqueness that distinguishes every human being from every other, the quality by virtue of which [the child] is not only a stranger in the world but something that has never been here before."[8] Yet by increasingly segregating children from adults and restricting the acceptable forms of adult-child relation, modern societies have gone a long way towards "freeing" most adults from the responsibility of having to face, respond to, and care for most children. Despite the perceived sense of progress in societal attitudes towards children, and the intensification of the responsibility for children of specially designated individuals (parents, child experts, and professionals) notwithstanding, we have eradicated most of the social and discursive spaces where relations between any adult and any child can occur. The extent of our failure to engage with children should give us pause.[9]

Confronted with the task of having to identify and respond to children's (often silent) demand, modern adults turn to expert knowledge. In so doing, we turn a moral question into a scientific problem. But does scientific knowledge help us solve beforehand the challenge of our encounter with the child? If, as I have argued, knowledge is implicated in all relations between people, what we must rethink, I suggest, is the relation between knowing the other and meeting the other. Knowledge may either precede or result from my encounter with the other. The knowledge produced by the human sciences fosters the illusion that we know the other before actually meeting him or her. We have seen, in some of the stories of wild children, how knowledge arrived at in a concrete relationship was transposed to a whole category of people. One instance of detailed and careful (and caring) observation of a child was transmuted into an excuse not to observe (attend or listen to) other children. Equipped with scientific, ready-made knowledge we approach the other as if we knew her or him already. And while we think the knowledge we bring to our encounter with the other/child eases our access to him or her, indeed it clouds our perception. Thinking I already know "the child" I foreclose the possibility of ever knowing and learning from *this* child. Knowledge about an abstract or generic other takes the place of a specific understanding of the other I meet. But it is an illusion: the continuing existence in the world of new, weak, dependent, demanding, and sometimes radically different people with whom we must nevertheless engage makes the challenge interminable.

Lists of Wild Children

SCHREBER'S LIST (*DIE SÄUGTHIERE*, 1:31–6)

1. a boy found in Hesse in 1544, who had been raised by wolves [Camerarius]
2. a twelve-year-old boy found in Wetterau in 1544, who lived among wolves [Camerarius]
3. a boy aged about nine who lived among bears, found in 1661 in Lithuania [Connor]
4. another child aged about ten found living with bears in Lithuania near the Russian border in 1694 [Valmont de Bomare, Connor]
5. a boy found in the wilderness in Ireland during the last century [Tulp]
6. a nineteen-year-old girl captured in August 1717 in a forest in Kranenburg near Zwolle [*Breslauer Sammlungen*]
7. two boys captured in 1719 in the Pyrenees [Linnaeus]
8. a boy aged about thirteen found near Hameln in 1724 [*Breslauer Sammlungen*, vol. 35]
9. a girl, nine or ten years old, captured in 1731 in Songi, near Châlons in Champagne [La Condamine]
10. Johann von Lüttich, lost when he was five and found sixteen years later [Boerhaave, Linnaeus]

BONNATERRE'S LIST (*NOTICE HISTORIQUE*, 182–93)

1. *Juvenis Lupinus Hessensis* (1544) [Camerarius, Rousseau] and another boy found the same year in Wétéravie [Camerarius]
2. *Juvenis Ursinus Lithuanus* (1661) [Valmont de Bomare] and another boy found among bears in Lithuania in 1694 [Connor, Rousseau, Condillac]
3. *Juvenis Ovinus Hibernus* [Tulp, Schreber]
4. *Juvenis Bovinus Bambergensis* [Camerarius]
5. *Puella Transisalana* (1717) [*Breslauer Sammlungen*]

6. *Pueri Duo Pyrenaïci* (1719) [Rousseau, Schreber]

7. *Juvenis Hannoveranus* [*Breslauer Sammlungen*]

8. *Puella Campanica* (1731) [L. Racine]

9. *Joannes Leodicensis* [Boerhaave, Linnaeus, Schreber]

10. *Puella Karpfensis* [*Dictionnaire des Merveilles de la nature*, vol. 2, art. "Sauvage"]

11. *Juvenis Averionensis*

TYLOR'S LIST ("WILD MEN AND BEAST-CHILDREN")

the two boys of Overdyke

Procopius's Ægisthus

two wild men seen by missionaries in Tahiti

Peter the Wild Boy

Sleeman's boys

the boy of Hesse [Dilich]

the boys of Lithuania [Connor, Koenig]

a wolf-child caught in the forest of Ardennes [Koenig]

a wild man caught in the forest of Compiegne [Koenig]

Tulp's Irish boy

the girl "caught living wild in Holland (of all places in the world), in 1717" (28)

the two boys seen in the Pyrenees

"Lord Monboddo's friend, the wild girl" (29) caught at Châlons-sur-Marne in 1731

the wild boy of Bamberg

RAUBER'S LIST (*HOMO SAPIENS FERUS*, 15–63)

1 and 2. The boys of Hesse (*Juvenes lupini Hessenses*)

3. The boy of Bamberg (*Juvenis bovinus Bambergensis*)

4. The Lütticher Hans (*Johannes Leodicensis Boerhavii*)

5. The Irish youth (*Juvenis ovinus Hibernus*)

6, 7, and 8. The Lithuanian boys (*Juvenes ursini Lithuani*)

9. The girl of Cranenburg (*Puella trans-isalana*)

10 and 11. The boys of the Pyrenees

12. Wild Peter of Hameln (*Juvenis Hannoveranus Linn.*)

13. The girl of Songi in Champagne (*Puella campanica*)

14. The Hungarian bear-girl

15. The savage of Kronstadt

16. The boy of Aveyron

SMALL'S LIST (A SUBSET OF HIS MUCH LONGER LIST OF EXAMPLES OF SOLITUDE AND ISOLATION, "ON SOME PSYCHICAL RELATIONS," 44–8)

...F. Caspar Hauser

G. Feral Men

    a. The Hessian Boy [Dilich, Rousseau]

    b. The Irish Boy [Tulp, Rauber]

    c. The Lithuanian Boys [3 cases, Connor]

    d. The Girl of Cranenburg [Rauber]

    e. Clemens of Overdyke [*Anthropological Review*, 1863]

    f. Jean de Liege [Rauber]

    g. The Savage of Aveyron [*All the Year*]

    h. The Wolf Children of India [2 cases described in *Chambers' Journal*]

    i. Peter of Hanover [*Penny Magazine*]

    j. The Savage of Kronstadt [Wagner, Rauber]

    k. The Girl of Songi [Rauber, *Histoire*, etc.]

"To the cases cited, there might be added: that of the Hungarian Bear Girl, the Boys of the Pyrenees, the Wild Boy of Mt. Pindus, and others less minutely described" (48).

HUTTON'S LIST ("WOLF-CHILDREN")

ancient legends (Atalanta, Romulus and Remus, Cyrus)

Procopius's child

the boy of Hesse

the bear-nurtured boys of Poland and Lithuania

the boy of Bamberg

the bear-child of Savoy

about a dozen Indian cases (including Sleeman's, the children at the Sikandra
    Orphanage, the wolf girls of Midnapur, the Maiwani boy)

the bear-girl of Jalpaiguri

the girl found with jackals

a tiger-child found in India

Stuart Baker's leopard-child

a monkey girl mentioned by Sir R.G. Burton

the South African boy

two children associated with lions in Africa

ZINGG'S FIRST LIST ("FERAL MAN," 1940)

[Linnaeus's cases:]

   1) First Lithuanian Bear-boy of 1661? (1657)

   2) Hessian Wolf-boy, 1344

   3) Irish Sheep-boy reported by Tulp, 1672

   3a) Bamberger Cattle-boy, end of the 16th century (a poor case)

   4) Wild Peter of Hannover, 1724

   5) The Pyrenees boys, 1719 (a most dubious case)

   6) Girl of Cranenburg, 1717 (*Puella trans-isalana*, Linn.)

   7) The Songi girl from Champagne, 1731 (*Puella campanica*, Linn.)

   8) Jean of Liège

[added by Schreber:]

   9) Second Wolf-boy from Germany, that of Wetterau, 1344

   10) Second Lithuanian Bear-boy, 1694

   11) Third Lithuanian Bear-boy

[Sleeman's cases:]

   12 to 17) Sleeman's Wolf-children

[other wolf children from India:]

   18) Wolf-child case reported from Sultanpur

   19) Wolf-boy of Shahjehanjur

   20) Dina Sanichar, the Wolf-child of 1867 at the Sikandra Orphanage

   21) Second Sikandra Wolf-child of 1872

[added by Tylor:]

   22) Second Overdyke wild-boy

   23) Clemens of Overdyke

[miscellaneous:]

   24) Swine-girl of Salzburg

   25) Wild-boy of Kronstadt

   26) Wild-boy of Aveyron

   27) Half-wild boy of Zips, Hungary

   28) Kaspar Hauser

   29) Amala, younger Midnapore girl

   30) Kamala, elder Midnapore girl

   31) Leopard-boy of India

ZINGG'S SECOND LIST ("FERAL MAN," 1942)

1) Wolf-children in India:

Cases I–VI. from *A Journey through the Kingdom of Oude*

Sleeman's seventh case, the "most doubtful" (in a footnote)

VII: Wild-child reported from Sultanpur

VIII: Wolf-boy of Shahjehanpur

IX: Dina Sanichar, the Wolf-child of the Sikandra (Secundra) Orphanage

X: Second Sikandra wolf-child of 1872

XI: Leopard-boy of India

XII: Jhansi Wolf-child

Maiwana boy

2) Early General Discussions of the Classic Cases of Feral Man:

XIII: Wild Peter

XIV: Clemens of Overdyke

XV: Swine-girl of Salzburg

XVI: Second Case from Overdyke

XVII: Case from ancient Rome

Two wild men seen by missionaries in Tahiti

3) Other Classic Cases of Feral Man, which showed no substantial recovery from early isolation:

XVIII and XIX: The two Hessian Wolf-boys

The Bamberger boy, *Juvenis bovinus Bambergensis* (Linn.)

XX: The Lütticher Hans (Jean of Liège) *Johannes Leodicensis Boerhavii*

XXI: The Irish Youth (*Juvenis ovinus Hibernus*)

XXII–XXIV: The Lithuanian boys (*Juvenes ursini Lithuani*)

XXV: The Bear-girl of Hungary

XXVI: Bear-girl from India

The Bear-boy of Denmark

XXVII: Recent reports of a girl rescued from a bear on Mt Olympus

XXVIII: Another possible Wild-boy from Greece

XXIX: The Wild-boys of the Pyrenees

Alleged Wild-man from Trebizond

4) Cases of Feral Man without Animal Nurture, and Similar Cases of Isolation of Children by Cruel or Insane Guardians:

XX: The Girl of Cranenburg (*Puella transisalana Linn.*)

XXXI: The Wild-boy of Kronstadt

XXXII: The Wild-boy of Aveyron

Anna of Pennsylvania and Isabelle of Ohio

5) Cases of Feral Man which Recovered from the Effects of Severe and Long-continued Isolation:

XXIII: The Girl of Songi in Champagne (*Puella Campanica* Linn.)
XXXIV: "Tarzancito" of El Salvador
XXXV: Tomko of Zips
Kaspar Hauser

MANDELBAUM'S LIST ("WOLF-CHILD HISTORIES FROM INDIA")

1: 1841 or 1842, Sleeman's first boy
2: 1843, Sleeman's second boy
3: 1843, Sleeman's third boy
4: about 1843, Sleeman's fourth boy
5: 1847, Sleeman's fifth boy
6: 1849, Sleeman's sixth boy
7: date of capture unknown, Sleeman's old man
8: youth seen by Mr Grieg in 1858 in Shahjahanpur
9: wolf boy seen by H.D. Willock in 1858
10: 1860–61, boy brought by police to H.G. Ross in Sultanpur
11: 1867, boy sent to the Secundra orphanage, came to be called Sanichar
12: 1872, second Secundra boy
13: 1887, girl found with bear near Jalpaiguri
14: 1893, boy found in jungle near Bazitpore, Bihar
15: 1895, two boys captured in Etawah and brought to Mr A.J. Broun
16: 1910 (?): Stuart Baker's leopard boy
17: 1916, Mr C.H. Burnett's wolf-boy
18: about 1923: girl rescued from jackals
19: 1927, boy found with wolves at Miawana
20: 1933, child found with wolves at Jhansi

MALSON'S LIST (*LES ENFANTS SAUVAGES*, 72–5)

1. The wolf-child [boy] of Hesse
2. The wolf-child of Wetteravie
3. The 1st bear-child of Lithuania
4. The sheep-child of Ireland
5. The calf-child of Bamberg
6. The 2nd bear-child of Lithuania
7. The 3rd bear-child of Lithuania
8. The girl of Kranenburg (Holland)

9–10. The two boys of the Pyrenees

11. Wild Peter of Hanover

12. The girl of Sogny, in Champagne

13. Jean of Liège

14. Tomko of Zips (Hungary)

15. The bear-girl of Karpfen (Hungary)

16. Victor the wild child of Aveyron

17. Gaspard Hauser of Nuremberg

18. The sow-girl of Salzburg

19. The child of Husanpur

20. The 1st child of Sultanpur

21. The 2nd child of Sultanpur

22. The child of Chupra

23. The 1st child of Lucknow

24. The child of Bankipur

25. Captain Egerton's child

26. Clemens, the pig-child of Overdyke

27. The wolf-child of Overdyke

28. Dina Sanichar, of Sekandra

29. The 2nd child of Sekandra

30. The child of Shajahampur

31. The 2nd child of Lucknow

32. The girl of Jalpaiguri

33. The child of Batzipur

34. The wolf-child of Kronstadt

35. The snow-hen of Justedal

36. The child of Sultanpur

37. Lucas, the baboon-child of South Africa

38. The Indian panther-child

39. Amala of Midnapore

40. Kamala of Midnapore

41. The 1st leopard-child

42. The child of Maiwana

43. The child of Jhansi

44. An Indian wolf-child

45. The child of Casamance

46. Assicia of Liberia

47. The 2nd leopard-child

48. Anna of Pennsylvania
49. Edith of Ohio
50. The gazelle-child of Syria
51. Ramu, the child of New Delhi
52. The gazelle-child of Mauritania
53. The ape-child of Teheran

WARD'S LIST ("FERALCHILDREN.COM," 22 SEPTEMBER 2003)
Traian Caldarar (Romania, 2002)
Sudam Pradhana (India, 2001)
Axel Rivas (Chile, 2001)
Edik (Ukraine, 1999)
Ivan Mishukov (Moscow, 1998)
Bello (Nigeria, 1996)
Oxana Malaya (Ukraine, 1991)
John Ssebunya (Uganda, 1991)
Andes boy (Peruvian Andes, 1990)
Jhansi leopard-girl (India, 1986)
Kunu Masela (Kenya, 1983)
Robert (Uganda, 1982)
Isabel Quaresma (Portugal, 1980)
Tissa (Sri Lanka, 1973)
Ramchandra (Uttar Pradesh, 1973)
Shamdeo (Sultanpur, 1972)
Rocco (Italy, 1971)
Genie (USA, 1970)
Marcos Pantoja (Spain, 1965)
Yves Cheneau (Saint-Brévin, 1963)
Djuma (Turkmenistan, 1962)
Saharan gazelle-boy (Mauritania, 1960)
Kevin Halfpenny (Ireland, 1956)
Ramu (India, 1954)
CauCau (Chile, 1947)
Syrian gazelle-boy (Syria, 1946)
Sidi Mohamed (N Africa, 1945)
Misha Defonseca (Europe, 1945)
Isabelle (USA, 1938)
Anna (USA, 1938)

Turkish bear-girl (Turkey, 1937)

Assicia (Liberia, 1930s)

Casamance boy (Guinea, 1930s)

Istoki (Hungary, 1930s)

Child of Užice (Serbia, 1934)

Tarzancito (El Salvador, 1933)

Jhansi wolf boy (India, 1933)

Maiwana wolf boy (India, 1927)

Jackal girl (India, 1923)

Indian panther-child (India, 1920)

Amala (India, 1920)

Kamala (India, 1920)

Satna wolf boy (India, 1916)

Leopard boy of Dihungi (India, 1915)

Goongi (Uttar Pradesh, 1914)

Lucas (South Africa, 1904)

Mauritanian gazelle boy (French Mauritania, c1900)

Batsipur wolf boy (India, 1893)

Jalpaiguri bear-girl (India, 1892)

Skiron (Greece, 1891)

Second Sekandra wolf boy (India, 1872)

Dina Sanichar (India, 1867)

Wild boy of Overdyke (Holland, ?)

Clemens (Holland, c1863)

Third Sultanpur wolf boy (India, 1860)

Shajehanpur wolf boy (India, 1858)

Chupra wolf boy (India, 1849)

Second Sultanpur wolf boy (India, 1848)

The Lobo Girl of Devil's River (USA, 1845)

First Lucknow wolf boy (India, 1844)

First Sultanpur wolf boy (India, 1843)

Bankipur wolf boy (India, 1843)

Hasunpur wolf boy (India, 1841)

Sow-girl (Salzburg, ?)

Kaspar Hauser (Nuremberg, 1828)

Isabella (Brazil, c1817)

Victor (France, 1799)

Wolf-boy of Kronstadt (Kronstadt, c1780)

Bear girl of Fraumark (Hungary, 1767)

M A Memmie LeBlanc (France, 1731)

Wild Peter (Germany, 1724)

Girl of Isseaux (Pyrenees, 1719)

Kranenburg girl (Holland, 1717)

Second Lithuanian bear boy (Lithuania, 1694)

Bamberg boy (Bavaria, c1680)

Irish sheep-boy (Ireland, 1672)

Joseph (Lithuania, 1660s)

Jean de Liège (Liège, 1630s)

Danish bear boy (Denmark, c1600)

Ardenne wolf boy (France, c1500)

Jostedalsrypa (Norway, 1350)

Wolf-boy of Wetterau (Wetterau, 1344)

Wolf-boy of Hesse (Hesse, 1341)

Aegisthus (Italy, 250)

Acknowledgments

Many people made the writing of this book possible. I am forever indebted to Deborah Britzman's gracious supervision and unfailing support. This work indeed grew out of, and benefited from, many conversations with her and with Paul Antze over several years, and I thank them both. Ian Hacking deserves very special thanks because, his work having had such a profound influence on my own, he honoured me greatly by being one of its first readers. I also wish to thank: Carole Carpenter, Lorraine Code, Natalie Zemon Davis, Julia V. Douthwaite, Barbara Godard, David McNally, Barbara Herrnstein Smith, Mike Sokal, Dror Wahrman, and John Willinsky; the participants in the conferences and seminars at which I presented parts of this work; and the staff of the libraries where I spent countless hours over the years it took me to write the dissertation and turn it into the book, including the libraries at York University, the University of Toronto, New York University, Columbia University, the University of British Columbia, Mount Saint Vincent University, and the University of Michigan; the Bibliothèque du Saulchoir, former site of the Centre Michel Foucault; the New York Public Library; Thomas Fisher Rare Book Library at the University of Toronto; the Osler Library of the History of Medicine at McGill University; and the Bibliotheca Albertina of the Universität Leipzig. The digital collections of the Bibliothèque Nationale de France (Gallica), the Bibliothèque Interuniversitaire de Médecine, and the Disability History Museum proved immensely useful. I am grateful to Glen A. Gildemeister of Northern Illinois University Libraries; the William Ready Division of Archives and Research Collections, McMaster University; the History of Medicine Division of the National Library of Medicine; the National Portrait Gallery; the Northeastern Association of Graduate Schools, and for help with translations from

Latin, Wayne Ingalls and Damián Fernández, and from German, Andre Porsch. I owe many thanks as well to everyone at McGill-Queen's University Press, and especially to John Zucchi, Joanne Pisano, Joan McGilvray, and Claire Gigantes. Financial support was generously provided by the Social Sciences and Humanities Research Council of Canada, the Killam Trusts, York University, and Mount Saint Vincent University. Special thanks to Victoria Heftler, Pamela Leach, Dennis Soron, Jeremy Stolow, and Betina Zolkower for lending an attentive ear, asking intriguing questions, pointing me to key sources, and most important, for enriching my life and my work with their friendship. My colleagues and friends at Mount Saint Vincent University have supported me in more ways than I can count, and so has Mark Phillips, who believed that this book should see the light of day and persisted until I did too. Lastly, I thank Stephen Barber, dearest friend and inspiration; my family, who have been with me across the distance; and Roni Gechtman (he knows why).

I dedicate this work to you, Roni.

Notes

INTRODUCTION

1 The first account is from Pistorius, *Illustrivm vetervm scriptorvm*, 1:264; translation modified from Zingg, "Feral Man" (1942), 205. The account of Djuma is in Sieveking, "Forteana."

2 See for instance Malson, *Wolf Children and the Problem of Human Nature*, originally published as *Les enfants sauvages*; Lane, *The Wild Boy of Aveyron*; Gineste, *Victor de l'Aveyron*; Candland, *Feral Children and Clever Animals*; and Masson, ed. and trans., *Lost Prince*. For examples of recent works that focus on individual cases or summarize several stories for a general readership, see Maclean, *The Wolf Children*; Shattuck, *The Forbidden Experiment*; Rymer, *Genie*; and Newton, *Savage Girls and Wild Boys*.

3 Ginzburg, "Checking the Evidence," 294. See also Ginzburg, *Clues, Myths, and the Historical Method*.

4 Ginzburg and Poni, "The Name and the Game," 4–5. On Italian microhistory, see Ginzburg, "Microhistory." In this article Ginzburg states once again that the theoretical sophistication of the microhistorical approach – "the definite awareness that all phases through which research unfolds are *constructed* and not *given*: the identification of the object and its importance; the elaboration of the categories through which it is analyzed; the criteria of proof; the stylistic and narrative forms by which the results are transmitted to the reader" – is not to be confused with postmodernist cognitive scepticism (32).

5 Foucault, *The Archaeology of Knowledge*, 117.

6 Foucault, ed., *I, Pierre Rivière*. In this work we see Foucault's interest beginning to shift from the analysis of discourses (archaeology) to the analysis of power (genealogy). See Forrester, "If *p*, Then What?" for a discussion of "reasoning in cases," which, Forrester suggests, may be added to the six styles of reasoning presented in Hacking, "Styles of Scientific Thinking or Reasoning." On Menocchio, see Ginzburg, *The Cheese and the Worms*. In "The Name and

the Game," 8, Ginzburg and Poni write: "If the sources are silent about or systematically distort the social reality of the lower classes, then a truly exceptional (and thus statistically infrequent) document can be much more revealing than a thousand stereotypical documents ... These marginal cases function, that is, as clues to or traces of a hidden reality, which is not usually apparent in the documentation."

7 Bakhtin, *Problems of Dostoevsky's Poetics*, 58; emphasis in the original.

8 Bakhtin, *Speech Genres*, 7; emphasis in the original. See also Todorov, *The Morals of History*.

9 On "history of the present," see Foucault, *Discipline and Punish*, 31, and "Questions of Method."

10 Todorov, *Les abus de la mémoire*, 31–2.

11 On contemporary understandings of childhood, see Benzaquén, "Childhood, the Sciences of Childhood, and the History of Science." See also Steedman, *Strange Dislocations*.

12 See Hacking, "Historical Epistemology," and *Historical Ontology*, especially pp. 1–26 (Hacking would not necessarily agree with my very unphilosophical use of "historical epistemology").

13 On humanism, see Todorov, *Imperfect Garden*. One way to envision the encounter between the civilized adult and the wild child is as an intersubjective re-enactment of the encounter between the Spaniards and the native peoples of the "New World." Both the encounter with the wild child (at the microscopic level) and the encounter with the American "Indians" (at the macroscopic level) provide the student of otherness and self-other relations with many examples of what actually happened when a culture, a society, an individual or a group of individuals confronted an *other* that could not be either recognized or ignored; see Todorov, *The Conquest of America*.

CHAPTER ONE

1 Foucault, *The Archaeology of Knowledge*, 44–5.

2 See below, chapters 8 and 5.

3 Quoted in Rymer, *Genie*, 184. See Curtiss, *Genie*, and Garmon, *Secret of the Wild Child*.

4 See Janer Manila, *La problemàtica educativa*, 81–2, on the use in Spanish of "*bravío*," "*selvático*," and "*silvestre*" as alternatives to the more straightforward "*salvaje*"; Tylor, "Wild Men and Beast-Children"; Tinland, *L'Homme sauvage*.

5 See below, chapter 2.

6 Hacking, "The Looping Effects of Human Kinds," 366.

7 See chapters 3, 4, and 7, below, and Newton, *Savage Girls and Wild Boys*, 14.

8 The examples are many, including the incessant references to Romulus and Remus and other legendary wild children in accounts and discussions of historical wild children; the name Itard gave to the wild boy of Aveyron, which, Gineste tells us, was taken from the play *Victor ou l'enfant de la forêt* (see chapter 5, below); the use of tropes from Kipling's *Jungle Book* in Gesell's psychological biography of Kamala, the wolf girl of Midnapore (see chapter 7, below), and the influence of Truffaut's *Wild Child* on the professionals who studied and treated Genie, mentioned above.

9 Franck Tinland, preface to Madame H...t, *Histoire* (1970), 12. The accounts of wild children have been collected in several specialized works. In English, the most consequential of these is Zingg, "Feral Man" (1942).

10 For instance, Ogburn and Bose carried out an inquiry on the wolf girls of Midnapore in 1951, and Maclean carried out another in 1975. The girls had been captured in 1920; Amala died in 1921 and Kamala in 1929 (see chapter 7, below).

11 Armen, *Gazelle-Boy*, 17.

12 Crowds of curious people are mentioned in Tulp's account of the Irish boy (see below), in reports of the wild boy of Aveyron's arrival in Rodez and Paris, and in Maclean's book on the girls of Midnapore. Some accounts of Indian wild children (the boys of Sekandra, the girl of Jalpaiguri, Ramu) make reference to hundreds of visitors.

13 Examples of this kind of criticism are Feydel's letters and articles in the *Journal de Paris* attacking the scientists and philosophers who defended the wild boy of Aveyron, and Evans's venomous comments on Gesell's and Zingg's infatuation with the wolf girls of Midnapore (see chapters 5 and 7, below).

14 Tylor, "Wild Men and Beast-Children," 23; McCartney, "Greek and Roman Lore," 31. See also Austin, "Autobiography and History," 55.

15 Procopius, *The Gothic War*, book 6 of *History of the Wars*, 11–15.

16 "Additiones ad Lambertvm Schafnabvrgensem appositæ ab Erphesfordensi monacho ignoti nominis, sed non indiligenti scriptore: in quibus res CCC annis post Lambertum gestæ breuiter explicantur," in *Illustrivm vetervm scriptorvm*, 1:264. In the third edition of Pistorius's collection of works of early German historians, *Rervm germanicarvm scriptores aliqvot insignes*, the account of the boy of Hesse is on 1:439. The unknown monk's entries cover the period 1068–1352.

17 Dilich, *Hessische Chronica*, 2:187.

18 Camerarius, *Operæ horarvm svbcisivarvm*, 345; emphasis in the original. English translation: *The Living Librarie*, 239–40 (in this edition the boy's capture is dated 1543); Le Loyer, *Discovrs, et histoires des spectres*, 140. The wolf boy does not appear in the earlier, shorter version of Le Loyer's treatise, *IIII. Ljvres des spectres*, or its English translation, *A Treatise of Specters*. Le Loyer wrote that

the boy was caught during Louis the Bavarian's empire (1328–1347) but did not name his source ("a certain German Historian who wrote the History of the Landgraves of Hesse"). On Le Loyer and the wolf boy, see also "L.," "Children Nurtured by Wolves" (3 April 1858).

19 "Additiones ad Lambertvm," in Pistorius, *Illustrivm vetervm scriptorvm*, 1:264; Camerarius, *Operæ horarvm svbcisivarvm*, 345, and *The Living Librarie*, 240; Webster, *The Displaying of Supposed Witchcraft*, 91–2. Camerarius introduced the Bamberg youth and his amazing "motions and tumbling tricks" in the chapter "Of the stone called Phengites. Also, of the strange agilitie and nimblenesse of some." The youth reminded him of other, similar cases, which he proceeded to narrate as well – the ancient myth of Habides, grandson of Gargoris king of the Curetes (told by Justin the Historian); other stories from antiquity, Scripture, and recent voyages about very fast or wild people, and then the boys of Hesse and Wetterau.

20 Ross, *Arcana Microcosmi*, 112-13; emphasis in the original. Ross cited *Les Diverses leçons de Loys Guyon, sieur de La Nauche …* (several editions between 1604 and 1625). In the same passage, Ross also recalled reading about "a man bred among Wolves, and presented to *Charls* the ninth of *France*" (who ruled from 1560 to 1574).

21 Digby, *Two Treatises*, 246–8 (the account is in the treatise on the nature of bodies, in the chapter "Of the motions of sense; and of the sensible qualities in generall; and in particular of those which belong to Touch, Tast, and Smelling"). On Digby (1603–1665), see Petersson, *Sir Kenelm Digby*.

22 Virey, "Homme sauvage," 264–5. Le Cat (1700–1768) gave an embellished version of Digby's account: the boy, "whom his Parents had brought up in a Forest, (whither they had fled to avoid the Calamities of War) and who had lived on nothing but Roots, had a Smell so delicate, that by this Sense he perceived the Approach of the Enemy, and apprized his Parents of their coming." Made prisoner, he lost "much of that surprizing Delicacy of Smell," but not all: "For being married, he could very easily by smelling distinguish his own Wife from another Woman, and even find her out by the Print of her Foot, as a Dog does his Master." Such a husband "would in *Italy* make an *Argus* still more terrible than the famous one in the Fable"; Le Cat, *A Physical Essay on the Senses*, 31–2, *Traité des sens*, 36. Interest in the senses and their relation to knowledge was intense throughout the eighteenth and early-nineteenth centuries (see chapters 4 and 5, below). According to Itard, Victor recognized Mme Guérin by smell.

23 Tulp, *Observationes medicæ*, 296–8 (the case of the *"Juvenis balans"* was not in the first edition of 1641); I quote from the translation of Tulp in Blumenbach, *The Anthropological Treatises*, 165–6n4. Another of Tulp's observations was the *"Satyrus Indicus,"* one of the first anthropoid apes examined by a European

scientist; *Observationes medicae*, 270–7 (on the relation between wild children and apes, see chapter 4, below).

24 Rauber, *Homo sapiens ferus*, 20; Blumenbach, *Anthropological Treatises*, 165.

25 Rzaczynski, *Historia naturalis curiosa*, 354. See also Rauber, *Homo sapiens ferus*, 21–3; and Zingg, "Feral Man" (1942), 211–12.

26 Kircher, *China monumentis*, 194; English translation: *China illustrata*, 186 (modified).

27 Gramont, "Relation de mon voyage en Pologne," 715–16 (this was a previously unpublished manuscript from the duke of Guiche's archives).

28 Birch, *The History of the Royal Society*, 1:378 (meeting of 3 February 1663–64).

29 Moreri, *The Great Historical, Geographical and Poetical Dictionary*, URI-URS, "Ursin (*Joseph*)." *Le grand dictionaire historique* first appeared in Lyon in 1674 and went through many editions and revisions by Moreri (1643–1680) and other authors.

30 Connor, *Evangelium medici*, 181–3, and *The History of Poland*, 1:342–50. See also "Account of a Book"; and Dalitz and Stone, "Doctor Bernard Connor."

31 Connor inserted both the French original and an English translation of Cleverskerk's letter; in the latter, the date is (misprinted?) 1661.

32 Cited in Connor, *History of Poland*, 1:346–9; emphasis in the original.

33 Ibid., 342–3, 349–50. Many years later, Monboddo heard from a Swedish gentleman in Edinburgh a story the latter had from Linnaeus himself, who told it in his class, about a human creature caught in the woods of Saxony in the time of Frederick Augustus King of Poland, running wild upon all fours with the bears and feeding chiefly on wild honey. He was taught to walk upright by hanging "weights to his shoulders," to counteract his propensity to fall prone, and learned to speak but "still retained his bearish love for honey, and inclination to rob the bees"; *Antient Metaphysics*, 3: 74–5. In turn, Blumenbach (*Anthropological Treatises*, 337–8), after slyly referring to "the imaginative Connor," mentioned a monograph by the elder Johann Daniel Geyer, *On the Lithuanian Bear-Men*, which offered several instances of Polish bear children, one of whom "King John III. met with, and had baptized; and who was made fife-player to the militia, notwithstanding that he preferred going on four feet instead of two"; see also Blumenbach, "Vom Homo sapiens *ferus* Linn.," 36–7. Here Blumenbach's English editor, Bendyshe, added a footnote (338n1) quoting this passage from David Durand, *La vie et les sentiments de Lucilio Vanini* (1714): "A man of credit assured me, that there was found in *Denmark*, a young man of about fourteen or fifteen years old, who lived in the woods with the bears, and who could not be distinguished from them but by his shape. They took him, and learned him to speak; he said then, he could remember nothing but only since the time they took him from amongst the bears." While Ben-

dyshe was obviously implying that this was yet another account of the ubiquitous Lithuanian boys, Zingg made of this brief passage a whole new "case," but one he deemed "of little or no scientific value"; "Feral Man" (1942), 222. More sources on the Lithuanian boy(s) are mentioned in Porchnev, "La lutte pour les troglodytes," in Heuvelmans and Porchnev, *L'homme de Néanderthal*, 132–4.

34 Cox, *The Gentleman's Recreation*, 133–4; P.H. McCormack to the editor of *The Times* (11 April 1927); Hutton, "Wolf-Children," 15. McCormack (or *The Times*) discreetly omitted the words "where in a venereal manner he had the carnal use of her Body." Cox's source could be the pamphlet published in 1605 and reprinted in Joisten, ed., *Récits et contes populaires de Savoie*, 120–5, which tells the "horrifying" story of Anthoinette Culet, kidnapped by a bear in 1602 and rescued in 1605. She told her rescuers that she gave birth to a half-bear, half-human "monster" who was accidentally killed by its bestial father.

35 Feijoo, *Teatro crítico universal*, 6:273–314; Macanaz, "Varias notas al Teatro critico," 53; Monboddo, *Antient Metaphysics*, 4:37n. I quote from Macanaz's version, as translated in *Antient Metaphysics*. On Macanaz (1670–1760), see Sotomayor, "Nota del editor." For a recent story of an "amphibian boy" – Ramchandra of the river Kuano in Uttar Pradesh, India – see *Fortean Times* 32 (Summer 1980) and 47 (Autumn 1986).

36 Kanold, ed., *Sammlung von Natur- und Medicin-*, January 1718, 546–50 and October 1722, 437–44, translated in Zingg, "Feral Man" (1942), 234–7. The girl's kidnapping was an intricate affair involving illicit loves, inheritances, and revenge.

37 Virey, "Homme sauvage," 266.

38 Rousseau, *Discours*, as translated in *The Basic Political Writings*, 84n3.

39 Virey, "Homme sauvage," 264; Monboddo, *Antient Metaphysics*, 3:46–7.

40 Leroy, *Mémoire sur les travaux*, 8–9n1; the account of the wild man is translated in *Annual Register* 21 (December 1778): 116, and *Gentleman's Magazine* 49 (supplement for 1779): 632.

41 Monboddo, *Antient Metaphysics*, 4:38n; Macanaz, "Varias notas," 57.

42 Sigaud-Lafond, *Dictionnaire des merveilles de la nature*, 2:292.

43 The anonymous account of the wild boy of Kronstadt appears in Michael Wagner, *Beiträge zur philosophischen Anthropologie und den damit verwandten Wissenschaften*, vol. 1 (1794), reprinted in Rauber, *Homo sapiens ferus*, 49–53, and translated in Zingg, "Feral Man" (1942), 237–40. The author mentions the *Histoire d'une jeune fille sauvage*, attributed to La Condamine. Another report, by the scholar Mihaly Frobenius, contains additional material on the circumstances of the boy's capture, his reaction to different stimuli, social behaviour, and changes after his return to "civilized" life; discussed in O.A. Vertes, "Egy XVII Szazadi Magyar Lelektani Dolgozat," *Magyar Pszichologiai Szemle* 17

(1960): 50–9, and in Friedman, "A Historical Note to 'The Wild Boy of Kronstadt,'" 284.

44 Report in the records of Zips, Hungary, 11 October 1793, reproduced in Wagner, *Beiträge*, and translated in Zingg, "Feral Man" (1942), 268–71.

45 Monboddo, *Antient Metaphysics*, 3:45, 3:48n, and 4:21n.

46 Tylor, "Wild Men and Beast-Children," 21–2; *Dusselthal Abbey*, 36–9 and 43–8. According to the unidentified author of *Dusselthal Abbey*, "the original situations of the reclaimed savages, mark a state of society similar to that of the darkest and most deplorable of the middle ages; when deserted infants, left to perish in the woods, were said to have been suckled by the beasts of the forest, after being forsaken by those in human form" (37).

47 Kinneir, *Journey through Asia Minor*, 335–6 (the wild man reminded Kinneir of "a similar circumstance of a woman having been discovered in the forests near Smyrna, who could neither walk nor speak, and, like a beast, was entirely covered with hair"; 336n); also cited in Zingg, "Feral Man" (1942), 231 (Zingg quotes Kinneir's passage but deems the evidence too slim to warrant a number and full "case" status); Feuerbach, *Caspar Hauser*, 307–8; also cited in Zingg, "Feral Man," 202. Feuerbach's source is Wilhelm Horn, *Reise durch Deutschland, Ungarn, Holland, Italien, Frankreich, Grossbritannien und Irland*, vol. 1 (1831), 138.

48 See chapter 7, below.

49 Mitra, "On a Wild Boy and a Wild Girl," in Zingg, "Feral Man" (1942), 220–1, and Frazer, ed. and trans., *The Fasti of Ovid*, 2:380–1; Baker, "The Power of Scent in Wild Animals," in Zingg, "Feral Man," 170–2; an article in *Illustrated Weekly of India*, 5 February 1933, cited in Hutton, "Wolf-Children," 24; Maranz, "Raised by a She-bear," in Zingg, "Feral Man," 222–6 (Maranz also discussed Istoki, the "beast-boy," found some time earlier in Hungary "much in the same manner as the hunters found the bear girl"); "La vie de Sidi Mohamed avec les autruches," 4–5 (this issue of *Notes africaines* contains two more stories of animal-nurtured children: "Histoire de Regaj Es-bou â: homme des lions," about a child who lived with lions, and "Histoire de Eddami, la biche," about a child nursed by a bitch, both by Dah ould Haïba of Dakar, 5–7); "Syria," 34, and Heuvelmans, *Les bêtes humaines*, 112; Sieveking, "News from the Wild Frontiers"; Poole, "Uganda's Wild Child," and Sieveking, "Feral News"; Newton, *Savage Girls*, 1–3; Isabel Ferrer, "John, el último niño salvaje del siglo," *El País*, 17 October 1999. On Lucas, the gazelle boy of the Sahara, and John of Burundi, see chapter 7, below.

50 Ornstein, "Wilden Menschen in Trikkala"; Zingg, "Feral Man" (1942), 259–68, and Krout, *Introduction to Social Psychology*, 111–13; Janer Manila, *La problemàtica educativa*, translated into English as *Marcos*.

51 See below, chapter 8.

52 Sieveking, "Forteana." Reports of wild children continue to appear in popular media; see the many articles and updates published in the British magazine of "strange phenomena" *Fortean Times* since the early 1970s (especially Sieveking, "Wild Things") and the accounts collected in Ward, "FeralChildren.com."

CHAPTER TWO

1 Mandelbaum, "Wolf-Child Histories from India," 43.

2 Linnaeus, *Systema naturae*, 10th ed., 1:20–4; 12th ed., 1:28 (in the 12th ed. Linnaeus changed the date of discovery of the boy of Hesse to 1544).

3 For Tinland, the very fact that Linnaeus created the class *Homo ferus* is an indication of how strange these children appeared to observers; see Tinland's preface to Madame H...t, *Histoire* (1970), 8.

4 Rousseau, *Discours sur l'inégalité*, as translated in *The Basic Political Writings*, 84; Linnaeus, *Anthropomorpha*, 65. Pointing to a finite number of known cases, Linnaeus's "multitude" does not contradict my claim that the examples of wild children exhaust the class "wild child."

5 De Pauw reproduced Linnaeus's list in *Recherches philosophiques sur les Americains*, 2:77n, and Delisle de Sales listed Rousseau's and Linnaeus's cases in *De la Philosophie de la nature*, 3:211–12 and 4:255–7. Sigaud-Lafond listed the child found with wolves near Cassel in 1334, the child found with bears in Lithuania in 1694 and later "taken to the Court of England," the two savages found in the Pyrenees in 1719, and the girl found with bears in Frauenmark in 1767 (*Dictionnaire des merveilles de la nature*, 2:291–2).

6 Schreber, *Die Saugthiere*, 1:31–7. See Scheber's list in the appendix. Schreber did not name Peter (the boy found near Hameln) but had him dying in London in 1727 (Peter died in 1785, ten years after Schreber published *Die Saugthiere*). On Schreber, see Goerke, "Linnaeus' German Pupils," 227–35.

7 Bonnaterre, *Notice historique*, 180–93, 210–11, and Virey, "Questions de Physiologie et de Métaphysique," 345. Bonnaterre listed eleven numbered cases but in the text referred to other wild children as well. Each child was identified with Linnaeus's (or a Linnaeus-style) Latin name followed by the French translation (see appendix). Virey listed the "young savages" of Hanover, 1724; Lithuania, 1661; Hesse, 1544; Transylvania, 1717; the Pyrenees, 1719; Bamberg; Champagne, 1731, "etc.; and Jean of Loudun discussed by Boerrhaave." In the entry "Homme sauvage" of *Nouveau dictionnaire d'histoire naturelle* (262–9), Virey discussed the boy found among wolves in Hesse in 1544; the savage found near Bamberg (Camerarius); the boys found in Lithuania in 1657 (Rzaczinsky) and 1694 (Connor); the Irish boy (Tulp); the two wild boys of the Pyrenees; Jean of Liège (Boerhaave); the boy of Hanover; the girl of Over-Yssel; the girl of Hungary

(Sigaud de la Fond); the wild girl of Sogny (Racine and La Condamine), and the boy of Aveyron.

8 The first and third editions of *De generis humani varietate nativa* (1775 and 1795), as well as "On the Homo Sapiens *Ferus* Linn.," are translated in Blumenbach, *Anthropological Treatises*. I cite from pages 165 and 336–9. See also "Vom Homo sapiens *ferus* Linn.," 32–40. That "there were never any wild sheep in Ireland" had also been pointed out by de Pauw in *Recherches philosophiques*, 2:77n.

9 Rudolphi, *Grundriss der Physiologie*, 1:24–6; Bory de Saint-Vincent, *L'Homme*, 1:17–19 and 1:57–9n7, and Tafel, *Die Fundamentalphilosophie in genetischer Entwickelung: mit besonderer Rücksicht auf die Geschichte jedes einzelnen Problems* (Tübingen, 1848), cited in Zingg, "Feral Man" (1942), 195–6. Bory's list comprises Linnaeus's cases and some additions: another youth captured among bears in Lithuania in 1694; the girl found among bears in Lower Hungary in 1767; Mlle Leblanc (Bory seems unaware that she is Linnaeus's *Puella Campanica*); and the wild boy of Aveyron.

10 Tylor, "Wild Men and Beast-Children," 21, 29, 32, and see the appendix. Tylor's list does not include Victor.

11 Rauber, *Homo sapiens ferus*, 15–63, and see the appendix.

12 Ireland, *The Mental Affections of Children*, 434–5. In the chapter "Wolf Boys: An Inquiry into some Accounts of Children being fostered by Wild Beasts," Ireland reviewed the legendary accounts of the "forbidden experiment" (see chapter 3, below) and the accounts of "children found straying in the woods, deserted by their parents, and feeding like wild animals" (the girl of Soigny, the boy of Aveyron, Peter) before moving on to a "still more curious subject of inquiry … stories of children, deserted by their parents, being fed and guarded by animals" (419–20). Once again he began with myth (Romulus and Remus, Cyrus) and then switched to the "real" cases: Ægisthus, Sleeman's boys, the boys at the Sekandra orphanage, a wolf boy then living in the Lucknow Lunatic Asylum, and Connor's Lithuanian boys. Ireland discussed Kaspar in an earlier chapter, "Idiocy by Deprivation."

13 Small, "On Some Psychical Relations," 48. See Small's list in the appendix. In the brief section "Wild Children" of his study of the child in "primitive culture" (originally delivered as lectures at Clark University under the presidency of "the *genius* of the movement for 'Child-Study' in America," G. Stanley Hall), Chamberlain included *two* full lists, Tylor's and Rauber's, and mentioned Sleeman's and Ball's wolf children; Chamberlain, *The Child and Childhood in Folk-Thought*, vii, 173–5.

14 Hutton, "Wolf-Children," 28, and see the appendix.

15 See Zingg's 1940 and 1942 lists in the appendix. In his 1942 list Zingg included all known cases but only numbered the "authentic" ones (Amala and Kamala,

given a privileged place in *Wolf-Children and Feral Man* as a whole, were not in the list).

16 Dennis, "The Significance of Feral Man," 425, 428; Mandelbaum, "Wolf-Child Histories from India," 26, 33. See Mandelbaum's list in the appendix. (Amala and Kamala, discussed at length in the article, are not in his list.)

17 Dennis, "A Further Analysis," 154; M.W. Smith, "Wild Children and the Principle of Reinforcement," 115–23. Dennis's list included Zingg's cases II, V, VI, VII, XI, and XXVI. Smith rearranged "Dennis's Data on Six Feral Children Reported by Singh and Zingg" in a table, retaining Dennis's categories of estimated age at isolation, estimated age at discovery, and recovery, and adding period (length) of isolation (116).

18 Malson, *Wolf Children*, 38, 39n4. In the French edition, *Les enfants sauvages*, the list is on pages 72–5. In the English edition the list is on pages 80–2 and contains even more mistakes, for which Malson cannot be held accountable, of course. The categories are: designation, date of discovery, age at discovery, and first important account; see the list of cases in the appendix. Malson found some of the cases (e.g., the Casamance child and Assicia of Liberia) in Demaison, *Le livre des enfants sauvages*. The story of the "little snow-hen of Justedal," which Malson found in Le Roux, *Notes sur la Norvège*, 16, is in fact a Norwegian legend that dates back to the Black Death. Janer Manila reproduced Malson's list in *La problemàtica educativa*, 114–16.

19 Favazza, "Feral and Isolated Children," 109, 105. Favazza restored Procopius's child and added some cases from Zingg's 1942 list (Denmark bear-boy, wild man from Trebizond, Greek sheep-boy, Tarzancito, bear-girl of Mt Olympus), Ogburn's wolf-boy of Agra, and a new case (Czech twins, seven years old, 1967). Favazza's is not the longest list, though. On 22 September 2003, Andrew Ward's "list of feral children" included *eighty-four* cases (see the appendix). As of 17 August 2004, Ward offers both a list of all "feral children" (now the total is 102 cases, fourteen of them "discovered" since 1990) and separate lists of children raised by animals (fifty-six cases, seven since 1990), confined children (twenty cases, six since 1990), isolated children (twenty-one cases, one since 1990), and hoaxes (five cases); see "FeralChildren.com."

20 McNeil, Polloway, and Smith, "Feral and Isolated Children," 70. The authors reviewed forty-six cases but discuss only a few examples selected as representative of each group: (a) Amala and Kamala; (b) wild boy of Aveyron, girl of Cranenburg, Songi Girl of Champagne, and Tarzancito; (c) Kasper Hauser, Anna, and Albert, and (d) Anne (Albert's older sibling) and Isabelle. Genie is not included.

21 More lists or list-type discussions of wild children, both scientific and popular, may be found in Miller, "The Wolf-Girls and the Baboon-Boy"; Magny, ed., *Les*

enfants célèbres; Demaison, *Le livre des enfants sauvages*; Broche, "Le secret des enfants sauvages"; Douglas, *The Beast Within*; and Candland, *Feral Children and Clever Animals*.

22 Occasionally it was suggested that a wild child might be the offspring of a human female and a male animal. This is how Feijoo explained the discovery of two boys among bears in Lithuania in 1661, in *Teatro crítico universal*, 6:304–7 (in the same discourse in which he recounted the story of the "amphibious" Francisco de la Vega) and in *Cartas eruditas y curiosas*, 3:334–7 (letter 30, "Philosophical Reflections, on the Occasion of the Recent Finding of a Human Creature in the Womb of a Goat"). According to Thomas (*Man and the Natural World*, 134), some English families traced their descent from wild animals, "like Siward, Edward the Confessor's Earl of Northumberland, whose grandmother had been ravished by a bear; or the Devonshire family of Sucpitches, who in the eighteenth century maintained that their ancestor had been found in the Prussian woods sucking a bitch."

23 "Peter the Wild Boy; and the Savage of Aveyron," 170.

24 The suspicion that idiocy or imbecility might be involved was voiced as early as the 1720s; see chapter 3, below.

25 Zingg, "Feral Man" (1942), 131.

26 Wild children are sometimes associated with "monsters"; see "Wild Men and Feral Children," in Fiedler, *Freaks*, 154–77, and "Philosophers Trim the Tree of Knowledge," in Darnton, *The Great Cat Massacre*, 193 (Darnton mentions "the wolf boy" as an example of monsters that "horrify and fascinate us because they violate our conceptual boundaries").

27 The prototype theory of categorization is explained in Lakoff, *Women, Fire, and Dangerous Things*, and Hacking, *Rewriting the Soul*. See also Wittgenstein, *Philosophical Investigation*, and Rosch, "Principles of Categorization."

28 Zingg, "Feral Man" (1940), 493; McNeil, Polloway, and Smith, "Feral and Isolated Children," 70. When "wolf child" is construed as the core of the class, it may be (misleadingly) used to designate wild children in general (e.g., the title of the English translation of Malson's book, *Wolf Children and the Problem of Human Nature*) or any wild child. Darnton follows his reference to "the wolf boy" with a footnote citing Shattuck's book on Victor; see Darnton, *The Great Cat Massacre*, 193 and 277n3, and Shattuck, *The Forbidden Experiment*. Similarly, Code discusses the "wolf boy of Aveyron" in *Epistemic Responsibility*, 65, 171, 178.

29 Malson, *Wolf Children*, 61 (*Les enfants sauvages*, 71); Rauber, *Homo sapiens ferus*, as translated in Zingg, "Feral Man" (1942), 192n23. Zingg agrees with Rauber: "It is certain that [Peter] does not represent the typical picture of an isolated being" (194).

30 Linnaeus, *Anthropomorpha*, 65–6; emphasis in the original.

31 There are widely divergent interpretations of the impact of diet on the wild child's life and health. For instance, Madame H...t blamed the change from a raw-meat diet to ordinary cooked food for the deterioration of Mlle Leblanc's health; Daumer, Kaspar Hauser's teacher, claimed that the introduction of meat in a previously vegetarian diet caused Kaspar to lose his special sensitivity and innocence; Dr Sarbadhicari, who treated Amala and Kamala, attributed their premature death to their inability to do without raw meat and failure to become accustomed to a more varied diet; and Zingg ("Feral Man" [1940], 507) wrote that "in the light of recent research in the effects of diet on the intelligence, there is but little doubt that the inadequate diet of feral man has something to do with his mental retardation."

32 Zingg, "Feral Man" (1940), 508, 509, 513.

33 Malson, *Wolf Children*, 47; Tinland, *L'Homme sauvage*, 84, 85; Tylor, "Wild Men and Beast-Children," 26. Mandelbaum found a striking uniformity in the twenty cases of animal-nurtured children inventoried in his article: most of them went on all fours, never learned to speak, ate only raw meat, and would not wear clothes, while some ate from the ground like dogs, gave off an offensive odour, and sniffed the food before eating it; see "Wolf-Child Histories from India."

34 Zingg, "Feral Man" (1940), 495.

35 Malson, *Wolf Children*, 55; Blumenbach, *Anthropological Treatises*, 339; Tinland, *L'Homme sauvage*, 81.

36 Tinland, preface to Madame H...t, *Histoire* (1970), 27; Malson, *Wolf Children*, 35–6 (*Les enfants sauvages*, 40); Zingg, "Feral Man" (1940), 514.

37 Hacking, "The Looping Effects of Human Kinds," 351–4. See Hacking's earlier and later takes on kinds of people in "Making up People" and *The Social Construction of What?*

38 Carroll made a shoddy effort to introduce statistics in a debunking discussion of wild children. Noting that "six, or 18 percent, of the thirty-three children in Table 1 [a list of children allegedly raised by animals] are female," a statistic "amazingly similar to Rutter and Lockyer's [1967] finding that twelve, or 19 percent, of the sixty-three young children diagnosed as psychotic (a category that included early infantile autism) in one particular hospital over an eight-year period were female," he proclaims that "the ratio of females to males in Table 1 is exactly what one would expect if the children listed were a representative sample of psychotic children"; Carroll, "The Folkloric Origins," 67. Representative of what?

39 Hacking, "Looping Effects," 374, and "Normal People," 69–70.

40 Hacking, *Rewriting the Soul*, 8.

41 On the strong tendency to "biologize" human kinds ("biological" standing for "biochemical, neurological, electrical, mechanical, or whatever is the preferred model of efficient causation in a given scientific community or era"), see Hacking, "Looping Effects," 372.

42 See Bonnaterre, *Notice historique*; Pinel, "Rapport fait à la Société des Observateurs de l'homme"; and chapter 5, below.

43 Tredgold, *Mental Deficiency*, 332–3.

44 "Peter the Wild Boy; and the Savage of Aveyron," 170; de Pauw, *Recherches philosophiques*, 2:76; Rauber, *Homo sapiens ferus*, 17; Mandelbaum, "Wolf-Child Histories from India," 34–5; Stark, *Antecedents of the Social Bond*, 105–6; Hutton, "Wolf-Children," 29; Bettelheim, "Feral Children and Autistic Children"; Money, *The Kaspar Hauser Syndrome*; Masson, ed. and trans., *Lost Prince*; Porchnev, "La lutte pour les troglodytes," in Heuvelmans and Porchnev, *L'homme de Néanderthal*, 132–6.

45 Curtiss (*Genie*, 7) ended her account of Genie's childhood and the circumstances that brought her to the attention of the social services and police with these words: "Genie was admitted into the hospital for extreme malnutrition. She had been discovered, at last." Genie's mother, father, and brother, presented as perpetrators or covictims, seem to be automatically excluded from the status of "discoverer" as well.

46 Elias, *The Civilizing Process*.

47 The wild child story-form replays some motifs found in the European myth of the "wild man," e.g., the capture ("Medieval writers are fond of the story which tells how hunters, venturing farther than usual into unknown parts of the forest, would chance upon the wild man's den and stir him up; and how, astounded at the human semblance of the beast, they would exert themselves to capture it, and would drag it to the local castle as a curiosity") and the response ("the wild man is dragged out of his habitat and brought to the castle, there confined, and immediately exposed to the efforts of his captors to return him to fullfledged human status"); Bernheimer, *Wild Men in the Middle Ages*, 16–17.

CHAPTER THREE

1 Gaspard Guillard de Beaurieu, *Cours d'histoire naturelle, ou tableau de la nature*, vol. 1 (1770), quoted in Douthwaite, "Rewriting the Savage," 184.

2 Cited in Defoe, *Mere Nature Delineated*, 10. Similar reports appeared in *St James's Evening Post*, 14 December 1725; *Applebee's Journal*, *British Journal*, and *Mist's Journal*, 18 December, and *Edinburgh Caledonian Mercury*, 21 December.

3 *Flying Post*, 30 December 1725, reprinted in *Caledonian Mercury*, 7 January 1726, in Monboddo, *Antient Metaphysics*, 3:58, and in Defoe, *Mere Nature Delineated*, 10.

4 *Weekly Journal, or The British Gazetteer*, 22 January 1726, in Norton, "Peter the Wild Boy"; "Wye's Letter" (London), 24 March 1726, in *Caledonian Mercury*, 29 March, in Monboddo, *Antient Metaphysics*, 3:59.

5 "Wye's Letter," 5 April 1726, in *Caledonian Mercury*, 11 April, in Monboddo, *Antient Metaphysics*, 3:59.

6 Countess Schaumburg-Lippe to Count Zinzendorf, 12 February 1726, cited in Spangenberg, *The Life of Nicolas Lewis*, 2:205.

7 *Edinburgh Evening Courant*, 12 April and 5 July 1726, in Monboddo, *Antient Metaphysics*, 3:60.

8 From the occasional paper "The Country Gentleman," no. 10 (11 April 1726), in *Edinburgh Evening Courant*, 8 August, in Monboddo, *Antient Metaphysics*, 3:60–1.

9 "Wye's Letter," in *Edinburgh Evening Courant*, 14 November 1726, in Monboddo, *Antient Metaphysics*, 3:61.

10 Saussure, *A Foreign View of England*, 147–50. Born in 1705 to a Huguenot family exiled in Switzerland, Saussure left home in the spring of 1725 and travelled for eleven years. His letters were lent to more than two hundred readers and in 1755 were praised by Voltaire. The account of Peter is in Letter 5, from East Sheen, near Richmond, 14 June 1726. Saussure also recounted Peter's appearance at court: "The youth did not appear put out or embarrassed at finding himself in the midst of such a fashionable assembly. He remained where he was, planted like a statue. The Princess of Wales wore that evening a sort of habit of black velvet, with fastenings and trimmings of diamonds, and at her girdle hung a gold watch that struck the hours. The chiming of this watch attracted the young savage, who ran towards the Princess to see from whence the sound came; without permission he examined the sparkling gems on the Princess's gown and also the watch, which she made chime several times for his pleasure. For some time he thus stood, much to the amusement of the whole circle, but unfortunately he could not be taught good manners, and he had to be removed" (ibid.). Since so much in Saussure's account is rumour and legend, one may legitimately wonder whether his claim that the king sent the boy to the school of a master "said to be patient and clever in teaching children" who nevertheless had "extreme difficulty in making him understand anything, his intellect being very dull and stunted," must be taken as serious evidence of additional educational efforts or a distorted reference to Arbuthnot.

11 Swift to Thomas Tickell (16 April 1726), in *Correspondence*, 3:128.

12 [Swift and/or Arbuthnot], *The Most Wonderful Wonder*, 4, 8. On the controversy regarding authorship of this and other pamphlets on Peter, and for a dis-

cussion of this literature as political satire, see Nash, *Wild Enlightenment*. See also Novak, "The Wild Man Comes to Tea," Bartra, *The Artificial Savage*, 171-8, 184-8, and Newton, *Savage Girls*, 39-49.

13 [Swift and/or Arbuthnot], *It cannot Rain but it Pours*, 5-8. Whereas most later commentators took *It cannot Rain but it Pours* as no more than a pleasant amusement, Monboddo saw it as a valid source of facts about Peter not mentioned anywhere else, "whatever we may think of the application [Swift] makes of them"; *Antient Metaphysics*, 3:61.

14 Defoe, *Mere Nature Delineated*, 3. Hereafter references to this work are in the text. Any emphasis is in the original.

15 No observer had seen Peter walking on all fours: "I do not find, that at any of the Times when he has, for Observation, been turn'd out a Grazing, as in the Park, or in the Paddock, or any where else, that he return'd to that Posture of going; but that he continu'd walking erect as at other Times" (12).

16 At first unsure ("I think it is granted he can laugh, tho', I confess, when I saw him, we could just make him Grin"), Defoe confirmed the fact a page later: "I am just now inform'd, that our wild Creature can really laugh out, as a Man should do, and has done so several Times, tho' himself cannot be said to understand what laughing is, or what is the proper Object of his Mirth" (19, 20).

17 Like Swift/Arbuthnot, Defoe found in Peter an excuse to make fun of the ladies of the court: they "are a little disgusted at him, in that he seems not yet capable of understanding what they are, or what the Intent and Meaning of Beauty is ... upon which, it is said, A certain Lady looking gravely upon him, shook her Head, and added, *'Tis pity he is not a little older, he would make an admirable ——— for he could tell no Tales*" (31). On Defoe's pamphlet and the debate on the nature of the soul, see Newton, "Bodies without Souls."

18 *An Enquiry*, 2-4; *The Manifesto of Lord Peter*, 3-4 (this pamphlet, signed by "Solomon Audrian," has also been attributed to Arbuthnot); *Vivitur Ingenio*, title page.

19 "The SAVAGE; occasion'd by the bringing to Court a wild Youth, taken in the Woods in *Germany*, in the Year *1725*," in Lewis, ed., *Miscellaneous Poems*, 305-6.

20 [Swift and/or Arbuthnot], *It Cannot Rain but It Pours*, 474.

21 "Reliable and truthful report of the wild boy, found in the fields near Hameln, the circumstances relating to him, how he behaved after his capture, and the conjectures which resulted; and also other interesting events that happened, written by a reliable person from Hameln to a friend, and now brought to print because of its interest," 18 March 1726, in *Breslauer Sammlung: Supplementum IV* ... von Joh. Kanold (Breslau, 1729), 69-78; reproduced in Rauber, *Homo sapiens ferus*, 33-5, and translated into English in Zingg, "Feral Man" (1942), 192-4n23.

22 Ibid. Blumenbach's account of Peter's discovery differed in some important
    respects and added some interesting points: a "naked, brownish, black-haired
    creature," about the size of a twelve-year-old boy, was met by Jürgen Meyer,
    a townsman of Hameln, on Friday, 27 July 1724, "by a stile in his field, not
    far from Helpensen"; just when "it" was found, the creature "had caught
    some birds, and eagerly dismembered them," yet was "happily enticed, by its
    astonished discoverer showing it two apples in his hand, into the town, and
    entrapped within the Bridge-gate"; first received by "a mob of street boys" who
    named him Peter, he was "placed for safe custody in the Hospital of the Holy
    Ghost, by order of the Burgomaster Severin"; once accustomed to life in soci-
    ety, he was allowed to move freely, "go about town and pay visits"; the cloth-
    maker with whom he was put to board, and to whom he became truly attached,
    accompanied him in October 1725 to the hospital (located by the House of Cor-
    rection) in Zell; around Advent King George summoned him to Hanover, and
    in February 1726 he was brought to London under the safeguard of a royal ser-
    vant named Rautenberg; "Vom Homo sapiens *ferus* Linn.," 13–18, and *Anthro-
    pological Treatises*, 329–31.
23 Countess Schaumburg-Lippe to Count Zinzendorf (undated), cited in Span-
    genberg, *The Life of Nicolas Lewis*, 2:206.
24 Peter's obituary appeared in *Gentleman's Magazine*, March 1785, 236. Little
    more than a year after Peter's arrival in London the *British Journal* had pub-
    lished an "Epitaph on PETER, the Wild Youth: Occasioned by the Report of his
    Death," in which the "dear departed Youth" was depicted as the "Glory" of the
    Yahoo race, who in life had been "solely rul'd by *Nature*'s Laws" and had "Dy'd
    a *Martyr* in her Cause!"; *British Journal*, 3 June 1727, in Norton, "Peter the Wild
    Boy." Also in 1727, another pamphlet announced that Peter the Wild Boy, "who
    appear'd so Sly and so Serious," had "play'd some of his Wild Pranks with a
    Dairy Maid at *Harrow* the *Hill*, whom he has got with Child"; *The Devil to pay
    at St. James's*, 9 (this pamphlet has also been attributed to Arbuthnot). Accord-
    ing to Samuel Parr (1747–1825), Peter was lodged in the boarding-house of a
    Mrs King in the early 1760s (Parr, then a student at Harrow School, also lodged
    there); *Bibliotheca Parrianna*, 705. A later author claimed that the wild boy had
    been sent to Mrs King because she was "the person most likely to kindle the
    dormant torch of reason in a totally untutored mind – a task, alas! found to be
    beyond mortal power"; Thornton, *Harrow School*, 151.
25 The extract from the parish register was reproduced in *Annual Register … For
    the Years 1784 and 1785* (1787), 43–5 and in *Gentleman's Magazine*, November
    1785, 851–3. It states that Peter was found in 1725 "in the woods near Hamelen
    … when his majesty George I. with his attendants, was hunting in the forest of
    Hertswold." Eighty years later the same discovery story was given a different
    emphasis: Peter had been found when "that shrewd cynical king, George the
    First, having got back for a time to his beloved country, was out hunting near

Hamelen with his hideous mistresses and motley court ... The cynical king and his ugly favourites, all rouge and black wig, gathered round the boy with extreme curiosity, and prettily assumed pity"; "Old Stories Re-told," 301.

26 Peter's legendary flights were reported in *Gentleman's Magazine*, November 1751, 522 and mentioned in Burgess's account (see below) and Blumenbach, "Vom Homo sapiens *ferus* Linn.," 25–6, and *Anthropological Treatises*, 333–4.

27 According to *An Enquiry*, 3, "the middle and 4th Finger of his Left hand are something web'd together like a Duck's Foot, but it seems rather to have been wounded and healed up again, than natural." Shortly before Peter's death, a reader of *Gentleman's Magazine* (April 1780, 171) declared him to be "an ideot, palmed on the public," whose "intellects are those of a child." In contrast, the writer who had reported on Peter's appearance before the royal family in London in 1767, after indicating that the wild man, "like Shakespear's Caliban, can fetch wood and water, but can speak no language articulately" and had been "kept for many years at the expence of 30 l.," insisted that "the tale in the papers of his being a poor Hanoverian idiot, sent here in a drunken frolic to be maintained, deserves contempt"; "Chronicle," 6 January, *Annual Register ... For the Year 1767* (1768), 47; also in *Gentleman's Magazine*, January 1767, 43; in other words, Peter was a "real savage": the Crown's honour (and yearly expenditure) must be defended. During his stay in London Peter's portrait was painted by Pierre-Etienne Falconet (1741–1791); on this and another portrait painted by John Alefounder (1757–1794) three years before Peter's death, see Blumenbach, "Vom Homo sapiens *ferus* Linn.," 31–2, and *Anthropological Treatises*, 335–6, and Burgess's account.

28 *Philosophical Survey of Nature*, 69–71n; Monboddo, *Antient Metaphysics*, 3:63–4. Monboddo's account of Peter was also printed in *Gentleman's Magazine*, February 1785, 113–14. Monboddo had already manifested his interest in Peter in *Of the Origin and Progress of Language*, 1:187: "a person who lived for a considerable time in the neighbourhood of a farmer's house where he was kept, and had an opportunity of seeing him almost every day" had informed him that Peter was "not an idiot, as he has been represented by some who cannot make allowance for the difference that education makes upon mens minds."

29 Burgess's account is in Monboddo, *Antient Metaphysics*, 3:368–73.

30 Ibid., 3:372–3, 377n.

31 Edgeworth and Edgeworth, *Practical Education*, 1:63–4. For Douthwaite (*The Wild Girl*, 27, 25) the Edgeworths "did not question [Peter's] humanity" but "merely saw him inhabiting a low level on the developmental continuum"; what their experiments attempted to show was "that Peter did think, but in a different way."

32 Blumenbach, "Vom Homo sapiens *ferus* Linn.," 20–5, and *Anthropological Treatises*, 332–4. Blumenbach consulted printed and manuscript sources in Hanover and England; on Peter's later life in England, "besides what I found out

there myself, many of my friends there, such as the ambassadors of Hanover, Dr. Dornford and M. Craufurd, have communicated to me accurate accounts, which they themselves got together on Hertfordshire itself" (335; 29–31 in the German original).

33 Tafel, *Die Fundamentalphilosophie*, 85, cited in Zingg, "Feral Man" (1942), 187n18; Rauber, *Homo sapiens ferus*, 40, and Zingg, "Feral Man," 182.

34 The inscription in the brass plate erected to the memory of Peter in the parish church of Northchurch notes that once he proved "incapable of speaking, or of receiving any instruction, a comfortable provision was made for him at a farmhouse in this parish, where he continued to the end of his inoffensive life"; *Gentleman's Magazine*, November 1785, 853. On the possible influence of Peter's story on Wordsworth's poetry, see Bewell, *Wordsworth and the Enlightenment*, 51–70. Examples of later popular interest in Peter are his inclusion in Wilson and Caulfield, *The Book of Wonderful Characters*, 133–40; the "special 'Peter the Wild Boy' exhibit" being prepared in April 1927 at the Berkhamsted School Museum (see C.T. Spurling's letter to the editor, *Times*, 18 April 1927); and Tennant's novel *Peter the Wild Boy*.

35 A new spate of attention has been directed at the wild girl in recent decades; see Tinland's preface to Madame H...t, *Histoire d'une jeune fille sauvage* (1970); Douthwaite, "Rewriting the Savage" and *The Wild Girl*; and Newton, *Savage Girls*.

36 "Lettre écrite de Châlons, en Champagne, le 9 Decembre 1731, par M. AM.N ... au sujet de la Fille sauvage, trouvée aux environs de cette Ville" and "Extrait d'une autre Lettre sur le même sujet," *Mercure de France*, December 1731, 2d vol., 2,983–91. Hereafter references to these letters are in the text.

37 According to Madame H...t, who was probably following the baptism record (see below), the girl was about nine years old. At first she was black, but repeated washings (or, for Racine, "the change of life") exposed her natural whiteness. She had large fingers and very large thumbs which, she said, had been useful during her life in the forests.

38 Reproduced in Madame H...t, *Histoire*, 50. Madame H...t guessed that the girl's precipitate baptism (which, Racine noted, Mlle Leblanc did not remember) was prompted by fear for her life during one of her illnesses.

39 Racine, *Eclaircissement sur la fille sauvage dont il est parlé dans l'Epître II sur l'homme*, in *Œuvres*, 6:580.

40 Luynes, *Mémoires*, 13:70–2.

41 Madame H...t, *Histoire* (1755), 49. In their reviews of the *Histoire*, both Grimm (*Correspondance littéraire*, January 1755) and Raynal (*Nouvelles littéraires* 125, 18 February 1755) attributed it to La Condamine; Tourneux, ed., *Correspondance littéraire*, 2:477–8 and 222–4. In a letter to M. de Boissy of the Académie française, La Condamine affirmed that the author was a widow living near

Saint Marceau who had met Mlle Leblanc after the death of the duc d'Orléans. He had only edited the manuscript (of which he still had the original), removed some unconfirmed facts, added his own conjectures regarding the girl's arrival in France, and facilitated the book's publication to attract attention to Mlle Leblanc's sad situation and help her secure an income from its sale; *Mercure de France*, April 1755, 74–5. La Condamine assured Monboddo that the facts in the *Histoire* "might be depended on" because he "knew the lady that wrote it"; *Antient Metaphysics*, 4:34. The *Histoire* was reprinted in 1761 and translated into English several times. On late-eighteenth- and early-nineteenth-century British chapbooks based on the *Histoire*, see Weiss, *A Book about Chapbooks*, and Douthwaite, *The Wild Girl*, 48–53.

42 Madame H...t, *An Account of a Savage Girl*. Monboddo also inserted an account of his meeting with Mlle Leblanc (to whom he had been introduced by La Condamine) in *Antient Metaphysics*, 4:403–8.

43 Racine, *Œuvres*, 6:582.

44 Madame H...t, *Histoire* (1755), 10–11.

45 Ibid., 26–7.

46 Luynes, *Mémoires*, 13:72.

47 Madame H...t, *Histoire* (1755), 28, 10, 40, 29.

48 Luynes, *Mémoires*, 13:72; Racine, *Œuvres*, 6:582. Like the author of the *Histoire*, Racine drew uplifting conclusions from Marie-Angélique's faith: "Those who first spoke to her about religion claim that they did not find in her any idea of a Supreme Being, but that it was easy for them to make her understand a Creator, and then a Mediator. Let those who so despise man explain this difference between man and the other animals" (580–1).

49 Monboddo, *Antient Metaphysics*, 4:408.

50 Madame H...t, *Histoire* (1755), 3, 9, 3, 5–7, 21, 20. Racine's version differs somewhat. The girl was first seen one night on top of an apple tree by servants of the castle, and when they tried to catch her she escaped by jumping from tree to tree. The lady of the castle asked for some water and showed her an eel, and thus she was seized, Mlle Leblanc told him. On the wild girl's attempts to escape, see Madame H...t, *Histoire* (1755), 9–10, and Monboddo, *Antient Metaphysics*, 3:80–1. Racine was mystified by her food preferences: "The blood of animals, so forbidden to men after the flood, was her nectar, and perhaps gave her that strength and agility that our ordinary foods made her lose ... She confessed to me that when she saw a child she was tormented by this desire. While she said this, my daughter, still young, was with me; she noticed in her face some emotion caused by the confession of such a temptation, and soon added, laughing, 'Do not fear anything, Mademoiselle, God has completely changed me'"; *Œuvres*, 6:578–9, 581–2.

51 Racine, *Œuvres*, 6:580.

52 Madame H...t, *Histoire* (1755), 14–15; Racine, *Œuvres*, 6:580.

53 Madame H...t, *Histoire* (1755), 17, 30, 32.

54 Ibid., 43, 31–2, 60–2. Madame H...t appended contemporary descriptions of "the Eskimo," including a letter sent her by Me. Duplessis of Sainte Helène, dated 30 October 1751, in which they are portrayed as "Savages among the Savages." They eat raw meat and human beings when they can catch them ("In the past they have eaten many of our compatriots"), seldom light fires, and speak a language that nobody understands. Eskimo girls captured to be used as domestic slaves "are very nice girls, white, neat and very Christian, retaining nothing of the savage." They speak good French but they die soon, and are thus very costly (64–8).

55 Racine, *Œuvres*, 6:577; Monboddo, *Antient Metaphysics*, 4:403–8, and his preface to Madame H...t, *An Account of a Savage Girl*, xv, xiii. See also Monboddo, *Origin and Progress*, 1:480–1, and *Antient Metaphysics*, 4:111.

56 Tinland's preface to Madame H...t, *Histoire* (1970), 11. Tinland also voices his scepticism in footnotes to the text of the *Histoire*, e.g., 75–6n8 and 80n9.

57 Madame H...t, *Histoire* (1755), 33.

58 When in August 1773 Johnson and Boswell visited Monboddo's former clerk Robertson (who had accompanied Monboddo to France) in Cullen, he told them that "he did not believe so much as his lordship did; that it was plain to him, the girl confounded what she imagined with what she remembered: that, besides, she perceived Condamine and Lord Monboddo forming theories, and she adapted her story to them"; Boswell, *The Journal of a Tour to the Hebrides*, 117.

59 Halbwachs, *On Collective Memory*, 37–8 (originally published as *Les cadres sociaux de la mémoire*). Halbwachs found the story in *Magasin pittoresque* (1849). On recent controversies on memory and identity, see Hacking, *Rewriting the Soul*.

60 Tourneux, ed., *Correspondance littéraire*, 2:223–4. Virey (*Histoire naturelle du genre humaine*, 2:305n1) took the description of the wild girl in Madame H...t's *Histoire* as an indication that she was European.

61 Itard, *De l'Éducation*, 3–4 and 4n1; Zingg, "Feral Man" (1940), 494.

62 Rauber, *Homo sapiens ferus*, 41; Douthwaite, "*Homo ferus*," 195–6.

63 Douthwaite, who in "Rewriting the Savage" favoured the view that the wild girl was originally European, reports (in *The Wild Girl*, 230n55) Franck Rolin's findings on Mlle Leblanc's early and later life. A Sioux from the Wisconsin region, the girl was bought in 1712 by a French woman who took her first to Labrador and then (in 1720) to Marseilles. "She escaped in May 1722 and made her way more than 1,000 kilometers north to Châlons, where she was captured." Mlle Leblanc received royal pensions at various points in the 1750s, 1760s, and early 1770s and died in Paris on 15 December 1775 (31).

CHAPTER FOUR

1 On the European myth of the "wild man," see Bernheimer, *Wild Men in the Middle Ages*, Husband, *The Wild Man*, and Bartra, *Wild Men in the Looking Glass*.

2 *Histoire de l'Académie royale des sciences* (1703), 18–19; the story had been reported by M. Felibien of the Académie des inscriptions. On the controversy on innate ideas and the ways in which the opposition between Descartes and Locke was construed and misconstrued by Enlightenment thinkers, see Schøsler, *John Locke et les philosophes français*; on sensationism, see O'Neal, *The Authority of Experience*.

3 La Mettrie, *Histoire naturelle de l'ame*, 378–9, 384, 387–9, and *Traité de l'ame*, in *Œuvres philosophiques*, 204–5.

4 Condillac, *Essai sur l'origine des connaissances humaines*, 198–9, 205, 207; emphasis in the original.

5 Condillac, *Traité des sensations*, 1:5–6, 2:222, 2:256. On the relation between the *Essai* and the *Traité*, see the chapter "Condillac's Speechless Statue" in Aarsleff, *From Locke to Saussure*.

6 Defoe, *Mere Nature Delineated*, 34, 38; Wolff, *Psychologia rationalis*, 378–80. Already in 1706, Bayle had suggested, in *Réponse aux questions d'un provincial*, 943, that the Chartres deaf-mute, himself proof that a man could not arrive at the idea of God by his own reflections, was, in not having received any instruction, equivalent to a child abandoned in a desert place and nurtured by beasts.

7 Condillac, *Traité des sensations*, 2:264, 2:262. Charles Bonnet (1720–1793) revisited the statue in *Essai analytique sur les facultés de l'âme*, while Buffon used a comparable discursive device in the chapter on the senses in the treatise *Histoire naturelle de l'homme*, in *Histoire naturelle*, 3 (1749): 363–70. Enlightenment philosophers called the isolation experiment a "natural experiment," "metaphysical experiment," or "experiment on man." I use Shattuck's term: the forbidden experiment.

8 Herodotus, *History*, 2.2–3, and Salimbene, *Chronicle*, in Coulton, ed., *From St. Francis to Dante*, 242.

9 Bayle, *Réponse aux questions d'un provincial*, 944 (immediately following the story of the deaf-mute of Chartres). According to Samuel Purchas (1577?–1626), Melabdim Echebar, the great Mogor, had thirty children raised in isolation and silence, "purposing to be of that Religion whereto they should addict themselves." But the children never spoke (*Purchas His Pilgrimage*, 40). According to Robert Lindsay of Piscottie (*The Historie and Cronicles of Scotland*, 1:237), another such experiment was conducted by James IV of Scotland (1473–1515), whose isolated children spoke Hebrew. See also Sułek, "The Experiment of Psammetichus."

10 La Mettrie, *Traité de l'âme*, in *Œuvres philosophiques*, 205–7 (see also *Histoire naturelle de l'ame*, 336–8 note a, and Arnobius of Sicca, *The Case against the Pagans*, 1:133–9).

11 Maupertuis, *Lettre sur le progrès des sciences*, 426–30; Formey, "Réunion des principaux moyens employés pour découvrir l'origine du langage, des idées et des connaissances des hommes," in *Anti-Emile*, 211–30 (I quote from page 216); Montesquieu, *Mes pensées*, in *Œuvres complètes*, 967–8. On Maupertuis, Formey, and the Berlin Academy of Sciences, see Aarsleff, *From Locke to Saussure*, and Terrall, *The Man Who Flattened the Earth*. The many fictive representations of "natural education" in the eighteenth century may be seen as disguised enactments of the forbidden experiment – or, for that matter, the alleged life experiences of wild children; see Racault, "Le motif de 'l'enfant de la nature,'" and Durand-Sendrail, "*L'Elève de la nature* de Gaspard Guillard de Beaurieu." Jeremy Bentham (1748–1832) envisaged the "Panopticon" (or "inspection-house") as the perfect site to recreate Psammetichus's experiment; *Panopticon*, 114–15.

12 Landucci, *I filosofi e i selvaggi*, 334–5; Racine, "Epître II sur l'homme," and *Eclaircissement sur la fille sauvage*, in *Œuvres*, 2:123–4 and 6:575.

13 Defoe, *Mere Nature Delineated*, 17; Montesquieu, *De l'esprit des loix*, 1:5; Tourneux, ed., *Correspondance littéraire*, 2:223.

14 Rousseau, *Discourse*, 34, 85n3; emphasis in the original. In another note Rousseau suggested that the great apes, so carelessly depicted by "unsophisticated travelers," might be the natural men, adding that these travellers might have described a silent and stupid creature such as the child found in Lithuania in 1694 as "a very curious beast who looked rather like a man" (98–9n10). On Rousseau's "natural man" see the chapter "The Supposed Primitivism of Rousseau's *Discourse on Inequality*" in Lovejoy, *Essays in the History of Ideas*, and Moran, "Between Primates and Primitives."

15 Tomko's guardian is quoted in Michael Wagner, *Beiträge zur philosophischen Anthropologie*, vol. 1 (1794), cited in Zingg, "Feral Man" (1942), 271; Friedman, "A Historical Note to 'The Wild Boy of Kronstadt,'" 284. The poet Jean-François de La Harpe (1739–1803) evoked Rousseau as well after Victor "played the savage" during his botched visit to Mme Récamier (see below, chapter 5). See Yousef, "Savage or Solitary?" for a reinterpretation of Rousseau's *Discours* in light of later writings on Victor.

16 Buffon, *Histoire naturelle*, 3: 492–3. On Buffon, see Roger, *Buffon*, and the many excellent articles collected in Gayon and Beaune, eds., *Buffon 88*, especially Franck Tinland, "Les limites de l'animalité et de l'humanité selon Buffon et leur pertinence pour l'anthropologie contemporaine," 543–55, and Claude Blanckaert, "La valeur de l'homme: L'idée de nature humaine chez Buffon," 583–600.

17 Buffon, "Les animaux carnassiers," in *Histoire naturelle*, 7 (1758): 26–30. Delisle de Sales, a great admirer of Buffon, asserted that wild children, in whom philosophers wanted to discern natural man, "were probably love children abandoned by wild beasts called parents, and nurtured by other wild beasts called bears." His conclusion: "The state of nature has ... never existed" (*De la Philosophie de la nature*, 1:236–7). The view that children found alone or with animals in the woods were not examples of natural man because man's natural state is a *social* state may also be found in Voltaire, *La Philosophie de l'histoire*, 105–7; Ferguson (1723–1816), *An Essay on the History of Civil Society*, 5–6; Schreber, *Die Saugthiere*, 1:31–7, and Zimmermann (1743–1815), *Zoologie géographique*, 203.

18 Blumenbach, *On the Natural Variety of Mankind*, 3d ed. (1795), and "On the Homo Sapiens *Ferus* Linn." (1811), in *Anthropological Treatises*, 165, 340; Tinland, *L'Homme sauvage*, 58.

19 On eighteenth-century human science, see Tinland, *L'Homme sauvage*; Moravia, *La scienza dell'uomo*, and "The Enlightenment and the Sciences of Man"; Duchet, *Anthropologie et histoire*; Gusdorf, *Dieu, la nature, l'homme*; Fox, Porter, and Wokler, eds., *Inventing Human Science*; P.B. Wood, "The Science of Man"; R. Smith, *The Fontana History of the Human Sciences*.

20 Rousseau, *Discourse*, 85n3; Herder, *Outlines of a Philosophy of the History of Man*, 68–9; Blumenbach, *On the Natural Variety of Mankind*, 1st ed. (1775), in *Anthropological Treatises*, 87–8; Monboddo, *Antient Metaphysics*, 3:74. A century earlier Samuel Butler (1612–1680) had commented on the use of wild children in the debate on man's natural gait: "For some *Philosophers* of late here, / Write, Men have four Legs by *Nature*, / And that 'tis Custom makes them go / Erroneously upon but two; / As 'twas in *Germany* made good, / B' a Boy that lost himself in a Wood, / And growing down t' a Man, was wont / With Wolves upon all four to hunt" (*Hudibras*, 1:322). In the note to this passage (1:322n), Zachary Grey (1688–1766) referred to the boy of Liège, the boy of Hesse, and "the Wild Youth who was found in a Wood near *Hanover*, when the late King was there, and by his order brought into *England* to be humaniz'd."

21 Monboddo, *Antient Metaphysics*, 3:57; *Origin and Progress*, 1:185, and *Antient Metaphysics*, 4:123. See also *Origin and Progress*, 1:184–95, where children, Orang Outangs, deaf-mutes, "savage nations," and wild children are all proffered as evidence that articulation is not natural to man.

22 Voltaire, "Poëme sur la loi naturelle," 2:505, and La Mettrie, *L'Homme machine* (1747), in *Œuvres philosophiques*, 44. During her visit to Versailles, Mlle Leblanc denied that she had eaten her companion, deploring the accusation as "very unjust" (Luynes, *Mémoires*, 13:71).

23 Defoe, *Mere Nature Delineated*, 7.

24 On perfectibility, see Rousseau, *Discours*, and Friedrich Melchior von Grimm's February 1755 article in Tourneux, ed., *Correspondance littéraire*, 2:492–4. See also Tinland, *L'Homme sauvage*, 165–226, and Lotterie, "Les Lumières contre le progrès?"

25 Robinet, *Considérations philosophiques*, 160.

26 Linnaeus, letter to Gmelin, 14 January 1747, cited in E.L. Greene, "Linnaeus as an Evolutionist," 25. In *Anthropomorpha* Linnaeus insisted that "it is difficult to draw any natural distinction" between apes and men: "Many may think that there is a greater difference between the ape and man, than between night and day. But if such persons were to institute a comparison between the greatest heroes of Europe and the Hottentots who live at the Cape of Good Hope, they would find it difficult to believe that they could have had common ancestors: or if they were to compare a noble court lady with a wild man abandoned to himself, they would scarcely guess the two to be of the same species" (*Anthropomorpha*, 65, as translated in Bendyshe, "The History of Anthropology," 449–50). This passage leads to the one on wild children cited above in chapter 2. For Linnaeus, there was an enormous difference between man and beast from the *moral* point of view. On eighteenth-century knowledge about apes, see Montagu, *Edward Tyson*; J.C. Greene, *The Death of Adam*; O'Malley and Magoun, "Early Concepts of the Anthropomorpha"; Wokler, "Tyson and Buffon," and "The Ape Debates"; and Schiebinger, *Nature's Body*.

27 *L'âme matérielle*, 84 (Niderst ascribes this pamphlet to César Chesneau Du Marsais [1676–1756] and dates it before 1734 but after 1720); La Mettrie, *Traité de l'ame*, and *L'Homme machine*, in *Œuvres philosophiques*, 202–3, 28.

28 Monboddo, *Antient Metaphysics*, 3:41; de Pauw, *Recherches philosophiques*, 2:52–3. That all groups of savages discovered by Europeans could speak proved, for de Pauw, that speech is natural to man when he lives with other men and depends much more on the soul than on the vocal organs.

29 On Linnaeus's classification of man, see Bendyshe, "The History of Anthropology," 421–48; Broberg, *Homo Sapiens L.*, and "Homo sapiens"; and Schiebinger, *Nature's Body*. Phillip Sloan compares the anthropologies of Linnaeus and Buffon in "The Gaze of Natural History," in Fox, Porter, and Wokler, eds., *Inventing Human Science*, 112–51.

30 Buffon, "L'asne," in *Histoire naturelle*, 4 (1753): 385, 384; Blumenbach, *Anthropological Treatises*, 150, 152, 129, 340, 294; emphasis in the original.

31 Voltaire, *La Philosophie de l'histoire*, 107. This passage was part of the discussion of savages in which Voltaire denied that wild children represented natural man.

32 Monboddo, preface to Madame H...t, *An Account of a Savage Girl*, xvi–xix. On Monboddo, see Cloyd, *James Burnett, Lord Monboddo*, and Verri, *Lord Monboddo*. Monboddo, like Rousseau, believed both that human history is progres-

sive ("human nature" is the result of a historical process) and that civilization was achieved at a cost (at least some aspects of the state of nature were preferable to it). On this tension, see the chapter "Monboddo and Rousseau" in Lovejoy, *Essays in the History of Ideas*.

33 Monboddo, *Antient Metaphysics*, 3:26–7, *Origin and Progress*, 1:ii, *Antient Metaphysics*, 3:377.

34 Monboddo, *Origin and Progress*, 1:x, *Antient Metaphysics*, 4:62, 4:367, 3:363, 4:22–33; emphasis in the original. Monboddo was keenly taken with Peter, whose life he deemed "a brief chronicle or abstract of the history of the progress of human nature, from the mere animal to the first stage of civilized life." He heralded the wild boy as "one of the greatest curiosities in the world, greater still than the wild girl I saw in France … more extraordinary, I think, than the new planet, or than if we were to discover 30,000 more fixed stars, besides those lately discovered" (*Antient Metaphysics*, 3:57, 62).

35 Samuel Johnson (1709–1784), quoted in Boswell, *The Life of Samuel Johnson*, 1:311; emphasis in the original; Tinker, *Nature's Simple Plan*, 14–15. Because Johnson's comment was registered during a dinner in September 1769, Lovejoy feels the need to indicate that even though Monboddo's theories "were not to be published to the world until four years later," they were "already notorious in the circles in which he moved in Edinburgh and London" ("Monboddo and Rousseau," in *Essays in the History of Ideas*, 40). But Monboddo had spelled out his key theoretical tenets in the 1768 preface to Madame H….t's *Account of a Savage Girl*. He discussed the project to publish a history of man "in which I would propose to trace him through the several stages of his existence" in a letter to James Harris dated 26 March 1766, that is, a year after his meeting with Mlle Leblanc; Knight, ed., *Lord Monboddo*, 50. Monboddo was not a stranger to wit. On Boswell, he said (according to a letter from Dorothea Gregory Alison to Elizabeth Robinson Montagu, dated 16 March 1791): "Before I read his Book I thought he was a Gentleman who had the misfortune to be mad; I now think he is a mad man who has the misfortune not to be a Gentleman"; quoted in McElderry, "Boswell in 1790–91," 268.

36 Monboddo, *Antient Metaphysics*, 3:366–7; Barnard, "*Orang Outang* and the Definition of Man," 108. Barnard relates Monboddo's views to those of twentieth-century scientists such as Raymond Dart, Phillip Tobias, and Richard Leakey. See also Montagu, *Edward Tyson*, 409n67.

37 Herder, *Outlines*, 69, 89; see also 285–6.

38 Immanuel Kant (1724–1804) was intrigued by the wild boy who appeared in Königsberg in 1764 in the company of a so-called "goat prophet." Since he had grown up in the woods and was uncorrupted by education, the boy seemed to Kant a perfect subject for the "experimental moralist" seeking to test Rousseau's hypotheses; "Ueber den Abenteurer Jan Pawlikowicz Zdomozyrskich Komar-

nicki" (1764), in *Sämtliche Werke*, 2:209. Yet another German philosopher who mentioned a wild child (Joseph) was Gottfried Wilhelm Leibniz (1646–1716), in *Nouveaux essais sur l'entendement humain* (written in response to Locke's *Essay* but first published in 1765); see *New Essays*, 316.

39 Defoe, *Mere Nature Delineated*, 61–3. See also Locke, *An Essay Concerning Humane Understanding*.

40 *Philosophical Survey of Nature*, 70–1n; Herder, *Outlines*, 92, 228; Roland, letter to Sophie, 1 August 1774, in *Lettres de Madame Roland*, 1:214–15.

41 Defoe, *Mere Nature Delineated*, 60–1; Herder, *Outlines*, 75. On critical periods, see below, chapter 8.

42 Defoe, *Mere Nature Delineated*, 58–9; Monboddo, *Antient Metaphysics*, 3:65, 373.

43 Monboddo, *Antient Metaphysics*, 4:28, 32–3.

44 Benedict, *Patterns of Culture*, 12–13; Lévi-Strauss, *The Elementary Structures of Kinship*, 4–5; Malson, *Wolf Children*, 9, 36, 8 (*Les enfants sauvages*, 7, 8). Lévi-Strauss replied to Malson's critique of his position on wild children in the revised edition of *Elementary Structures*, xxvii. Like Lévi-Strauss, D.J. Cunningham pictured wild children as "a curious belief entertained in the eighteenth century" definitively dispelled by Blumenbach; "Anthropology in the Eighteenth Century," 24. See the discussion of the dehumanization of wild (isolated) children in Chauchard, *Le langage et la pensée*, 81–6.

45 Kellogg, "Humanizing the Ape," 160; Kellogg and Kellogg, *The Ape and the Child*, 11; Kellogg, "Humanizing the Ape," 168. Kellogg reported on the girls of Midnapore in the *American Journal of Psychology* in 1931 and 1934 (see chapter 7, below). For more on the Kelloggs' experiment, see Desmond, *The Ape's Reflexion*. Twentieth-century researchers endeavouring to teach spoken or sign language to apes often refer to wild children in similar ways. According to the Gardners, who taught sign-language to the chimpanzee Washoe, in cross-fostering "the young of one species are reared by foster parents of another species": "So deep is the belief in the effect of rearing conditions on human behavior that even alleged but unverified cases of cross-fostering such as the wolf children of India ... and the monkey boy of Burundi ... attract serious scholarly attention. For obvious ethical reasons it is unlikely that we shall see any experimental account of a human child reared by nonhuman foster parents. But in the twentieth century, the Kelloggs with Gua and the Hayeses with Viki pioneered the logical alternative, a form of cross-fostering in which the subjects are chimpanzees and the foster parents are human beings" (Gardner and Gardner, "Cross-Fostered Chimpanzees," 220). Young used wild and isolated children and the Gua-Donald experiment as evidence that "human nature is the product of society and culture" (*Sociology*, 2–15; I quote from page 2). Wild children and apes are brought together in arguments concerning the difficul-

ties intrinsic to scientific attempts to demarcate human beings and animals in Horigan, *Nature and Culture in Western Discourses*, and Candland, *Feral Children and Clever Animals*.

46 Zingg, "Feral Man and Extreme Cases of Isolation," 504; Stark, *The Social Bond*, 103–4; Giddens, *Sociology*, 60. Not all twentieth-century human scientists dismissed the forbidden experiment as inherently unethical. Clarence Leuba, professor of psychology at Antioch College, berated "public opinion" for refusing to allow scientists "to let a few typical human beings grow up together from earliest infancy completely separated from any traditions, schooling, or other cultural influences" in order to learn about "the natural man out of which all civilizations develop." A few "unwanted or abandoned children, perhaps in some famine-striken section of the world," could be taken to "an isolated tropical island" and monitored from "observation towers connected by tunnels." Although "democratically trained people justly recoil at the thought of exploiting one human group for the benefit of another," they should not object to "the human, scientific use of a relatively tiny group of people for the benefit of all the peoples in the world." In the meantime, Leuba examined "indirect sources of information": wild children, apes, and primitive peoples (*The Natural Man*, 2–3, 6–12).

CHAPTER FIVE

1 "The Savage," in Lewis, ed., *Miscellaneous Poems*, 305.
2 See Hacking, "Normal People."
3 The reconstructed dossier is presented and analyzed in Moravia, *La scienza dell'uomo*; Gayral, Chabbert, and Baillaud-Citeau, "Les premières observations"; Bernard, ed., "Autour du Sauvage de l'Aveyron," and "Un dossier sur Victor"; Lane, *The Wild Boy*; Soda, "Biography of the Wild Child"; Shattuck, *The Forbidden Experiment*; Gineste's many articles and his *Victor*; and Chappey, *La Société des Observateurs*. While some authors, like Gineste and Shattuck, for the most part specify what is documented fact and what is personal conjecture in their accounts, Lane sprinkles his narrative with imaginative embellishments that are not identified as such, e.g., the supposed first meeting between Itard and the wild boy in the Luxembourg Gardens, which opens *The Wild Boy*. Gineste's scathing criticism of Lane's book is nevertheless directed not at its historical inaccuracies but at its interpretation of the story's scientific and practical significance; Gineste's review thus exemplifies the territorial controversies to which the story gives rise; see Gineste, "A propos de *L'enfant sauvage de l'Aveyron*." Dates in the French Republican calendar have been converted to their Gregorian equivalents.

4 See Gusdorf, *La conscience révolutionnaire*; Staum, *Minerva's Message*; Chappey, *La Société des Observateurs*; Goldstein, *Console and Classify*; Weiner, *The Citizen-Patient*; Swain, "Une logique de l'inclusion: les infirmes du signe" (1982), in *Dialogue avec l'insensé*, 111–30; Lane, *When the Mind Hears*; Rosenfeld, *A Revolution in Language*.

5 Paul Foulquier-Lavergne, *Le sauvage de l'Aveyron*, in *L'enfant sauvage de l'Aveyron*, 126. Barring this instance, the wild boy, like Peter and unlike Marie-Angélique, was recognized (or imagined) as the child of "a father and mother like one of us."

6 One version is that the widow mistreated him from fear that he would set her house on fire: he was beginning to imitate others, and "seeing that his teacher used straw to light the fire, heat being very agreeable to him, he set fire to the attic with straws just to warm himself"; see Marie-Jacques-Philippe Mouton-Fontenille, "Notice sur le Sauvage du Dt. de l'Aveiron" (August 1800), reprinted in Gineste, *Victor*, 214.

7 Guiraud to Randon, 2 February 1800, in Gineste, *Victor*, 121; Virey, *Histoire naturelle*, 2:329–30. See also Ritson, *An Essay on Abstinence*, 192. The wild boy's food preferences and eating habits occupy a central place in all the accounts, both because the observers privileged food and eating as distinctive markers of the boundary between savagery and civilization and because the boy himself was exceedingly concerned with them.

8 Foulquier-Lavergne, *Le sauvage*, in *L'enfant sauvage*, 127.

9 Guiraud's report is reprinted in Gayral et al., "Les premières observations," 467–9.

10 On 10 January, in a letter to the administrators of the Saint-Affrique hospice, Constans had written that "now that he is somewhat civilized" he eats baked potatoes, while "right after he was found" he used to eat raw potatoes and roots; in Gineste, *Victor*, 114. Is this a hint that Constans was aware that what had taken place at the tanner Vidal's was not strictly a discovery but the latest (and decisive) episode in a more complex history of recent relations with the local people?

11 Constans to Randon, 31 January 1800, and to the administrators of the Saint-Affrique hospice, 10 January 1800, in Gineste, *Victor*, 117–20, 113–14. On Jacques-Jean Constans-Saint-Estève (1757–1833), see Foulquier-Lavergne, "Étude historique et statistique," 187–8, and Affre, *Biographie Aveyronnaise*, 125–6. According to Foulquier-Lavergne (*Le sauvage*, in *L'enfant sauvage*, 130, 135), when in his old age Constans recalled the episode in casual conversation, he became animated, manifesting a singular emotion and compassion towards the wild boy. He "had never been able to forget the first intelligent look the child cast at him, with an ineffable expression." Congratulating himself on having brought him to the scientists' attention and saved him from the dangers and anguish of

a condition so opposed to human well-being, Constans nevertheless regretted not having solved the mystery of his origin: "He had traveled, he said, up and down the region of the forest of La Bassine. He had visited the cottages and the castles in the neighbourhood. He had spoken to the eminent men of Lacaune and Pierre-Ségade to find out the first traces of the child and the date of his abandonment," all in vain.

12 Nougairoles to the editor of *Journal des Débats*, 11 January 1800; D. Bourgoug-non to the Municipal Administration of Toulouse (the author wanted to pub-licize the story to see if the boy's family could be found), in *Clef du Cabinet*, 30 January; Guiraud to Randon, 2 February, all in Gineste, *Victor*, 114–15, 127–8, 121–3.

13 Itard to the prefect of Aveyron, 9 June 1801, and the prefect of Aveyron to Itard, in Gineste, *Victor*, 267–8, 268–70. Bonnaterre mentioned the rumour that the boy was the legitimate son of D... N..., of M..., abandoned six years earlier by "inhumane parents" because "he was deprived of speech" (*Notice historique*, 198). The prefect told Itard that since then Constans had found out that this rumour had no basis.

14 Randon to the central commissioner of Tarn, 13 February 1800, in Gineste, *Victor*, 125–6.

15 Guiraud to Randon, 2 February 1800, in Gineste, *Victor*, 121–2; Bonnaterre, *Notice historique*, 199; Foulquier-Lavergne, *Le sauvage*, in *L'enfant sauvage*, 133. Virey devoted a long and melodramatic note to the boy's scar, the dire conse-quences of society's notion of honour, and marriages of convenience (*Histoire naturelle*, 2:311–4n3).

16 Nougairoles to *Journal des Débats*, 11 January 1800 (printed on 25 January together with Constans's 10 January letter cited above and reprinted in other newspapers and journals), and Randon to Constans and Guiraud, 23 January, in Gineste, *Victor*, 114–15, 116–17.

17 Randon to Guiraud, 5 February 1800, and to Constans, 5 February, in Gineste, *Victor*, 470, 124–5.

18 L. Bonaparte to the central administration of Rodez, 1 February 1800, and the central administration of Rodez to Bonaparte, 14 February, in Gineste, *Victor*, 130, 131–2.

19 Sainthorent to Bonaparte, 7 June 1800, in Gineste, *Victor*, 135–6. Sainthorent's claim that the boy did not have a name is significant since, according to Virey (*Histoire naturelle*, 2:301), he had already been christened Joseph – which Virey thought "quite singular," that also being the name given to the Lithuanian savage found with bears in 1657, mentioned by Rzaczynski. An article in *Jour-nal de l'Aveyron*, 12 July 1843, stated that, when the boy was conditionally bap-tized in mid-March 1800, Sainthorent gave him a gown and Melle Bonnaterre made him "a bonnet and 'a shirt *à colorette* and cuffs'" (Gineste, *Victor*, 49n69).

20 Jean-Antoine Chaptal to the administrators of the Institute, 6 October 1802; the administrators of welfare institutions to the minister of the interior, Montalivet, 13 July 1810, and the administrators of welfare institutions to Mme Guérin, 5 April 1811, all in Bernard, "Un dossier," 47, 58, 65. This phenomenon must be related not only to the crowds, curiosity seekers, and visitors mentioned in other stories of wild children but also to the regular public demonstrations by educated deaf-mutes at the Institute, initiated by the abbé de l'Épée and continued with great success by Sicard. On spectacle in early modern human science, see Christopher Fox, "How to Prepare a Noble Savage: The Spectacle of Human Science," in Fox, Porter, and Wokler, eds., *Inventing Human Science*, 1–30.

21 Bonnaterre to Sainthorent, 2 September 1800, and article in *Publiciste*, 2 September, in Gineste, *Victor*, 145–6, 477; "Souvenirs d'une dame du palais impérial," in Wairy, *Mémoires de Constant*, 3:48–51. Among the guests who shared the table with Victor and Itard at Mme Récamier's were Degérando, his friends Mathieu de Montmorency and Camille Jordan, and the astronomer Joseph-Jérôme de Lalande.

22 R. Vaysse to the editor of *Journal de Paris*, 23 May 1800, in Gineste, *Victor*, 473–5.

23 Lemaistre, *A Rough Sketch of Modern Paris*, 115 (dated 17 January 1802); Warren, *The Journal of a British Chaplain*, 147–8 (dated 31 December 1801). Besides summarizing Itard's "interesting little pamphlet" and noting that the doctor-teacher assured him "that he entertained no doubt of his ultimate speaking," Lemaistre rapturously described Sicard's remarkable achievements and those of his star pupil Massieu: "Of all which I have yet beheld at Paris, this is to me the most interesting sight. Other objects strike the imagination, but this moves the heart" (114, 73). Warren was less enthusiastic: "I was not pleased at the appearance and contrivance in the exhibition. It lessened the effect. I could not help thinking that the pupil whose acquirements were displayed was particularly prepared to deliver his answers" (145). See also the account of Victor and of Sicard's "curious and delightful" demonstrations in Wilmot, *An Irish Peer on the Continent*, 71 (dated 19 June 1802).

24 Feydel's articles and the letters they inspired, printed in *Journal de Paris* from August to early November 1800, are in Bernard, "Autour du Sauvage," 84–9, and in Gineste, *Victor*, 146–80. Vaysse contributed several letters insisting that the boy was a true savage with "all the attributes and all the habits of the state of nature" (13 August). The witness who claimed that the boy was an imbecile signed "M...n, octogenarian" (24 October). Feydel (who, it seems, never even bothered to visit the wild boy) lost the bet.

25 "Romance du Sauvage de l'Aveyron," reprinted in *L'enfant sauvage*, 48 (a manuscript note in the copy held at the Société des lettres de l'Aveyron attributes it to Pierre-Jean Bonnet de Jalenque [1741–1812]); Robinson, "The Savage of Avey-

ron," in *The Poetical Works*, 2:2, 8; reviews of *Le Sauvage de l'Aveyron ou il ne faut jurer de rien* in *Journal de Paris*, 30 March 1800, in Gineste, *Victor*, 133–4, and in *Magasin encyclopédique* 5th year, vol. 6, no. 23 (March–April 1800): 417–18; Rousseau, *Du contract social*, 36. Samuel Taylor Coleridge (1772–1834), a friend of Robinson's, wrote in his notebooks that the "Savage Boy of Aveyron in Itard's account" might be a "fine subject" for Wordsworth's poetry because of "his restless joy and blind conjunction of his Being with natural Scenery; and the manifest influence of Mountain, Rocks, Waterfalls, Torrents, & Thunderstorms – Moonlight Beams quivering on Water, &c on his whole frame – as instanced in his Behavior in the Vale of Montmorency – his eager desires to escape, &c." Coleridge saw the wild boy (who "seems clearly a *man* / & his conduct nearer derangement than absolute Imbrutement") as both a subject for poetry and an object of science: "How deserving this whole account of a profound psychological examination / & comparison with wild animals in confinement" (*The Notebooks*, vol. 3, note 3,538; see also vol. 1, note 1,348). The Aveyronnais R.J. Vaysse de Villiers (1767–1834), who had defended the boy's valuable wildness in the press, wrote the comedy *Le Sauvage de l'Aveyron*, appended to the 1806 Rodez edition of Bonnaterre's *Notice historique* (Vaysse had the boy recover both speech and his parents). At the public meeting of the Société d'agriculture et des arts of Boulogne-sur-Mer held on 28 April 1802, Citizen Wyant read an "Epître en vers au Sauvage de l'Aveyron"; *Magasin encyclopédique* 8th year, vol. 2, no. 3 (1802): 379. Gineste (*Victor*, 39) sees the origin of the name Itard gave the wild boy in the huge success of a play by Guibert de Pixérécourt staged around the time of the boy's arrival in Paris. The play was based on the popular novel by Ducray-Duminil, *Victor, ou L'enfant de la forêt*. For more literary references to the wild boy, see Bernard, *Surdité, surdi-mutité et mutisme*, 179–82.

26 Bonnaterre, *Notice historique*, 181, 183, 198–9, 206–7, 209, 202. The *Notice historique*, completed in Rodez, was published in Paris in September 1800. Bonnaterre worked in Paris with Daubenton on the *Encyclopédie méthodique ou par ordre de matières* from 1788 to 1792. During the Terror he returned to Aveyron, where he was later appointed professor at the Central School (founded in 1796); see Affre, *Biographie Aveyronnaise*, 63–5.

27 Bonnaterre, *Notice historique*, 207–9, 203–4. The trip lasted from 20 July to 6 August. During a stop at Lyon the boy was examined by Mouton-Fontenille (1769–1837), professor of natural history at the Central School, who restated that "in external appearance [this child] does not differ from an ordinary child at all" and rendered his character as "a mixture of intelligence and imbecility, vivacity and inaction, joy and sorrow, whose cause it would be very difficult to guess." He registered the boy's obsession with food ("I have seen him laugh on seeing the many foods offered him and become angry if anyone tried to

take them away") and escape (three attempts while at Lyon); in Gineste, *Victor*, 212–15. See also Girard, "L'histoire véridique," 361–7.

28 Bonnaterre, *Notice historique*, 202–3, 211.

29 See Gayral et al., "Les premières observations," 485; Soda, "Biography," 43, and Gineste, *Victor*, 27.

30 A letter published on 4 February 1865 in the *Napoléonien de l'Aveyron*, denouncing Bonnaterre's cruelty and accusing him of exhibiting the boy "like a bizarre beast in Paris, where he died, pining for his forests and the old oaks of La Caune," instigated an inquiry in which the Société des lettres, sciences et arts de l'Aveyron undertook Bonnaterre's defence while some old citizens testified that the boy had been exposed in chains in the streets of Rodez: "To eat, he was given the livers of cattle and other coarse meats. He was small, with frizzy hair and enormously long nails"; quoted in *L'enfant sauvage*, 51–2.

31 Jauffret to the administrators of the Saint-Affrique hospice, 29 January 1800; Jauffret to the editors of *Journal de Paris*, 26 February; Vaysse to the editors of *Journal de Paris*, 29 February, all in Gineste, *Victor*, 129, 471–2. Besides directing the Institute for Deaf-Mutes since 1790, the abbé Roch-Ambroise Cucurron (1742–1822), known by his mother's maiden name, Sicard, had taught the grammar course at the short-lived Normal School and was a founding member of the Society of Observers of Man. He came very close to being executed during the Revolution for his religious convictions. While in "La crèche ou le tombeau" Gineste contended that the attention directed at the wild boy in January 1800 was part of a conspiracy orchestrated by Constans to reinstate his old friend Sicard at the head of the Institute, Chappey proposes that the very creation of the Observers was a "coup de force" by Sicard and Jauffret to profit from the discovery of the boy (*La Société des Observateurs*, 31).

32 *Gazette de France*, 9 August 1800, in Gineste, *Victor*, 142–4. This article, which may have been written by Sicard himself, was reprinted widely in the Parisian press.

33 Virey's "Dissertation, Sur un jeune Enfant trouvé dans les forêts du département de l'Aveyron, comparé aux sauvages trouvés en Europe à diverses époques, avec des remarques sur l'état primitif de l'Homme" is in *Histoire naturelle*, 2:289–350 (I quote from pages 290, 315, 320). On Virey, see Benichou and Blanckaert, eds., *Julien-Joseph Virey*.

34 Virey, *Histoire naturelle*, 2:297, 332, 347–9. For Virey, the savage of Aveyron, like the wild girl of Champagne, was French and had not "crossed the seas" or "come out of the forests of Africa" (2:305n1).

35 "Réflexions sur le *Sauvage de l'Aveyron*," 13, 16, 18, 9; emphasis in the original. This article has been attributed to Virey (Gineste) or Pierre-Charles Lévesque (1736–1812); see Régaldo, *Un milieu intellectuel*, 230.

36 Pinel, "Rapport fait à la Société des Observateurs de l'homme," 383–98 and 441–54; *Mercure de France*, 5 June 1801, in Gineste, *Victor*, 485. Pinel's report has been reprinted several times (e.g., by Gineste in *Victor* and by Copans and Jamin in *Aux origines de l'anthropologie française*), and translated into English by Lane in *The Wild Boy*. Yet Humphrey believed it was lost, and as recently as 1993 Candland stated (on Humphrey's authority) that it "remains missing"; see Humphrey, "Introduction," vii; Candland, *Feral Children and Clever Animals*, 373n20. As Shattuck puts it, Pinel's observations "do not always ring true" (*The Forbidden Experiment*, 33). They often contradict the prior accounts, e.g., Pinel claims ("Rapport," 443) that the boy revealed "a great deal of clumsiness in his manner of seizing various foods with his hand" and that he "defecates even in his bed." Moreover, as I noted in chapter 2, time erodes the reliability of any evidence in stories of wild children. Girard, in "L'histoire véridique," 365, maintains that, for us, Pinel's observations of idiots are as inadequate and incomplete as Bonnaterre's accounts of savages were for Pinel. See also Lane, *The Wild Boy*, 172.

37 "Aux Rédacteurs de la Décade Philosophique," *Décade philosophique* 30, no. 32 (August 1801): 312–13. The editors added that they had lately seen the child, who uttered only meaningless cries but recognized his caretakers and showed "a certain preference for a young lady, the daughter of one of our leading astronomers," whom he sometimes met in his walks in the gardens of the Observatory: "He obeys her almost the way a dog obeys his master: it is an attachment mixed with fear. Does she signal him to sit down next to her? He comes running. But soon distracted by another object, he gets up, and it requires a struggle to make him stay there" (313).

38 Hervé, "Le sauvage de l'Aveyron," 389–90; Itard to the *Mercure de France*, 20 June 1801, in Gineste, *Victor*, 278–9. Itard's first report, *De l'Éducation d'un homme sauvage*, was translated as *An historical account of the discovery and education of A SAVAGE MAN, or of the first developments, physical and moral, of THE YOUNG SAVAGE caught in the woods near Aveyron, in the year 1798* (London: Richard Phillips, 1802). It was reprinted together with Itard's 1806 report (see below) as *Rapports et mémoire sur le sauvage de l'Aveyron, l'idiotie et la surdi-mutité*, ed. D.M. Bourneville (Paris: Alcan, 1894), and more recently by Malson in *Les enfants sauvages* and by Gineste in *Victor*. Itard's biography remains to be written. For the mainstream version, see Groff, "Jean Marc Gaspard Itard." Gineste presents his research on Itard's life in *Victor* (but see below, chapter 6, on the shortcomings of his interpretation).

39 Itard, *De l'Éducation*, 1, 5–6; emphasis in the original. As mentioned in chapter 4, the epigraph to *De l'Éducation* was Condillac's (indeed Fontenelle's) "The greatest source of ideas among men is in their dealings with each other."

40 Itard, *De l'Éducation*, 21–2, 6. On the relation between Itard's work and Pinel's moral treatment of the insane, see Rose, *The Psychological Complex*, 23–30. It is simplistic and historically inaccurate to reduce the disagreement between Itard and Pinel to an opposition between competing theories of the role of heredity and environment, between "essentialism" ("biologism") and "relativism" ("culturalism") or between "naturalists" and "artificialists"; see Humphrey, "Introduction," xv; Métraux, "Victor de l'Aveyron"; Leary, "Nature, Art, and Imitation." Lane singles out Itard's adherence to Condillac's philosophy: "Because Itard believed in Condillac's analysis of the origin of human knowledge, he was thoroughly opposed to the prevailing explanation of the wild boy's inabilities" (*The Wild Boy*, 73). Yet not only Itard but also Pinel and Sicard were followers of Condillac. Furthermore, Itard accepted Pinel's medical views, and both Pinel and Sicard backed Itard's endeavour. In a postscript to Itard's letter to the prefect of Aveyron, 9 June 1801, Sicard observed that the prefect would certainly hasten to fulfill "this request so important to the perfectibility of our species ... for the glory he will thus have by aiding the progress of human knowledge" (in Gineste, *Victor*, 268).

41 Itard, *De l'Éducation*, 95n1, 10, 98–9; emphasis in the original. Itard recognized that the boy had *regressed* in his first months at the Institute for Deaf-Mutes: "A sudden change in his way of life, the frequent pestering of curious people, some bad treatment, the inevitable effect of cohabitation with children his own age, seemed to have extinguished all hope of civilizing him. His petulant activity had insensibly degenerated into a dull apathy that had produced even more solitary habits" (22–3).

42 Ibid., 25–7, 36, 49–50. More examples of Victor's pleasure in nature: when the light of the full moon penetrated into his room, "he rarely failed to waken and place himself before the window," and according to Mme Guérin he stayed there for a long time in a "contemplative ecstasy" (27); when Itard took the boy to Montmorency, "it was a most curious sight, and I dare say most touching, to see the joy painted in his eyes, in all the movements and the attitude of his body, at the sight of the little hills and woods of that laughing valley" (46); Coleridge was struck by this passage, as noted above. Interestingly, upon his return to the Institute in January 1800 Sicard had implemented a strict disciplinary regime in which the punishment for a student found in the garden alone was dismissal; see Weiner, *The Citizen-Patient*, 238.

43 Degérando's report was published posthumously as "Considérations sur le sauvage de l'Aveyron," *Annales de l'éducation des sourds-muets et des aveugles* 5 (1848): 110–18; reprinted in Gineste, *Victor*, 324–30. Despite his enthusiasm, Degérando did not entirely discard the hypothesis of organic lesion or damage, and Lévesque (secretary of the class) held on to the less positive alternative: "If one discovers that he is an imbecile, then one could suspect that he did not live

long in the forests; he would be an idiot escaped from the hands that deigned to care for him. Those who had sustained his useless existence would not have reclaimed him once they learned he was receiving assistance" (Lévesque, "Notice des travaux," 257).

44 "Rapport fait au Ministre (et rédigé par le C^en Sicard) de l'examen du Sauvage de l'Aveyron quant à ses facultés intellectuelles avec prière au Ministre d'ordonner que l'essai de son éducation soit encore prolongé, d'après l'espoir qu'a fait concevoir ledit examen, cijoint deux notices du C^en Itard, Médecin, chargé de l'éducation physique et morale de cet enfant," in Bernard, "Un dossier," 43–6. Among the tasks Victor performed for the examiners (and not mentioned in Itard's published reports) were threading a needle and sewing a few stitches. The extant correspondence makes reference to several manuscript reports by Itard that have not been found.

45 Itard, "Vésanies," 598, 600, 603–5; emphasis in the original. Many later writers, echoing Lane, faulted Itard for not using sign language to instruct Victor once he realized that the boy's difficulties with articulation could not be overcome. This text invalidates this criticism. The manuscript was discovered by Gineste, who dates it between 1801 and 1805, and most likely 1802. See also Gineste, "Les écrits psychiatriques." Itard's examples of the effects of social deprivation were the earlier wild children. He was perplexed by the fact that Mlle Leblanc was caught and "tamed" at the time when (and, he says, even in the same village where) Condillac worked on his treatises on sensations and the origin of ideas, and yet he seemingly did not care to observe her, since he did not mention her in his works.

46 Chaptal to the Administration of Welfare Institutions, 2 May and 20 June 1804, and the administrators to Chaptal, 21 July, in Bernard, "Un dossier," 47–50.

47 Itard, *Rapport*, 12. Champagny's letter to Itard, 13 June 1806, is reprinted on pages 1–2.

48 Ibid., 83–4. If one had "dared to unveil to this young man the secret of his restlessness and the aim of his desires, one would have derived from it an incalculable advantage." But Itard did not attempt the experiment, fearing the consequences of "making known to our Savage a need which he would have sought to satisfy as freely and publicly as the others, and which would have led him to acts of revolting indecency!" (87–8).

49 Ibid., 91. See Gineste, *Victor*, 42–3, for Itard's subsequent attempts to apply what he learned in his work with Victor to the physical and moral education of other small groups of deaf children. Gineste ("Jean Marc Gaspard Itard," 66–7) offers a psychological/symbolic explanation for Itard's loss of interest in Victor: for Itard, the only survivor of five siblings, working with Victor was a mourning offering to his mother for the children she had lost (the inconsolable mother being unconsciously close to the mother as unforgivable murderer of

her children). After his mother's death in 1805, the offering became useless. Kincaid, who addresses the relationship between Victor and Itard in the context of the sexualization of children in the last two hundred years, maintains that the "love story" ended when Victor grew up and "ceased to be mesmerizing" (*Erotic Innocence*, 62).

50 Itard, *Rapport*, 13, 14; Dacier, permanent secretary of the Class of History and Ancient Literature of the National Institute, to Champagny, 19 November 1806, and Champagny to Itard, 26 November, in Itard, *Rapport*, 7–9, 5–6. Following Napoleon's restructuring of the National Institute in 1803, the second class was eliminated and many of its members (including Degérando) were transferred to the third class.

51 Alphonse Leroy (1742–1816), professor of medicine at the School of Medicine of Paris and author of *Médecine maternelle*, to whom Itard had sent a copy of the report, enthusiastically affirmed that Itard's wise observations might contribute to the creation of "a method for the development of the intellectual faculties," a "new science" whose importance for "the happiness of the human species" could not be overemphasized; see Alphonse Leroy, "Réflexions sur le rapport," 518.

52 The Administrators of welfare institutions to Montalivet, 13 July 1810, in Bernard, "Un dossier," 56–60. The letter retraced the boy's stay at the Institute, intimating that Chaptal might have been right in believing that his proper place was the hospice. The background information was gathered in a report dated 15 June 1810; in Bernard, "Un dossier," 51–5. About Victor's present the report said that "in growing up he slowly returned to his earlier brutish state: because, what is surprising, after his first success, he has not yet acquired the idea, not even by imitation, he is unable to turn a tap to fill the pitcher with which he comes to get water; he waits, with a stupid look, for someone to come and turn the tap" (52).

53 The prefect of Drôme to Montalivet, 26 June 1811; Montalivet to the Administration of deaf-mutes, 13 July, and the Administration of Welfare Institutions (Sicard, M. Montmorency, Demeunier, Malus, Garnier) to Montalivet, 26 July, all in Gineste, "Post-scriptum à l'immaculée conception," 130–7. The young man was arrested in Valence, but when it was ascertained that he was not pretending and had no known relatives, he was freed and placed in the hospice. The prefect would prefer that he enter a public institution for deaf-mutes to be educated (133). On 20 August, Montalivet conveyed the administrators' verdict to the prefect: "We have an example of the meagre success one could expect on this occasion in a poor wretch of the same class found several years ago in the forests of Aveyron, and who, brought to the Institution where he received all kinds of help, did not benefit from it at all" (137).

54 Saint-Simon, *Mémoire sur la science de l'homme* (1813), 119, 127. Written when Saint-Simon was recovering from a breakdown and in dire poverty, the *Mémoire* was not published until 1858. Saint-Simon's account was not very accurate. According to him, Sicard, "better versed in theology than in physiology," was disturbed by the boy's ignorance of God and religion and for that reason neglected and mistreated him (121–2). Itard, to whom Saint-Simon sent a copy of the manuscript, denied these claims and asked him to withdraw them; see Manuel, *The New World of Henri Saint-Simon*, 390n22.

55 Gall and Spurzheim, *Anatomie et physiologie*, vol. 2 (1812): 41–4. Their description of Victor's behaviour was not too distant from Itard's except in tone: "We have not been able to convince ourselves that he can hear; no one could get his attention in our presence either by calling him or by striking a glass behind his ears. He has a quiet character; his attitude and way of sitting down are correct; one notices only that he rocks his trunk and head back and forth incessantly; he greets people who arrive by bowing slightly, and is visibly pleased when they depart ... He knows a few written characters, and even indicates the objects these characters designate. Besides, his favourite occupation is to restore objects to their proper places when they have been disarranged" (2:42–3). Gall and Spurzheim theorized what would later be called phrenology.

56 Virey, "Homme sauvage," 269.

57 Itard, *De l'Éducation*, 9. At Bonnaterre's suggestion, Lucien Bonaparte granted Clair two hundred francs in recognition of his good care of the wild boy. Some observers took the boy's seeming lack of concern at his separation from Clair (as earlier from the woman who cooked for him in Rodez) as a sure sign of his unresponsiveness and self-centredness. But how could he have *expressed* that concern, and to whom? It is however a well-attested fact that in his first few months at the Institute he grew increasingly unhappy.

58 Itard, *De l'Éducation*, 64–5. Another of Victor's words, the exclamation "*oh Dieu!*," "which he lets escape frequently in moments of great joy," was directly lifted from Mme Guérin (65–6).

59 The Administrators of Welfare Institutions to Mme Guérin, 5 April 1811, in Bernard, "Un dossier," 64–6. Not only must Victor not be exposed to curious people but also, since the measures adopted ensured that all his needs would be covered, "the public's pity need not be concerned with him." If Mme Guérin lapsed from her obligations he would be "taken away from you immediately and placed in a hospice for indigents." On 2 May, the widow accepted her new duties under the conditions prescribed by the authorities, only asking that "the child known as the Savage of Aveyron" be allowed to keep his bed and clothing. On 10 July she acknowledged receipt of an old oak bed with bars, a straw

mattress, a mattress, a bolster, and a woollen blanket, to be returned when his charge no longer lived with her; Bernard, "Un dossier," 66–7.

60 The Administrators of welfare institutions to Montalivet, 13 July 1810, and Itard's report to the Administration, 8 July 1825, in Bernard, "Un dossier," 59, 67–8.

61 Shattuck, *The Forbidden Experiment*, 53–5; François Truffaut, in Flatley, "So Truffaut Decided"; emphasis in the original.

62 Itard, *Rapport*, 45–6.

63 Itard, "Vésanies," 606. For a contemporary description of the department of Aveyron noting its backwardness and "savagery," see Monteil, *Description de l'Aveyron*; see also the reviews of this work in *Décade philosophique* 33, no. 26 (June 1802): 481–4 and *Magasin encyclopédique* 8th year, vol. 3, no. 12 (October–November 1802): 557–9. On the perception of French peasants as savages and the attempts to "civilize" them that were part of the project of nation-formation in this period, see de Certeau, Julia, and Revel, *Une politique de la langue*; Weber, *Peasants into Frenchmen*; and Bourdieu, *Language and Symbolic Power*. Recent accounts of the wild boy of Aveyron have raised the question of his relationship with the peasants; see Soda, "Biography," 128; Shattuck, *The Forbidden Experiment*, 18; and *L'enfant sauvage*, 46.

64 The catalogue of the exhibition, *L'enfant sauvage*, offers a balanced presentation of the story, which privileges the documents originating in Aveyron and takes into account different points of view, including the boy's, and essays – by Gineste, child psychiatrist Annette Delbès, Alain Hirt (inspector of National Education), and psychiatrist André Gassiot – that reproduce various scientific/professional appropriations of the story. For local histories that include accounts of the wild boy, see Maldinier, *Lacaune-les-Bains*; Plancke, *La vie quotidienne*; and Bedel, *Sent-Sarnin*.

65 The testimonies are reproduced (in Occitan, the language of the region) in Bedel, *Sent-Sarnin*, 103, and also (in Occitan and French translation) in *L'enfant sauvage*, 52–3, and Plancke, *La vie quotidienne*, 83.

CHAPTER SIX

1 Lieberman, "Itard," 566.

2 Esquirol, "Idiotisme," 510–11, and *Des Maladies mentales*, 2:375, 333; Jean-Baptiste Bousquet, "Eloge historique de M. Itard, lu dans la séance publique annuelle de l'Académie royale de médecine, du 1er décembre 1839," in Itard, *Traité des maladies de l'oreille*, 1:xvi.

3 Delasiauve, "Le sauvage de l'Aveyron," 209–10. Delausiave's article was partly motivated by Dr Mesnet's account of the "savage of Var" (thirty-nine-year-old Laurent L...), who, unlike the wild children, had full use of his faculties and

voluntarily pursued isolation, self-sufficiency, and a natural existence; Dela-siauve, "Le sauvage du Var." Bory de Saint-Vincent agreed that the Savage of Aveyron was "a true idiot, dirty and disgusting" but he saw no reason to praise Itard: "In our day people tormented by the obsession to write want to make [him] famous to become famous themselves" (*L'Homme*, 1:59).

4 Séguin, *Traitement Moral*, 4–10, and "Origin of the Treatment and Training." See also Lane, *The Wild Boy*, 257–80.

5 The entrenchment of the story of Victor and Itard took place in Europe and North America in the context of the growth, diversification, and institutional-ization of the human sciences; the rise of statistics and professional expertise grounded on the organizing concept of normalcy; the anthropological preoc-cupation with race and its relation to the medical and psychiatric concern with degeneracy, and the gradual expansion of schooling; see Hacking, *The Taming of Chance*, and Rose, *The Psychological Complex*. With regard to "idiocy," the nineteenth century witnessed two tendencies: from the 1840s on, the medico-philanthropic movement to educate idiots (led by Séguin) as an attempt to recuperate them for humanity; a little later, the institutionalization of the men-tally defective as a means to protect society from the danger they were believed to pose. By the end of the century, rising intolerance and fear found an outlet in eugenic ideas and policies; see Kanner, *A History*, and Trent, *Inventing the Feeble Mind*.

6 Ireland, *The Mental Affections of Children*, 419–20; Barr, *Mental Defectives*, 28; and Pichot, "French Pioneers," 130. Ireland was medical superintendent of the Scottish Institution for the Education of Imbecile Children and medical officer of Miss Mary Murray's Institution for Girls at Preston. Barr, chief physician of the Pennsylvania Training School for Feeble-Minded Children, elaborately in-scribed Victor into the history of idiocy (*Mental Defectives*, 30–1): "The savage of Aveyron might be likened to a guide-post reading two ways. Standing at the beginning of the nineteenth century, a literal symbol of the parting of ways for his caste, in this uncouth figure is represented all the cruelty of the past and the beneficent influences of a new era. The last of those of whom history or tradi-tion speaks as, either through neglect or through wilful desertion, driven from the haunts of men; he is also the first example recorded of an idiot reclaimed from the life of a mere animal to be trained to a human existence." Similar appraisals may be found in texts by special educators. For Eugene E. Doll (who taught special education at the University of Tennessee), "the combination of scientific sagacity, affectionate humanism, and practical resourcefulness with which Itard labored over his '*sauvage*' for five years makes epic reading." Although mistaken ("Victor was, indeed, an imbecile, quite incapable of any-thing beyond the most elementary stages of learning") Itard "proved the edu-cability of imbeciles" and devised a training program "in terms of the child's

organic needs – mental, moral, social, and esthetic" ("A Historical Survey," 24–5). For Paul F. Cranefield, Itard's failure was "a victory in disguise, if looked at correctly," because it showed the world "that a rather seriously retarded boy could be enormously improved and could be brought to a very much higher level of function than anyone would have supposed" ("Historical Perspectives," 9).

7 Tredgold and Soddy, eds., *Tredgold's Textbook*, 350. See also Shuttleworth, *Mentally-Deficient Children*, 1; Binet and Simon, *Mentally Defective Children*, 3; and Kanner, "Itard, Seguin, Howe."

8 In his classification of idiocy (see *Children with Mental and Physical Handicaps*, 134), J.E. Wallace Wallin included idiocy caused by social deprivation or isolation (mental atrophy through disuse), exemplified by wild children (Victor, Kamala and Amala). For instances of Victor's case being offered as illustration in general discussions of idiocy or imbecility, see Tredgold, *Mental Deficiency*, 107; Wallin, *Children with Mental and Physical Handicaps*, 60; and Kirk, *Early Education of the Mentally Retarded*, 2–3.

9 Gaynor, "The 'Failure' of J.M.G. Itard," 442.

10 Ball, *Itard, Seguin and Kephart*, ix, 3–4, 5, 9, 35; emphasis in the original. Itard "anticipated the modern concept of imitation training" and discovered "what Kephart calls *training in generalization rather than specificity*"; the "practical techniques" he worked out are "almost identical to those employed 160 years later" (5). Itard and Séguin "evolved treatment applications of escape-avoidance conditioning many years before the *births* of Watson, Thorndike, or Pavlov" (83). In "Training Generalized Imitation," 140, Ball outlined the "fading" technique *he* would have used, and which, in his view, would have allowed Victor to achieve vocal speech. Lane, who followed Ball in seeing Itard as the inventor of behaviour modification, also affirmed that Victor "could have learned to speak with the proper conditioning technique" and gave his version of it (based on Lovaas's work) in *The Wild Boy*, 153–4. For yet another behaviourist appropriation of Itard, see Forness and MacMillan, "The Origins of Behavior Modification."

11 Sarason, *Psychological Problems* (1949), 336, and Sarason and Tomas Gladwin, "Psychological and Cultural Problems in Mental Subnormality: A Review of Research," in Sarason, *Psychological Problems* (1959), 577. In 1949 Sarason hailed Itard as having produced "one of the most detailed and illuminating reports dealing with an attempt to rehabilitate a defective child" (327); in 1959, Sarason and Gladwin credited him with "the best description yet made of the behavior of a severely defective individual" (577). For Michael H. Stone (associate director of the General Clinical Service at the New York State Psychiatric Institute), Itard was "the most celebrated pioneer" of the "humanist tradition in the psychotherapy of children." Itard's "empathic sensitivity and extraordi-

nary devotion" towards the "severely retarded" wild boy of Aveyron "set him apart as someone uniquely 'tuned in' to the feelings of a child" ("Mesmer and His Followers," 660).

12 Case and Cleland, "Eminence and Mental Retardation," 20. With 3,049 lines, Victor easily outdid the other contenders for the title, J.H. Pullen (702 lines), Gottfried Mind (forty-one lines), and "Blind Tom" (only four lines). *Mental Retardation* is the practitioner's journal of research, reviews and opinions of the American Association on Mental Retardation, the *American Journal of Mental Retardation* being its scholarly research journal. The American Association on Mental Retardation is the latest incarnation of the Association of Medical Officers of American Institutions for Idiots and Feeble-Minded Persons, founded in 1876, of which Séguin was the first president.

13 S.A. Warren, "Letter from an Editor."

14 Lieberman, "Itard," 566–8. Similar arguments are offered in Graham, "Wild Boys and Idiots," and Hunter, "Heritage from the Wild Boy of Aveyron." See Lamberts and Miller, "Itard and Language Pedagogy," for a discussion of the relevance of Itard's philosophy, procedures, and errors to speech-language professionals.

15 Lane, *The Wild Boy*, 170, 178, and Mannoni, "Itard et son sauvage" (in English: "Itard and His Savage"). For Gayral, Chabbert, and Baillaud-Citeau ("Les premières observations," 488), the boy's state was most likely imputable to lack of cultural matrix and of sensory and social stimuli, perhaps accompanied by a speech impairment.

16 Bettelheim, "Feral Children," 455. Bettelheim's method paralleled Pinel's: he compared the recorded characteristics, behaviours, and symptoms of wild children (his main examples were Amala and Kamala) with present, observable cases of a serious disorder with which he purported to be very familiar.

17 See Kanner, "Itard, Seguin, Howe," and *A History*. Kanner first described autism in "Autistic Disturbances of Affective Contact."

18 Bettelheim, *The Empty Fortress*, 371. Bettelheim had ended his 1959 article with a ruthless indictment of mothers: "Feral children seem to be produced not when wolves behave like mothers but when mothers behave like non-humans. The conclusion tentatively forced on us is that, while there are no feral children, there are some very rare examples of feral mothers, of human beings who become feral to one of their children" ("Feral Children," 467). In *The Empty Fortress* he softened his language somewhat, but the damage had already been done, and he became anathema to most experts on autism – and, understandably, to parents of autistic children.

19 Wing and Wing, "A Clinical Interpretation," 185, 186. In the second edition of *Early Childhood Autism* John Wing hinted that the shortcomings of Itard's theory combined with his eventual acceptance of "Pinel's opinion that the

child was an idiot" were partly to blame for the late recognition of autism. Itard descried "nearly all the behavioural characteristics" that Kanner would list in 1943, but since Itard "had not realised that he was dealing with a separate syndrome ... the chance of helping other children with the same behaviour pattern had been missed" ("Kanner's Syndrome," 6, 10).

20 Lane, *The Wild Boy*, 176-8.

21 Frith, *Autism*, 20-1, 26, 24.

22 Ibid., 16, 154-5. Even though Victor did not speak, witnesses concur that he communicated effectively by other means (gestures, expressions, signs). For analyses of Victor's forms of communication, see Léonetti, "Victor de l'Aveyron" (1986, 1987, and 1990). Whereas Frith distinguished between the autistic Victor and the non-autistic Kaspar, a more recent text absorbed Kaspar too: "Many earlier descriptions of unusual children such as those of Victor, the 'Wild boy of Aveyron' whom Itard studied ... and of Kaspar Hauser reportedly discovered in 1828 ... insofar as they can be taken as reliable accounts, are suggestive of the condition which Kanner so lucidly described" (Trevarthen, Aitken, Papoudi, and Robarts, *Children with Autism*, 4).

23 Mitchell, *Introduction to Theory of Mind*, 61, 57. On autism and theory of mind, see Baron-Cohen, Tager-Flusberg, and Cohen, eds., *Understanding Other Minds*. The idea that the study of autistic children can lead to knowledge about children in general is not new. John Wing stressed this relation (through Itard) in 1976: "It is likely that further study will help not only the affected individuals and their relatives but our understanding of the development of normal children, particularly their acquisition of speech. Itard was conscious of this aspect of his work" ("Kanner's Syndrome," 13).

24 Silberstein and Irwin, "Jean-Marc-Gaspard Itard," 314. The labels change, but the evaluation of Itard's achievement and Victor's condition does not. Silberstein and Irwin on Itard: "Knowing nothing of autism, childhood schizophrenia, anaclitic depression, childhood depression, childhood psychosis, or even about neonatal brain injury, or the essentials of a neurological examination, Itard's approach to Victor's problem was one of love" (ibid.). And on Victor: "The boy was at first more animal than human ... If Victor had anything like an identification, his identification must have been with an animal, not a human being" (315, 316).

25 Brauner and Brauner, "Le 'Sauvage' psychotique de l'Aveyron," and *L'enfant déréel*. For other attempts to situate Itard and Victor within the field of French child psychiatry, see Duche and Dugas, "La psychiatrie de l'enfant," and Gayda, "A l'avènement."

26 McDermott, "Jean Itard," 59, 60, 70. McDermott (then coordinator of the child and youth worker program at St Lawrence College in Kingston, Ontario) "translated" Itard's ideas and actions into modern terms: "Many of Itard's

methods and concerns sound quite modern. At one point, for instance, he uses backrubs to comfort Victor and then begins to worry about the sexually arousing effect they might have – a situation many modern-day CYCs [Child and Youth Counsellors] have had to confront" (61). As McDermott pointed out, Itard fitted Gilmour-Barrett and Pratt's 1977 definition of child and youth work as "the whole collage of skills involved in getting a disturbed child happily through the day": he worked with a clearly disturbed child, and his orientation (focus on fulfilling the child's needs) and methods (therapeutic use of daily routines, child management skills, and activities) were truly "child care" (66). For related uses of Itard to raise the status of professions and practitioners, see E. Wood, "The Wild Boy of Aveyron"; Fein, "Clinical Child Psychology"; and Routh and del Barrio, "European Roots of the First Psychology Clinic."

27 Séguin, *Idiocy*, paragraph 68.

28 Montessori, *The Montessori Method*, 34; emphasis in the original.

29 Fynne, *Montessori and Her Inspirers*, 127. See also Boyd, *From Locke to Montessori* (Boyd and Fynne taught education at the universities of Glasgow and Dublin respectively), and Lane, *The Wild Boy*, 278–86. Another early childhood educator and reformer influenced by Itard and Séguin in this period is Margaret McMillan; see Steedman, *Childhood, Culture and Class*.

30 Montessori, *The Montessori Method*, 44, 153; emphasis in the original.

31 Brown, *Words and Things*, 4, 19. For other uses (and misuses) of Victor and Itard in psycholinguistics and philosophy of language see Lebrun, "Victor of Aveyron," and Gill, *If a Chimpanzee Could Talk.*

32 M. Mannoni, "A Challenge to Mental Retardation," in *The Child, His "Illness," and the Others*, 207, 208. This chapter first appeared in a special issue of *Esprit* on "L'enfance handicapée" in November 1965, a month after the publication of O. Mannoni's "Itard et son sauvage" and a year after Malson reissued Itard's reports in *Les enfants sauvages.*

33 Biklen, *Communication Unbound*, 180, 182. Facilitated communication has been attacked as unscientific and invalid by the experts in the other camp, who cannot accept that autistic people may be the real authors of the communications reported by facilitators (especially since, were these communications authentic, they would give the lie to the "theory of mind" account of autism). For attempts to answer these charges and validate facilitated communication through empirical studies, see Biklen and Cardinal, eds., *Contested Words, Contested Science*. Regardless of the truth of their respective theories, the contrast between the representation of autistic people by cognitive scientists and by supporters of facilitation is striking.

34 O. Mannoni, "Itard and His Savage," 40–1, and Ernct, "Un admirable echec." See also Gineste and Postel, "J.M.G. Itard."

35 Gineste, "Jean Marc Gaspard Itard," 64–6, and *Victor.*

36 Gineste, "Les écrits psychiatriques de J.-M.-G. Itard," 185.

37 Gineste, "Jean Marc Gaspard Itard," 66, and *Victor*, 17. See also Gineste, "Naissance de la psychiatrie infantile." For another version of the historically informed psychiatric appropriation of Itard, see Carrey, "Itard's 1828 Mémoire." Carrey claims that since Itard was the first to differentiate mentally retarded children from children "who would now be considered to have autism or pervasive developmental disorders," he "should be considered as one of the earlier contributors to the field of child psychiatry and developmental disabilities" (1,655, 1,661). Itard's discovery, which anticipated Kanner's, remained unknown and its full implications unrecognized because the debate between Pinel and Itard on the wild boy of Aveyron "prejudiced future generations of medical practitioners" (1,660). Here Victor is seen as simultaneously enabling and hindering the progress of child psychiatry.

38 Shattuck, "How Much Nature, How Much Nurture?" 30. It is difficult to escape the allure of the legend. Thus, even as Lane forewarned readers that the "legend of the wild boy captures a certain conception – or one should rather say, misconception – of the pupil and the teacher, the child and the pedagogue," he availed himself of it when he introduced his book as "a moving story about how a man and a boy helped each other in the search for knowledge, and how that search changed their lives and ours" (*The Wild Boy*, 163, 6). For Gineste, Itard was "a monument of kindness" (*Victor*, 75). Humphrey exclaimed: "Happy the child, normal or deficient, whom chance had brought to such a master!" ("Introduction," xiii).

39 Truffaut, *Truffaut par Truffaut*, 115, 116. The script of *L'enfant sauvage* is in *Aesculape* (1970). It must be kept in mind that while barely fictionalized, Truffaut's film is not (and was never intended to be) a historical document. For other fictionalized treatments of the story of Victor and Itard, see Castan, *Le babou ou l'enfant sauvage*, a play for children, and the two books by Gerstein mentioned in chapter 1.

40 Jauffret, "Introduction aux mémoires," 482, and "Prix proposé par la Société des Observateurs de l'homme, pour l'an 11," *Magasin encyclopédique* 6th year, vol. 2, no. 8 (August–September 1800): 533–5. In his July 1801 paper Jauffret proposed "an experiment on natural man," which is none other than the forbidden experiment. On Jauffret's formulation of the experiment (the only instance I know of in which it was presented, to a scientific society that could possibly muster the resources necessary to put it into practice, as both feasible and desirable) and more generally on the "science of childhood" advanced by Jauffret and the Observers, see Benzaquén, "Childhood, Identity, and Human Science." The relation between the study of wild children and the new interest in the scientific study of children in general was noted by the philosopher Dietrich Tiedemann (1748–1803) in the introduction to his observations of the mental development of his son: "The fact that experience and practice teach us

to use our senses and perceive correctly has been proved by Chesselden's blind man; observations on persons who were found in forests, speechless, reared by animals, have shown that the mental faculties develop slowly, successively, and confusedly. Yet that part of mental philosophy which purports to teach the development of the mind's powers, important though it be both for pedagogy and for a rightful understanding of the soul, has been little pursued; undoubtedly for the reason that there is a dearth of exact and sufficiently numerous observations upon children's souls" ("Tiedemann's Observations," 205).

41 Verri, *Lord Monboddo*, 126. For J.C. Greene (*The Death of Adam*, 214), it is unfortunate that Monboddo died in 1799: "With what interest would Monboddo have viewed the boy as he first appeared in Paris ... With what joy would he have learned of the steady progress of the boy's education, with what heartbreak of Itard's failure to teach him to speak. And with what satisfaction would Monboddo have read Itard's conclusions." See also Formigari, "Language and Society."

42 Egle Becchi gave Victor a prominent place in the history of childhood in the West because he was "not just a savage or a pathological individual; he was a child"; see "Le XIXe siècle," in Becchi and Julia, eds., *Histoire de l'enfance en Occident*, 2:148. The notion that the child was born as a scientific object in the guise of, or as an epistemological replacement for, the savage needs to be further queried. The human sciences reinforced the correlation between child and savage throughout the nineteenth century in what would later be known as the theory of recapitulation, i.e., ontogeny recapitulates phylogeny, or the development of the individual from childhood to adulthood is analogous to the evolution of the race from animality to humanity or the progress of humanity from savagery to civilization; see Gould, *Ontogeny and Phylogeny*.

43 Hacking, "Normal People," 59, 64 (this paper was originally presented at a workshop hosted by the Ontario Institute for Studies in Education in 1993), and *The Taming of Chance*, 1–2. On the "coming into being" of scientific objects, see Daston's "Introduction" to Daston, ed., *Biographies of Scientific Objects*, 1–14. The rise of normality as a key concept in thinking about people, like the merging of knowledge and intervention and the growing interest in childhood and educability, must be related to the changing role of the modern state in the welfare of people (as individuals and as a population) outlined by Foucault in the first volume of *The History of Sexuality*, especially part 5, "Right of Death and Power over Life" (135–59).

44 Itard, trans. and ed., *Hygiène domestique*, 2:530–3 (the sixth of Itard's "critical and explanatory notes"). In "Vésanies" (599) Itard wrote: "A great defect in education is to believe that it must be the same for every individual. It must be as variable as is the human mind in its modifications and its stage of development."

45 Lane, *The Wild Boy*, 165, and Alain Hirt, "Pour une réflexion sur les connaissances actuelles de la pédagogie," in *L'enfant sauvage*, 73–6.

46 Shattuck supports Itard's decision not to give Victor information about sex on the grounds that "[Itard] had the courage to remain firm in observing the difference between a scientific experiment of reeducation and tampering with the life of another human being" (*The Forbidden Experiment*, 154). But was there *anything* about Itard's experiment that did not involve "tampering with the life of another human being"?

47 Sicard, *Cours d'instruction*, 4–5, ix–x, xiv. See also Sicard, "Chapitre préliminaire." On Sicard and his school, see Lane, *When the Mind Hears*, and Rosenfeld, *A Revolution in Language*.

48 "Notice sur l'enfance de Massieu, sourd-muet de naissance," in Sicard, *Théorie des signes*, 2:634, 637, and Sicard, *Cours*, 20; emphasis in the original. The program of the Observers' public meeting on 6 August 1800 included "*The Childhood of Massieu*, deaf-mute from birth, written by himself, then expressed by him at the meeting with the help of signs" ("Société des Observateurs de l'homme," *Magasin encyclopédique* 6th year, vol. 2, no. 8 [August–September 1800]: 532). Massieu, a close friend of Jauffret's, became an instructor at the Parisian school for the deaf following Sicard's appointment as director. His account of his childhood was first published by Jauffret in *La Corbeille de fleurs* ... (Paris: Perlet, 1807). Jauffret and his older brother, Gaspard-Jean-André (1759–1823) – a priest, later bishop of Metz, and himself a member of the Society of Observers of Man – interviewed Massieu to learn about his ideas before his education. G.-J.-A. Jauffret asked Massieu whether he had any idea of God before he met Sicard, and Massieu said he did not: "Before coming to the institution for deaf-mutes I was a wild man." G.-J.-A. Jauffret also asked Massieu's opinion regarding his brother's project to raise four children in isolation until the age of fifteen, nursed by deaf-mute women and without any other communication with people, "to discover whether they would have any idea of God, of providence, of the immortality of the soul." Massieu believed those children would have no idea of God, because "no child can raise himself to have knowledge, and another person is needed for one to be raised, to be led to knowledge. It would be a divine child, not a human child, who could raise himself" ("Conversation avec un sourd-muet de naissance," in Reboul, ed., *Les cartons d'un ancien bibliothécaire*, 56, 59). Sicard addressed criticisms of his view of the uneducated deaf as savages in *Théorie des signes*, 1:xii–xiv. On the friendship between the Jauffrets and Sicard, see Chappey, *La Société des Observateurs*.

49 Sicard, *Cours*, iv, and Itard, *De l'Éducation*, 83. Truffaut assigned some suggestive words to his Mme Guérin: "Mme Guérin: 'His tantrums, doctor, are your fault! You make this child work from morning to evening. You turn his only pleasures into exercises; meals, walks, everything ... it seems you want him to catch up in one fell swoop. He works ten times more than a normal child.' Itard: 'You are right, Madame Guérin, I will make his walks longer.'"

Critics have questioned the false optimism of the ending of Truffaut's film (e.g., Shattuck, *Forbidden Experiment*, 213). Victor, who has escaped back to the forest, returns of his own will after a few days and is greeted like the prodigal son. Mme Guérin leads him up the stairs to his room, while Itard, who remains downstairs, says: "Soon, we'll resume our exercises." Yet to my mind, when opposed to Mme Guérin's imagined speech the film's ending appears more ambiguous, if not directly ominous. Itard's single-minded concern with the boy's instruction (which turns pleasures into exercises) foretells the break in the pedagogical relation that marked the end of the experiment in real life (Truffaut, *L'enfant sauvage* [second part], 2, 14, 47).

50 Itard, *De l'Éducation*, 66–7, 69, 71, 62–3; O. Mannoni, "Itard and His Savage," 43.

CHAPTER SEVEN

1 Gesell, *Wolf Child and Human Child*, 5.

2 According to McCartney ("Greek and Roman Lore," 38), the ancient stories were created "to show that evidences of divine favor and omens of future greatness attended the hero or god even in youth." See also Dunn, *The Foundling and the Werwolf*. For the same theme in a different cultural context (the one in which some of the stories of "real" wolf children emerged), see the tales in Bompas, ed. and trans., *Folklore of the Santal Parganas*. Many accounts of animal-raised children cite this passage from Shakespeare's *Winter's Tale* (act 2, scene 3, line 185): "ANTIGONUS: '... Come on, poor babe: / Some powerful spirit instruct the kites and ravens / To be thy nurses! Wolves and bears, they say, / Casting their savageness aside have done / Like offices of pity.'" For discussions of wolf children in relation to werewolves, see Gilbert N. Smith, "Wolves Nursing Children," and Lysart, "Wolf Boys," in *Notes and Queries* 7, 1st series (9 April 1853): 355, and 11, 6th series (11 April 1885): 286; Burton, "Wolf-Children and Werewolves"; and Douglas, *The Beast Within*.

3 "L." was mystified by the idea of animals nurturing children but did not seem troubled by their reported condition: Sleeman's account of his first wolf boy (see below) "leaves no doubt that he was an idiot, and that he exhibited unmistakeable marks of mental imbecility" ("Children Nurtured by Wolves in India" [22 July 1854], 62).

4 Sleeman's report on Oude was an official document not intended for publication; hence the account of wolf boys came out separately and anonymously in the pamphlet *An Account of Wolves Nurturing Children*. The report appeared posthumously as *A Journey through the Kingdom of Oude*. The account of wolf boys, dated 28 December 1849, is in 1:206–22; it was also reprinted in

The Zoologist, organ of the London Linnaean Society, in March 1888. Sleeman (lieutenant-colonel 1843, colonel 1853, major general 1854), renowned for his role in the suppression of the Thugs, was resident at the Court of Lucknow from 1849 to 1856. Despite the state of turmoil and widespread violence in which he found Oude, he advised against British annexation. His recommendation was not heeded, and the annexation of Oude in 1856 was one of the main causes of the 1857–58 Sepoy Mutiny. This is how Sleeman was portrayed by his unidentified biographer: "He was one of those superior men which the Indian service is constantly producing, who have rendered the name of Englishman respected throughout the vast empire of British India, and whose memory will endure so long as British power shall remain in the East ... [He] won the respect and love particularly of the natives, who always regarded him as their friend, and by whom his equity was profoundly appreciated"; see "Biographical Sketch," in Sleeman, *A Journey*, 1:xiv–xv.

5 In later stories of wolf and animal-raised children, the children were taken to orphanages or mental hospitals.

6 Sleeman, *A Journey*, 1:216, 218–19. One of the later stories was that of the boy found by Mr H—, magistrate and collector of the Etawah District, given in "Wolf-Children," *Chambers's Journal*, 598. The one "wolf boy" Sleeman explicitly claimed to have met was the seventh case, an old man then living in Lucknow who had been found as a boy "by the hut of an old hermit who died": "He is supposed to have been taken from wolves by this old hermit. The trooper who found him brought him to the King some forty years ago, and he has been ever since supported by the King comfortably. He is still called the 'wild man of the woods.' He was one day sent to me at my request, and I talked with him ... He is very inoffensive, but speaks little, and that little imperfectly; and he is still impatient of intercourse with his fellow-men, particularly with such as are disposed to tease him with questions. I asked him whether he had any recollection of having been with wolves. He said 'the wolf died long before the hermit'; but he seemed to recollect nothing more, and there is no mark on his knees or elbows to indicate that he ever went on all fours" (221).

7 Sleeman, *A Journey*, 221–2. On reading about the Sekandra wolf boys (see below), A.B.W. was "disturbed only by this sceptical thought, viz., If so many of the specimens have been discovered at an early age, what becomes of the undiscovered ones that make up the average? Do they progress to manhood on all-fours, and remain so?" ("Wolf Boys," *Notes and Queries* 11, 6th series [6 June 1885]: 454–5). Sleeman did not comment on the absence of wolf *girls*, noted by Tylor and explained with reference to girls' "natural weakness" in the 1882 article in *Chambers's Journal* ("It is not easy to assign a sufficient reason for the fact that females have never been so discovered, unless we suppose that, being less vigorously constituted, they have been unable to withstand the terrible hardships of such an existence, and have very soon sickened and died")

and by Neilson ("I have never heard or read of a girl wolf-child having been found. The reason for this may be that they have soon broken down under the strain of so terrible an existence, and have perished in the jungle, where the stronger male child has survived"); Tylor, "Wild Men and Beast-Children," 26; "Wolf-Children," *Chambers's Journal*, 597; Neilson, "Wolf-Children," 253.

8 "Wolf-Children," *Chambers' Edinburgh Journal*, 34. This article was the first to use the term "wolf-children" and to relate the Indian boys to some of the European wild children (Peter, the girl of Songi, and the boy of Aveyron).

9 Quoted in Murchison and Egerton, "On Wolves Suckling Children," 153. Sir Roderick I. Murchison reproduced an extract (dated 14 February 1851) from the Indian journal of the Honourable Captain Francis Egerton, R.N. Egerton recounted some of the wolf boy stories, which he had from Sleeman. Murchison's communication is to my knowledge the first published reference to Indian wolf children (in the West). Egerton's diary was also quoted in "Children Suckled by Wolves." By July 1854 the wolf boys had crossed the Atlantic; see "Wolf Nurses in India" (a summary of Sleeman's pamphlet).

10 Smith, "Wolves Nursing Children," 355; "L.," "Children Nurtured by Wolves in India" (22 July 1854), 64; Tylor, "Wild Men and Beast-Children," 26, 31, 32; emphasis in the original. "L." contributed two more letters on wolf children to *Notes and Queries*, 20 February and 3 April 1858. During a later debate on wolf children, W.F. Prideaux proposed that "L." was the late Sir George Cornewall Lewis; see "Wolf Boys," *Notes and Queries* 12, 6th series (29 August 1885): 178. Sir Francis Galton (1822–1911) resorted to Sleeman's boys to back his claim that the nursing of children was a further way in which domesticated animals could be put to good use: "It is marvellous how soon goats find out children and tempt them to suckle. I have had the milk of my goats, when encamping for the night in African travels, drained dry by small black children who had not the strength to do more than crawl about, but nevertheless came to some secret understanding with the goats and fed themselves. The records of many nations have legends like that of Romulus and Remus, who are stated to have been suckled by wild beasts. These are surprisingly confirmed by Gen. Sleeman's narrative of six cases where children were nurtured for many years by wolves in Oude" ("The First Steps," 135–6). Many decades earlier, the French physician Alphonse Leroy (who in 1807 would write an enthusiastic letter to Itard on his second report on Victor) had recommended that babies be fed directly from the udder of a goat when a woman's milk was not available. He had introduced this method in the 1770s at the Aix foundling hospital: "Each goat, having just grazed, enters bleating and goes to find the infant that has been given to it, removes the covering with its horns, straddles the crib to suckle the child" (*Médecine maternelle*, 52).

11 These questions were first posed by "L." in "Children Nurtured by Wolves in India" (22 July 1854), 64–5.

12 "Wolf-Children," *Chambers' Edinburgh Journal*, 36; emphasis in the original.

13 V. Ball, *Jungle Life in India*, 458 (Ball reproduced the report of the Sekandra Orphanage published in Indian newspapers in late 1872), 459–61, 455, 466, 465; emphasis in the original. Ball, MA, of the Geological Survey of India, was a fellow of Calcutta University and member of several scientific societies. Why did wolves steal so many children in Oude but not in other places? Ball suggested that "the Oude wolves are a local race of man-eaters" with "an exceptional liking for human flesh" (457). See also the letter from Professor J.H. Seelye of Allahabad, India – who, like Ball, visited the orphanage, heard the story of the two boys from Mr Erhardt, and saw the surviving one – dated 25 November 1872 and printed in *Amherst Student*, reproduced in Ireland, *The Mental Affections of Children*, 425–6, and the review of Ball's work in Giglioli, "Ragazzi allevati e conviventi con lupi." In 1927 a reader of the London *Times* wrote that when he was a youth in India a "charming old man called Raj Keshwa Lal," his "Gamaliel in all matters of Indian lore and custom," told him the story of a wolf boy and his "theory" about his survival: "He suggested that the small baby had, as is common in India, been left lying on a mat by its mother in the vicinity of the jungle; that the she-wolf had picked it up to be a morsel of food and deposited it in her lair amongst her own cubs; that something had disturbed her before she had broken her meal up, and that when she resumed, the human scrap, by close proximity to her cubs, had become saturated with their smell, and that she was unable to distinguish it from her own litter. As she curled up over her whelps, the human infant proceeded to feed from her alongside her own cubs; and that from the first feed the child became hers, as it was henceforth impregnated with both the scent of her own cubs and that of her own milk" ("Wolf Children," letter to the editor by Lionel James, *Times*, 7 April 1927, 12).

14 *Notes and Queries* (29 August 1885): 178, and (11 April 1885): 286; Modi, "Recorded Instances," 144; Mr Theobald, quoted in Stockwell, "Wolf-Children," 123. In his letter to Prideaux (reproduced in *Notes and Queries* [29 August 1885], 178), Lewis noted that Sanichar had made some progress: "He cannot talk, and though undoubtedly *págal* [imbecile or idiotic], still shows signs of reason, and sometimes actual shrewdness." When Modi saw him in 1887, "he was asked by a boy of the Orphanage, by means of signs, to walk like a wolf. He did so on his hands and feet. Then he made me some signs which were interpreted to me as a desire to have some money for smoking cheroots, of which I was told he was very fond ... He is very ugly in appearance" ("Recorded Instances," 143). The orphanage continued to attract visitors for decades (Sanichar died in 1895). Some of them recounted what they saw, and what they were told, in the 1927 and 1939 series of letters to the London *Times* (see below). Zingg reprinted material provided by the orphanage in 1938, including Sani-

char's photograph and obituary, in "Feral Man" (1942), 159–69. Ireland received the following reply (dated 19 January 1874) from Dr John Whishaw, of the Lucknow Lunatic Asylum, to his inquiries about a "wolf boy" in his care: "The boy is fourteen and an impostor; he was made up to get money under false pretences. I found him out. He was certified to be dumb, but after he had been ten days with me he talked very well, argued, and described his life in the wolves' den ... He showed me the way in which he used to play with the young wolves. When the papa and mamma went out in search of food for the family he usually remained behind. Sometimes, however, he was allowed to go with them; and if one could judge of the pace he could go by the specimen of it I made him show the visitors of the asylum, the wolves would have had but poor sport and a bad dinner on the day this gentleman joined in their wild sports. I believe never in this world has there been an instance of a child being brought up by wolves, and I cannot understand how anybody can believe in such a thing. The majority of wolf-boys are idiots, taken by their parents and left near some distant police station"; quoted in Ireland, *The Mental Affections of Children*, 428.

15 Quoted in Ball, *Jungle Life in India*, 459 (my emphasis); Ireland, *The Mental Affections of Children*, 432.

16 *Notes and Queries* (29 August 1885): 178.

17 Ball, *Jungle Life in India*, 466. The philologist Max Müller (1823–1900) did not "pronounce any opinion, either adverse or favourable," on Sleeman's and Ball's wolf children. In his view, "the work of the comparative mythologist" could only begin after natural historians and practical sportsmen settled whether children "could be suckled and kept alive" in a wolf's den and after the value of the "documentary evidence" (which "might exercise the ingenuity of some of our cleverest lawyers") was ascertained ("Wolf-Children," 513).

18 See Neilson, "Wolf-Children"; Stockwell, "Wolf-Children"; Crooke, *Things Indian*; R. Kipling, *The Jungle Book*; Burroughs, "Tarzan of the Apes." Burroughs went on to publish many Tarzan novels. The first of numerous Tarzan films opened in early 1918. Kipling's father mentioned wolf children too: "India is probably the cradle of wolf-child stories, which are here universally believed and supported by a cloud of testimony, including in the famous Lucknow case of a wolf boy the evidence of European witnesses"; J.L. Kipling, *Beast and Man*, 281.

19 "2 Little 'Wolf Girls' in Den with Wolf Cubs; Rescued, 1 Dies; 1 Is Humanized Slowly," *New York Times* (hereafter *NYT*), 22 October 1926, 1. See also "Two Children Live in a Wolf's Lair – Bishop's Amazing Story – Girl Who Barked – Ate with Mouth in the Dish," *Westminster Gazette*, 22 October 1926, 1.

20 "Fight in London Club over 'Wolf Girl' Tale: Members Use Fists in Heated Argument on Report of Two Found in Den," *NYT*, 23 October 1926, and "E.A.J.," "Jungle's Laws Still Hold," *NYT Magazine*, 30 January 1927, 14. See also "Wolf

Girls," 25; "Mowgli in Real Life in News from India: Details of the Remarkable Story of Wolf Girls Revealed in the Jungle in West Bengal," *NYT*, 26 December 1926; Maclean, *The Wolf Children*; and Benzaquén, "Kamala of Midnapore."

21 "Indian Boy Found Living among Wolves," *Times*, 5 April 1927; "Find Boy in Wolf's Den: Evidently Nurtured by Animal, Ten-Year-Old Proves Savage," *NYT*, 6 April; "'Wolf-Child' Puzzles Physicians in India: Lad Found in Cave Reveals Further Signs of Having Been Nurtured by Animals," *NYT*, 27 April; "Wolf-Children," *NYT*, 2 May; and "New Wolf Child Found in India: Even Kipling Is Moved to Join the Dispute Over the Authenticity of Such Strange Jungle Beings – Many Other Cases Reported," *NYT*, 10 July. See also "Wolf Children of India," and "India's 'Wolf-Children' Found in Caves."

22 Letters to the editor, *Times*, 5–28 April 1927, and *NYT*, 17 July 1927. None of the correspondents cited the 1926 news reports on the wolf girls, but two of them – G.C. Blaxland (11 April) and A. Shewan, ICS, Retired (12 April) – mentioned personal letters from friends describing two wolf children recently rescued by a missionary.

23 Letters to the editor, *Times*, 27 June – 26 July 1939.

24 Foley, "The 'Baboon Boy'" (22 March and 28 June 1940); Zingg, "More about the 'Baboon Boy.'" Zingg apologized for the "premature" publication of the evidence (455–6). His purpose was to forestall objections to the documentation on Amala and Kamala, which he was in the process of editing for publication. For more on Lucas, see Heuvelmans, *Les bêtes humaines*, 113–25.

25 The later Indian wolf children failed to rival the Midnapore girls in celebrity, at least among Western scientists. Ramu, found in 1954 in the waiting-room of the Lucknow station and "identified" as a wolf boy, spent fourteen years at the Balrampur hospital in Lucknow (he died in April 1968) and showed no recovery. Hundreds of people every day paid a small fee to see him. According to Dr Sharma, who cared for him at the hospital, Ramu "began to die when people wanted to turn him into a human being"; quoted in Broche, "Le secret des enfants sauvages," 50. See also Prasad, "Ramu" (from the available medical evidence, Prasad, head of the Department of Philosophy and Psychology at the University of Lucknow, drew the preliminary conclusion that Ramu was not a wolf boy after all), and Kapoor, "Socialization and Feral Children." On Parasram of Agra, see Ogburn, "The Wolf Boy of Agra" (Ogburn's debunking of Parasram's case prompted Bettelheim's general reinterpretation of feral children as autistic children). Shamdev (or Shamdeo), found in the early 1970s in the forest of Musafirkhana playing with wolf cubs, was eventually taken to Mother Teresa's Mission of Charity in Lucknow, where he was renamed Pascal by the sisters and lived for seven years until his death in February 1985. Douglas noted that photographs of Shamdev "show him to have been in an advanced state of emaciation" (*The Beast Within*, 191); see also Chatwin, "The Quest for the Wolf Children."

26 Zingg, "Feral Man" (1942), 133. A native Bengali but unflinchingly loyal to the British, Singh (1873–1941) was a missionary with the Society for the Propagation of the Gospel in Foreign Parts. Finding many orphans in the jungle villages he periodically visited during his missionary work, he opened an orphanage for them in Midnapore (Bengal). It usually housed about twenty children and was in constant financial distress.

27 Singh and Zingg, *Wolf-Children and Feral Man*, xxxii–xxxiii; Bishop H. Pakenham-Walsh, "Preface," in ibid., xxv–xxvii; Zingg, "India's Wolf-Children." Excerpts from the correspondence between Singh and the scientists are in Squires, "'Wolf Children' of India"; Kellogg, "More about the 'Wolf Children' of India," and "A Further Note."

28 See Hutton, "Wolf-Children," and "Wolf-Children and Feral Man"; Zingg's introduction to *Wolf-Children and Feral Man*, xxxviii–xxxix; and Maclean, *The Wolf Children*.

29 In letters to Zingg, Kellogg and Squires vented their doubts concerning Singh's testimony and character. For Kellogg, "the chief difficulty is that Singh is not only a layman and a missionary, but a man who is not capable of expressing himself in English with accuracy and precision." Squires exclaimed that Singh's diary was "a hopelessly ignorant piece of drivel by a religious fanatic"; quoted in Maclean, *The Wolf Children*, 239, 238.

30 Singh and Zingg, *Wolf-Children and Feral Man*; Montagu, review of *Wolf-Children and Feral Man*, 469 (later reprinted in Montagu's *Anthropology and Human Nature*, 240–5); and Mandelbaum, "Wolf-Child Histories from India," 38. See also Gesell, "Wolf-Children and Genetic Psychology," 14. Flaws and controversies notwithstanding, *Wolf-Children and Feral Man* was deemed important enough to deserve a second edition (1966).

31 Ogburn and Bose, "On the Trail of the Wolf-Children," 191, 189. What Mrs Jana, Singh's daughter, told Ogburn's research assistant clashed with her father's more uplifting version of Kamala's last days: "It seems that her nature did not change much ... She died of typhoid fever. While she was sick Dr. Sarbadhi-kari told father to feed her with raw blood, as that would be the only thing she could digest at that time. A man would be sent to bring a glass of blood from where the goats are cut for meat. When Kamala caught sight of the blood her eyes would shine in joy. The blood would dry up and pieces were cut and fed to her. It made her very happy. She also ate a lot of earth. Mother could not prevent her from it. Sometimes she relieved herself in the rooms and earthworms would crawl out of her. Such sights made us nauseated, but what could we do? People take good care of cats and dogs, and this was a human child. Right after she was captured her body let out a strong bad odor. Mother bathed her every day. Nearer the end the smell had died down some" (ibid., 143). For Singh's account of Kamala's last illness and death, see Singh and Zingg, *Wolf-Children and Feral Man*, 112–13.

32 Maclean, *The Wolf Children*, 3. Maclean's portrayal of Singh underscored the missionary's ambivalent response to Amala and Kamala, his sense of guilt for having killed the "mother wolf" and perhaps deprived the girls of the only life they had come to desire, and his failure to restore them to the human community and even to ensure their survival. I have been unable to find any information about Maclean's professional or institutional affiliation (if any) nor about how his investigation was funded.

33 As I claimed in chapter 2, sceptics always demand that *one more condition* be fulfilled – or reject the evidence in principle. Bergen Evans contended that even if Singh had *really* rescued the girls from a wolves' den, "it would not have been positive proof that they had been reared by those or any other wolves": perhaps they had "fled into the den in fear. Or they may even have lived there independently. It would have been a strange situation, but nowhere nearly so strange as the one alleged" (*The Natural History of Nonsense*, 97).

34 Ogburn, "The Wolf Boy of Agra," 450; Stratton, "Jungle Children," 597; Dennis, "The Significance of Feral Man," and "A Further Analysis"; Lenneberg, "The Natural History of Language," 234; and Montagu, review of *Wolf-Children and Feral Man*, 469, 471. Environmentalist readings of wolf and wild children appeared in many textbooks, e.g., Krueger and Reckless, *Social Psychology*; Anastasi, *Differential Psychology*; Chapple and Coon, *Principles of Anthropology*; Krout, *Introduction to Social Psychology*; Ruch, *Psychology and Life*; Anastasi and Foley, *Differential Psychology*; Sargent, *Social Psychology*; and Giddens, *Sociology*. For a semiotic analysis of the story of Kamala, see Léonetti, "Analyse d'un cas d'observation clinique"; for an attempt to use the story to complicate the Lacanian model of the subject in language, see Wicke, "Koko's Necklace."

35 Jack Harrison Pollack, "Meet Dr. Gesell – The Man Who Knows Children," *Parents Magazine* (March 1954): 80, cited in Ames, *Arnold Gesell*, 195. *Wolf Child and Human Child* came out in March 1941, preceded by an abridged version, "The Biography of a Wolf-Child." Gesell completed his doctoral studies in psychology at Clark University under G. Stanley Hall and moved to Yale in 1911 to teach in the education department and direct the Juvenile Psycho Clinic, a small research facility that grew into the large, famous, and well-funded Yale Clinic of Child Development. He pursued medical studies at Yale and in parallel worked as a school psychologist (the first to hold that position in the United States) for the State Board of Education of Connecticut. Gesell's painstaking charting of normative development was hugely influential within paediatrics, psychology, education, and child welfare, while his popular child-rearing manuals for parents turned him into something of a household name. His publications were lavishly illustrated with photographs from his films; see Gesell, Thompson, and Amatruda, *An Atlas of Infant Behavior*; Gesell et al., *The First Five Years of Life*; Gesell and Amatruda, *Developmental Diagnosis*;

and Gesell, *How a Baby Grows*. On his life, work, and influence, see Ames, *Arnold Gesell*; Thelen and Adolph, "Arnold L. Gesell"; Marchese, "The Place of Eugenics"; Zusne, *Biographical Dictionary*, 155–6; Morss, "Gesell"; and the entry by Benjamin Harris in Garraty and Carnes, eds., *American National Biography*, 8:877–8.

36 Gesell to Zingg, 30 September 1940, quoted in Maclean, *The Wolf Children*, 266; Gesell, *Wolf Child and Human Child*, ix (hereafter references to this work are in the text).

37 Gesell used passages from *The Jungle Book* as epigraphs to chapters 3, 5, 6, and 7. This is the epigraph to chapter 3: "'How little! How naked, and – how bold!' said Mother Wolf softly. The baby was pushing his way between the cubs to get close to the warm hide. 'Ahai! He is taking his meal with the others. And so this is a man's cub ... Come soon,' said Mother Wolf, 'little naked son of mine; for, listen, child of man, I loved thee more than ever I loved my cubs'" (15). And to chapter 7: "'When we met at Cold Lairs, Manling, I knew it,' said Kaa, turning a little in his mighty coils. 'Man goes to Man at the last, though the Jungle does not cast him out'" (59).

38 Kipling, *The Jungle Book*, 25. As mentioned above, Gesell used this passage as the epigraph to chapter 3.

39 The emphasis is Gesell's. In response to the negative reviews of *Wolf Child and Human Child*, Ames tried to salvage Gesell's reputation with the argument that his analysis of Kamala's life depended on his sincere belief that the story was authentic and Singh trustworthy. Gesell's conviction derived from the diary's internal veracity: "Unless the clergyman was a total scamp and at the same time highly versed in the details of growing human behavior, he could not possibly have produced a diary so true to the ways in which young children develop" (*Arnold Gesell*, 195).

40 To lend force to his humanistic view of Kamala, Gesell used as his epigraph to chapter 1 Terence's dictum "I am a human being. To me nothing human can be alien (*Homo sum, humani nihil a me alienum pute*)" (1).

41 Emphasis in the original. For Singh's version of this episode, see Singh and Zingg, *Wolf-Children and Feral Man*, 76–7. See ibid., 65–7, on the exercises devised by the Singhs to teach Kamala to stand on her knees. Gesell's positive take on Singh's text is evident in his account of Kamala's "religious conversion": by 1927 she "had so far transcended wolf ways that she came regularly to the morning religious service, where she knelt in line with her fellow orphans who no longer called her 'heathen'" (42). Here is the corresponding passage in Singh's diary: "*March 9, 1927*: It was noticed at this time that Kamala joined in the singing in the service. In this singing mood of hers, she used to disturb the singing of the hymns very much. At times, she used to shout at the top of her voice in a shrill irregular note"; *Wolf-Children and Feral Man*, 106.

42 Just before her death, "the general level of her intelligence as evidenced by language and social behavior was comparable to that of a 3½-year-old child" (72–3), and since she still had "a considerable quota of developmental reserves which had not been drawn upon" (84), had she lived longer she might have progressed much further: "It is at least within the range of biologic possibility that if Kamala's life span were prolonged to the age of thirty-five years, she might have achieved a mental maturity level of ten or twelve years, not far below the average adult level of many villagers in India" (80). A troublesome consequence of "mental age" understandings of development is that the adults of other cultures seldom get to be *real* adults. Amala and Kamala were seriously ill during long stretches of their stay at the orphanage. The doctor who treated the girls, Dr Sarbadhicari, noted that when he first saw them, in September 1921, they were suffering from emaciation and loss of appetite. Attributing their illness to their refusal to eat a mixed diet, he treated them for worms. Amala died of nephritis and general oedema. "Curiously enough," remarked the doctor, "the older girl Kamala died also of the same disease"; statement reproduced in Kellogg, "A Further Note."

43 Gesell and Amatruda, *Developmental Diagnosis*, 318–19. In his review of *Wolf Child and Human Child*, Watson, for whom environmentalists "have had no other evidence so compelling as the experiences of the wolf-children," commented: "The power of habit is evident throughout the tale, but nowhere more clearly than in Professor Gesell's own effort to conclude that his traditional view of human growth as determined by natural maturation needs no modification in the light of this extraordinary observation" ("Life History of the Wolf Girl," 15). The most scathing review of Gesell's book was Evans, "Wolf! Wolf!," reprinted in an expanded version in *The Natural History of Nonsense*. Noting that Gesell's "'illuminating conclusions' regarding heredity, environment and the capacity of the human mind to accept things" by "rare good luck ... confirm certain theories which he has long maintained," Evans warned Gesell that his researches "may lead him to the oldest of all wolf stories, Aesop's tale of the man who said he saw a wolf when he didn't and later discovered that reputation is a high price to pay for notoriety" ("Wolf! Wolf!," 734–5). See Zingg's reply to Evans (followed by Evans's reply to Zingg), "The Wolf Child." See also "Even Nurture in the Wild Will Not Destroy Intelligence: From Study of Story of Kamala, 'Wolf Girl' of India, Psychologist Concludes She Was Not Feeble-Minded," *Science News Letter* (22 March 1941): 182, and "Wolf-Child Stories Are Doubted by Psychologist: Evidence Entirely Hearsay; Idiots Display Many of Same Behavior Characteristics, It Is Pointed Out," *Science News Letter* (26 April 1941): 261. Even though Gesell insisted on *Kamala's* normality, his textbooks were full of authoritative, deprecating, and dehumanizing descriptions of abnormal, deviant, and "deficient" children (who, in his view, had been born that way and not made abnormal by extraordinary circumstances). Gesell and

Amatruda wrote: "By application of the norms set up and described in the preceding chapters, we are able to compare the developmental status of any child with the norms appropriate to his age, and to determine whether he deviates from the norms, in what direction he deviates, and how much he deviates. In other words, we ascertain the completeness as well as the rate of his development; we make qualitative and quantitative comparisons" (*Developmental Diagnosis*, 111). The task of the child expert was to identify the abnormal child and make sure that parents accepted the child's defect: "All too frequently, parents, abetted by undue professional encouragement, cling for years to the faith that something can and will be done to make their defective child normal. This misplaced faith deepens and becomes an unhygienic method of escape from the realities of the situation ... It is the physician's duty to help the parents to face reality as early and as steadily as possible" (351). For Gesell and his collaborators in the 1930s and 1940s, facing reality meant agreeing to institutional confinement and "special" education (i.e., reduced to vocational training only).

44 Thelen and Adolph, "Arnold L. Gesell," 372, 375. Thelen and Adolph do not discuss *Wolf Child and Human Child* and Gesell's interest in Kamala.

45 See Appendix A, "Examination Technique," in Gesell and Amatruda, *Developmental Diagnosis*.

46 Lane and Pillard, *The Wild Boy of Burundi*, 4 (hereafter references to this work are in the text). The news article, reprinted in Lane and Pillard, 3–4 and 7–12, conveyed a standard story of a strange boy found by soldiers with a troop of monkeys and taken to an orphanage. He went on all fours, had thick calluses on hands and knees, and, according to Nurse Elizabeth Noigenegene, "was covered with a fine coat of dark hair on his back and legs" (10). The Russian psychiatrist who treated him stated that he was not a deaf-mute "as the hospital at first thought. Clinically he is an idiot with an IQ of a one-year-old. It is impossible to say whether he was born abnormal or became abnormal during his life ... The saddest thing is that he will never be able to communicate his experiences to us" (11). It was assumed that the wild boy's fate was linked to the 1972 civil war between Tutsis and Hutus.

47 This is how Lane presented his case to the director of the William T. Grant Foundation (which, he thought, was the appropriate sponsor for the project because it was then funding the study of Genie): "If John is a feral child, his discovery can be one of the most important in the behavioral sciences in this century. The opportunity may not arise again for another century and a half, if ever. If John is not feral, we need to know that, too; the case must be closed" (26–7). Lane was encouraged by Genie's purported progress, which showed that "we have learned a few things since Itard's day": "In Genie's dismal story we can find a ray of hope for John" (77, 80). On Genie, see chapter 8, below.

48 John resisted the procedures but was overpowered by the adults: "Hold him. You two take the right. You two take his shoulders. (Harlan and I took his

head.) Now, go! We quickly get six films [X-rays]. It is possible to overpower a ten-year-old boy; it's a question of numbers" (125).

49 Lane mentioned John's death in passing in *The Mask of Benevolence*, 31 (while discussing how, as a result of this adventure, he became involved with deaf education in Burundi). On John, see also Heuvelmans, *Les bêtes humaines*, 126–8.

CHAPTER EIGHT

1 Quoted in Rymer, *Genie*, 43.

2 "Girl, 13, Prisoner Since Infancy, Deputies Charge; Parents Jailed," *Los Angeles Times*, 17 November 1970. See also "Mystery Shrouds Home of Alleged Child Prisoner," *Los Angeles Times*, 18 November, and "Father Accused of Keeping His Daughter a Prisoner Ends Life," *Los Angeles Times*, 21 November, 1. Genie's father, Clark Wiley, shot himself on 20 November, "moments before he was to be arraigned on felony child abuse charges."

3 Summaries of Genie's story may be found in Curtiss, Fromkin, Krashen, Rigler and Rigler, "The Linguistic Development of Genie"; Fromkin, Krashen, Curtiss, Rigler, and Rigler, "The Development of Language"; and Curtiss, *Genie*. Curtiss noted that the name Genie was meant to protect the girl's identity and privacy while "captur[ing], to a small measure, the fact that she emerged into human society past childhood, having existed previously as something other than fully human" (*Genie*, xii). For more detailed accounts see Rymer, *Genie* (an expanded version of the two-part article "A Silent Childhood") and Garmon, *Secret of the Wild Child*. Genie was "the most profoundly damaged child" James Kent had ever seen. Jay Shurley spent a week examining her clinically: "I determined for myself that she was the genuine article – that she had suffered the most extreme long-duration social isolation of any child that had been described in any literature I could find"; quoted in Rymer, *Genie*, 40, 42. On Kaspar Hauser, see below. Anna and Isabelle, found in conditions resembling those of Genie's early life, were contemporary with the great spurt of interest in wild children in the late 1930s and early 1940s; see Davis, "Extreme Social Isolation" and "Final Note." Anna made some progress but remained retarded and died of hemorrhagic jaundice in August 1942. In contrast, Isabelle completely recovered; see Mason, "Learning to Speak." On Anne and Albert, "two youngsters who were reared by their psychotic mother in virtually total isolation from one another as well as the rest of the world," see Freedman and Brown, "On the Role of Coenesthetic Stimulation" (I quote from page 418). On Yves Cheneau, kept locked in a cellar for eighteen months by his stepmother, see Malson, *Wolf Children*, 56–7.

4 In Garmon, *Secret*, and quoted in Rymer, *Genie*, 57.

5 Curtiss, *Genie*, xii.

6 Ibid., 9, 7. Fromkin et al. had recourse to the same rhetoric: "Genie was first encountered when she was 13 years, 9 months. At the time of her discovery and hospitalization she was an unsocialized, primitive human being, emotionally disturbed, unlearned, and without language" ("The Development of Language," 84).

7 Curtiss, *Genie*, 208. See also Fromkin et al., "The Development of Language," 82, and Rymer, *Genie*, 3-6.

8 Curtiss et al., "The Linguistic Development of Genie," 529.

9 Fromkin et al., "The Development of Language," 83.

10 Curtiss, *Genie*, 11, xii. The linguists would of course contend that these questions are as crucial to the human sciences as those raised by Enlightenment philosophers and naturalists. On the critical-age hypothesis, see Lenneberg, *Biological Foundations*. Genie's story is inseparable from Chomsky's linguistic revolution. Rymer cited Chomsky's formulation of yet another version of the forbidden experiment: "Suppose that a child hears no language at all ... There are two possibilities: he can have no language, or he can invent a new one. If you were to put prelinguistic children on an island, the chances are good that their language facility would soon produce a language. Maybe not in the first generation. And that when they did so, it would resemble the languages we know. You can't do the experiment, because you can't subject a child to that experience" (quoted in *Genie*, 37-8). Looking back on the significance of the research on Genie, Curtiss told Rymer (in Rymer, *Genie*, 202) that it was "one of the first times scientists had used a case of an atypical child to understand the typical," a statement that runs counter to everything we know about the history of the sciences of childhood.

11 The book is based on Curtiss's dissertation, "The Case of Genie: A Modern Day 'Wild Child'" (November 1976). Curtiss's adviser was Victoria Fromkin, dean of linguistics at UCLA. In 1971 Jean Butler, a special educator at the rehabilitation centre of Childrens Hospital, applied to become Genie's foster parent. Butler's application was rejected and Genie moved in with the Riglers. The scientists resented Butler's disapproval of the research, which in her view was exhausting Genie. Curtiss said that they felt anxiety and anger at being "kicked out of Genie's house ... Why? [Butler] was crazy, and she didn't want the other attachments" (in Garmon, *Secret*). For David Rigler, Butler "was as destructive as she knew how. She became the Wicked Witch of the West from then on, as far as we were concerned"; but Shurley told Rymer that "to several of us, it seemed a pity that Genie could not be with someone like [Butler], who would bond to her as a person and not as a scientific case" (in Rymer, *Genie*, 107, 211). Butler died in 1988, and thus her own version of the events could not be included in Rymer's and Garmon's accounts.

12 Fromkin et al., "The Development of Language," 94.

13 Curtiss, *Genie*, 38, 102. Its stress on testing and neglect of teaching accounts for why Curtiss's work, while often cited in textbooks as evidence for or against various developmental and linguistic theories, has had no wide-ranging educational applications.

14 Fromkin et al., "The Development of Language," 85; Curtiss, in Rymer, *Genie*, 121. For Curtiss, "emotion has little to do" with language acquisition: "Certainly Genie was an emotionally disturbed child, but that wasn't relevant to my concerns"; ibid., 121.

15 Curtiss, *Genie*, 204.

16 Ibid., 42. According to Curtiss et al., "despite the tragic isolation which she suffered, despite the fact that she had no language for almost the first fourteen years of her life, Genie is equipped to learn language and is learning it. No one can predict how far she will develop linguistically or cognitively. The progress so far, however, has been remarkable, and is a tribute to the human capacity for intellectual achievement" ("The Linguistic Development of Genie," 544). This positive assessment of Genie's progress was widely echoed. Frith affirmed that, unlike autistic Victor, Genie, "who was normal in early childhood and could not be considered autistic even when seen at her worst soon after discovery, improved dramatically ... [I]t seems that there is an excellent prognosis for the victims of early deprivation provided that there is no organic damage" (*Autism*, 35). As mentioned in chapter 7, for Lane Genie's progress proved how much science had advanced since Itard's day and how much John of Burundi could expect from his and Pillard's intervention. But Aitchison suggested that Genie's "slow progress" could be interpreted as "clear evidence in favour of there being a 'cut-off' point for language acquisition" (*The Articulate Mammal*, 73).

17 Miner, quoted in Rymer, *Genie*, 154. The NIMH averred that the researchers had accomplished little and that their ambitious goals were not being met. Shurley saw Genie from time to time at the home for retarded adults where she was living in the early 1990s. In the photographs Shurley showed him Rymer saw "a large, bumbling woman with a facial expression of cowlike incomprehension"; *Genie*, 212.

18 In later articles Curtiss continued to use the linguistic data on Genie but reinterpreted them as evidence *for* the existence of a critical period for first language acquisition (i.e., assuming that Genie had not acquired language – or that most important aspect of language in linguists' view, grammar – after all). See Curtiss, "Dissociations between Language and Cognition," "The Development of Human Cerebral Lateralization," and "Abnormal Language Acquisition." In a more recent article Peter E. Jones calls into question the scientific import and validity of the linguistic research on Genie. He discerns "serious

discrepancies and inconsistencies" in the published accounts of Genie's language acquisition. While the earlier accounts (up to Curtiss's book) portrayed a slow but steady progress, the later ones, none of which furnishes "any details about Genie's life, behavior or circumstances since the Summer of 1975," are different in tone and display a more negative attitude towards Genie's language, partly grounded on "a *highly selective and misleading misrepresentation of the earlier findings*." Jones argues that the discrepancies require urgent clarification. As the matter stands, "the extent of Genie's progress in language acquisition ... remains ... *unknown*" ("Contradictions and Unanswered Questions," 261, 267, 278; the emphases are Jones's).

19 Quoted in Rymer, *Genie*, 58, 104.

20 During her stay at the rehabilitation centre of Childrens Hospital, Genie befriended the cooks. At the May 1971 conference, a scientist is said to have asked one of them: "So Genie responds well to your intrasupportive initiatives?" to which the cook replied, "I just gives her love"; quoted in Rymer, *Genie*, 55. Shurley, the expert in isolation, told Rymer (in *Genie*, 215): "I resolved that if I lived long enough I would do a case study that would show how things should be approached in cases like this ... None of the wild children have been handled well. All of them were handled the way Genie was. She *could* have been handled well. She would have been a disappointment in some ways, but the outcome would have been happier, certainly." While it is true that Genie could have been handled better, I hope to have shown that other wild children were dealt with more responsibly. The scientists most closely involved with Genie reacted strongly to what they saw as "misrepresentations" in Rymer's "A Silent Childhood" and *Genie*, as well as in Natalie Angier's review of Rymer's book; see Angier, "'Stopit!' She Said," Fromkin's and Curtiss's messages to the Linguist discussion list, April 1992 and May 1993, and D. Rigler's letter to the editor of the *New York Time Book Review*.

21 All in Garmon, *Secret*. Curtiss also asserted that Genie elicited extraordinary responses from strangers: "The gifts [strangers would buy for Genie] were chosen with such uncanny accuracy and were tendered in such silence that Curtiss became convinced that she was witnessing a preternatural communication – an explicit, unvoiced understanding – that her careful notebook analysis was unequipped to explain. 'Genie was the most powerful nonverbal communicator I've ever come across,' Curtiss told me" (Rymer, *Genie*, 93).

22 Curtiss, *Genie*, xvi; Curtiss, quoted in Rymer, *Genie*, 219; Miner, quoted in ibid., 181; Curtiss, in Garmon, *Secret*.

23 Simon, "Kaspar Hauser's Recovery and Autopsy," 210, 217.

24 The standard account is Feuerbach's *Kaspar Hauser*, reprinted in Singh and Zingg, *Wolf-Children and Feral Man*, and also in Masson, ed. and trans., *Lost Prince*. Both volumes contain English translations of additional documents.

For a selection of Kaspar's own writings and Daumer's comments on them, see *Kaspar Hauser Speaks for Himself*. See also Kitchen, *Kaspar Hauser*. Kitchen does discuss Genie but argues that Kaspar, "like Genie, was not a truly wild child" (14).

25 Kaspar was said to be the son of Stéphanie Beauharnais (1789–1860), Napoleon's stepdaughter, and Karl, grand duke of Baden (1786–1818). Born in 1812, he was presumably kidnapped and a dying child put in his place by the countess of Hochberg (Luise Geyer von Geyersberg, 1768–1820), second wife of Karl Friedrich of Baden (1728–1811), to permit the accession to the throne of her own eldest son, Leopold (1790–1852; he became grand duke in 1830). On how this theory has been disproved by DNA testing, see Weichhold, Bark, Korte, Eisenmenger, and Sullivan, "DNA Analysis." If Kaspar was not the heir of Baden, and if he was not an impostor, then who was he and what caused his strange behaviour? Kitchen, following recent German scholarship, suggests that he was "an epileptic and mentally retarded child whose parents or guardians had decided to rid themselves of a tiresome burden." Kaspar may indeed have spent his childhood confined in a dark cellar, which was "typical treatment meted out to the mentally ill" (Kitchen, *Kaspar Hauser*, 192, 193). Many writers and artists have been inspired by Kaspar's stirring yet mysterious fate, e.g., Verlaine, "Je suis venu, calme orphelin"; Wassermann, *Caspar Hauser*; Handke, *Kaspar*; and the films *Every Man for Himself and God Against All* by Herzog, and *Kaspar Hauser* by Sehr. On the figure of Kaspar Hauser in literature, see Sampath, *Kaspar Hauser*, Joshua Kendall, "Kaspar Hauser in Literature," in Money, *The Kaspar Hauser Syndrome*, 213–49, and Kitchen, *Kaspar Hauser*, 175–88. See also MacKenzie, "Kaspar Hauser in England." The interpretation proposed by Rudolf Steiner, founder of anthroposophy, and his followers is no doubt the wackiest: Kaspar's short life was "one of the most significant in the history of mankind"; he entered European history with a "great mission ... as a spirit active from its beginning in the true, hidden Rosicrucian stream"; his soul, "one of the greatest helpers for the whole world," leads us "into a new age of spiritual light" (Adam Bittleston, "Introduction," in *Kaspar Hauser Speaks for Himself*, 3, 18, 24). See also Baruch Luke Urieli, "Man's Approach to the Spirit Today and the Sacrifice of Kaspar Hauser," in ibid., 51–67.

26 Feuerbach, *Caspar Hauser*, 286, 293; on Dr Preu, see Bance, "The Kaspar Hauser Legend," 202.

27 Binder's proclamation, written on 7 July 1828 and published on 14 July, is in Masson, *Lost Prince*, 161–72 (I quote from pages 162, 169, 165, 163, 170–1). See Kaspar's own fascinating account of his early days in Nuremberg, in *Kaspar Hauser Speaks for Himself*, 38–44, and also in Masson, *Lost Prince*, 192–5.

28 Quoted in Gemünden, "The Enigma of Hermeneutics," 144.

29 Feuerbach, *Caspar Hauser*, 312; Shengold, "Kaspar Hauser and Soul Murder," 457; Wassermann, *Caspar Hauser*, xvii. Like Feuerbach, Shengold discarded any connection between Kaspar and wild children: "There can be little doubt (based on the work of observers of children) that there must have been some approach to adequate mothering in Kaspar's infancy. He is not one of those feral children who had so little human contact that they can never be taught to achieve even a semblance of human identity" ("Kaspar Hauser and Soul Murder," 463).

30 On the history of child abuse, see Hacking, "The Making and Molding of Child Abuse," and "World-Making by Kind-Making." The possible impact of abuse and neglect on the wild child's state was underlined by Zingg: "Whatever Wild Peter's mentality was, imbecile and tongue-tied as he is represented to us, we cannot today think but that the tragic abuse that he had received from an unnatural parent and from his step-mother must have been some factor in his retardation" ("Feral Man" [1940], 490). Even earlier, Rauber had suggested that Peter's limited mind might have been the lasting outcome of deep scars caused by his early and extraordinary neglect (*Homo sapiens ferus*, 40).

31 Money, *The Kaspar Hauser Syndrome*, 19, 26. Money did not mention Genie, whose history and condition would perfectly have fitted his definition of the "Kaspar Hauser syndrome." Money criticized the recent "shift in focus from brutality to sexual molestation as the primary manifestation of child abuse," in which Masson had a major role (see ibid., 251–63). One purpose of Money's "syndrome" was to account for the discrepancy between Kaspar's real age (he was sixteen in 1828) and his retarded growth. In the case of Genie, whose date of birth is known, appearance did not match real age. In other stories, in which the children's date of birth was not known, their age was estimated based on their appearance. Thus Victor was believed to be twelve or thirteen, but for Money he may have been older, "even as old as nineteen or twenty," for "under prolonged conditions of extreme deprivation and abuse, failure of statural growth may be accompanied by failure of the onset of puberty" (25). This theory might have impressed Sleeman and the many readers of his account of wolf children who were puzzled by the absence of *adults* found living with wolves. For a sharp critique of Money's sex and gender research, see Colapinto, *As Nature Made Him*.

32 Masson, *Lost Prince*, 3, 54.

33 Marcus, "The Wild Boy of Nuremberg"; Masson, *The Assault on Truth*, and *Lost Prince*, 60. In *The Assault on Truth*, Masson "revealed" and denounced Freud's reconceptualization of adults' sexual memories (from evidence of abuse during childhood to mere fantasies).

34 Masson, *Lost Prince*, 55, 61–2, 58, 228n139, 63, 61, 64.

35 Masson, *Lost Prince*, 65, 70–1, 66, 68, 71. Although Masson did not mention Genie either, he did relate Kaspar to the other wild children (39–41) and inserted an appendix on wolf children (203–9). This time too, the deep truth about wild and wolf children is abuse. Masson had something to say about Kipling's *Jungle Book*: "Perhaps if we understand why the theme recommended itself to Kipling we will come closer to understanding humanity's constant preoccupation with wolves and feral children. For obvious reasons this theme had deep emotional resonances for Kipling" (208). Why? Because he had been abused as well: "For mysterious reasons Kipling's parents took him and his sister to Southsea in England, and left them both for six years in a dreary boarding-house, with complete strangers who were committed to destroying the creativity of these unusually vivacious and open youngsters" (209). Masson also had something to say about one of the Salpêtrière patients to whom Pinel compared the wild boy of Aveyron: "It is of course merely speculation, but it is at least possible that these same so-called symptoms could derive from the fact that this girl was sexually abused, and learned early on that there was no point in resisting, that she could do nothing except signal her sorrow by crying" (40). Kincaid's critique of the uses of the "story" of child molesting in the contemporary adult imagination is to the point, as is his injunction to replace it by a new story, in which "the focus would be on the responsibilities of the present and on the grown-up. No more inner children! We are adults and need to tend to the children outside" (*Erotic Innocence*, 292).

36 Fairfax, "The other child?," in *Wild Children*, 45.

37 The correspondence between Auger and Monod is in Auger, "Un enfant-gazelle" (I quote from page 60n2).

38 Armen, *L'enfant sauvage du Grand Désert*, 6, 7 (Monod's preface is not in the English edition, *Gazelle-Boy*).

39 Armen, *Gazelle-Boy*, 17, 28, 13, 34, 44, 55. Monod regretted the lack of photographs, which would have "lifted all ambiguity regarding the materiality of the account" (in Armen, *L'enfant sauvage du Grand Désert*, 6). Armen wrote that he could not take any pictures because the boy ran away from the camera every time he tried.

40 Armen, *Gazelle-Boy*, 30, 32, 35, 58, 101, 75, 78, 80, 94. In 1963 Armen went again in search of the gazelle boy, in the company of a French captain stationed in the region and his aide-de-camp. He found the herd and the child and for a while resumed his observations and attempts at communication. As he became more familiar with the herd's internal organization, he realized that the boy was not "totally free *à la* Rousseau": "he too has to conform to the social pattern" (85).

41 Ibid., 93.

42 Freud, *Civilization and Its Discontents*. See also Elias, *The Civilizing Process*.

43 Armen, *Gazelle-Boy*, 95.

44 "Ostrich boy" and "The wild boy is taught," in Fairfax, *Wild Children*, 31, 40. See also Malouf, *An Imaginary Life*; Apted, *Nell*. Paton Walsh's representation of the wild child in *Knowledge of Angels* is much more ambiguous, emphasizing the lack of morality and consciousness inherent to the wild state. The nuns who are in charge of Amara, the ex-wolf girl, find out that she once had a twin sister and ask what happened to her: "'I killed her,' she said." When the abbess asks her why, Amara says: "'Not remember why'" (*Knowledge of Angels*, 213).

45 Armen, *Gazelle-Boy*, 93.

46 A new, sad form (or figure) of the wild child appears to be taking shape. Several so-called wild or feral children were found in recent years living with stray dogs in the contemporary wilderness, the dangerous and uncaring urban jungle, in Moscow and Ukraine, Chile and Romania, Manila and Kenya (see above, chapters 1 and 2).

EPILOGUE

1 Bakhtin, "From Notes Made in 1970–71," in *Speech Genres*, 134.

2 Ariès, *Centuries of Childhood*, 128 (originally published as *L'enfant et la vie familiale*). That Ariès's work continues to inspire and intrigue historians of childhood and the family is evident in the long passages devoted to it in Heywood, *A History of Childhood*, and Ozment, *Ancestors*. For more on the historiography of childhood's indebtedness to Ariès, see H. Cunningham, "Histories of Childhood," and Benzaquén, "Childhood, the Sciences of Childhood, and the History of Science."

3 Curtiss, *Genie*, 7.

4 DeMause, "The Evolution of Childhood," in *The History of Childhood*, 1, 6, 7. DeMause's assessment of the history of childhood (like Masson's rendering of Kaspar's story) relies heavily on an anachronistic and decontextualized understanding of abuse, and his "psychogenic theory of history" – which postulates that historical change is caused by "'psychogenic' changes in personality occurring because of successive generations of parent-child interactions" (3) – is rigid and simplistic at best. For a retrospective look by deMause himself on his work and the reactions it provoked, see his "On Writing Childhood History."

5 Elias, *The Civilizing Process*, 518.

6 Ibid., xiii. Elias wrote: "The more 'natural' the standard of delicacy and shame appears to adults and the more the civilized restraint of instinctual urges is taken for granted, the more incomprehensible it becomes to adults that children do not have this delicacy and shame by 'nature.' The children necessarily touch again and again on the adult threshold of delicacy, and – since they are not yet adapted – they infringe the taboos of society, cross the adult shame frontier, and penetrate emotional danger zones which the adult himself can

only control with difficulty" (137). A concern with the "civilization" of children was evident in child development textbooks and child-rearing manuals since at least the second half of the nineteenth century. One example: "From birth onwards, children feel the pressures of urgent body needs and powerful instinctive urges (such as hunger, sex and aggression) which clamour for satisfaction. Soon afterwards, the child encounters demands for restraint, and the prohibition on wish-fulfilment, which comes from the parents, whose task it is to turn their children from unrestrained greedy and cruel little savages into well-behaved, socially-adapted, civilized beings"; Edith Buxbaum, *Your Child Makes Sense: A Guidebook for Parents* (London: Allen and Unwin, 1951), quoted in Hardyment, *Dream Babies*, 230.

7 "Only in relation to other human beings does the wild, helpless creature which comes into the world become the psychologically developed person with the character of an individual and deserving the name of an adult human being. Cut off from such relations he grows at best into a semi-wild human animal. He may grow up bodily; in his psychological make-up he remains like a small child"; Elias, "The Society of Individuals – 1" (late 1930s), in *The Norbert Elias Reader*, 70.

8 Arendt, "The Crisis in Education," in *Between Past and Future*, 176, 185, 189.

9 The privatization (within the nuclear family) and professionalization of child care is a central feature of modern Western societies. Ever more exclusive and proprietary parent-child relations are complemented or, when parents are found wanting, supplanted by relations between children and professionals of childhood (educators, physicians, caregivers, social workers, psychologists, psychoanalysts). Paradoxically, this narrowing trend in adult-child relations has intensified with the rise of the concept of child abuse. Even though in most cases of child abuse the perpetrators are the parents, other close relatives, or child professionals, the actual effect of the panic surrounding child abuse on child-adult relations has been the almost total disappearance of informal relations between *any* adult and *any* child.

Bibliography

Aarsleff, Hans. *From Locke to Saussure: Essays on the Study of Language and Intellectual History.* Minneapolis: University of Minnesota Press, 1982.

"Account of a Book." Review of *The History of Poland*, by B. Connor. *Philosophical Transactions* 20, no. 238 (March 1698): 98–103.

Affre, H. *Biographie Aveyronnaise.* Rodez: H. de Broca, 1881.

Aitchison, Jean. *The Articulate Mammal: An Introduction to Psycholinguistics.* London: Hutchinson, 1976.

L'âme matérielle (ouvrage anonyme). Edited by Alain Niderst. Paris: Presses Universitaires de France, 1973.

Ames, Louise Bates. *Arnold Gesell: Themes of His Work.* New York: Human Sciences Press, 1989.

Anastasi, Anne. *Differential Psychology: Individual and Group Differences in Behavior.* New York: Macmillan, 1937.

Anastasi, Anne, and John P. Foley. *Differential Psychology: Individual and Group Differences in Behavior.* New York: Macmillan, 1949.

Angier, Natalie. "'Stopit!' She Said. 'Nomore!'" Review of *Genie*, by R. Rymer. *New York Times Book Review*, 25 April 1993, 12.

Annual Register, or a View of the History, Politick, and Literature, For the Year ... London: J. Dodsley, 1758–1787.

Apted, Michael. *Nell.* Beverly Hills: FoxVideo, 1995. Videocassette. Originally released as motion picture in 1994.

Arendt, Hannah. *Between Past and Future: Six Exercises in Political Thought.* New York: Viking, 1961.

Ariès, Philippe. *L'enfant et la vie familiale sous l'Ancien Régime.* Paris: Plon, 1960.

– *Centuries of Childhood: A Social History of Family Life.* Translated by R. Baldick. New York: Vintage, 1962.

Armen, Jean-Claude. *L'enfant sauvage du Grand Désert: Découverte d'un enfant-gazelle observé dans son milieu naturel.* Neuchâtel: Delachaux & Niestlé, 1971.

– *Gazelle-Boy: A Child Brought Up by Gazelles in the Sahara Desert.* Translated by S. Hardman. London: Bodley Head, 1974.

Arnobius of Sicca. *The Case against the Pagans.* Translated and edited by G.E. McCracken. 2 vols. Westminster: Newman, 1949.

Auger, Jean-Claude. "Un enfant-gazelle au Sahara Occidental." *Notes africaines* 98 (April 1963): 58–61.

Austin, N.J. "Autobiography and History: Some Later Roman Historians and their Veracity." In *History and Historians in Late Antiquity,* edited by B. Croke and A.M. Emmett, 54–65. Sydney: Pergamon, 1983.

Baker, E.C. Stuart. "The Power of Scent in Wild Animals." *Journal of the Bombay Natural History Society* 227 (July 1920): 117–18. In R.M. Zingg. "Feral Man and Cases of Extreme Isolation of Individuals," 170–2.

Bakhtin, Mikhail. *Problems of Dostoevsky's Poetics* (1929). Edited and translated by C. Emerson. Minneapolis: University of Minnesota Press, 1984.

– *Speech Genres and Other Late Essays.* Translated by V.W. McGee. Edited by C. Emerson and M. Holquist. Austin: University of Texas Press, 1986.

Ball, Thomas S. "Training Generalized Imitation: Variations on an Historical Theme." *American Journal of Mental Deficiency* 75, no. 2 (1970): 135–41.

– *Itard, Seguin and Kephart: Sensory Education – A Learning Interpretation.* Columbus: Charles E. Merrill, 1971.

Ball, Valentin. *Jungle Life in India; or the Journeys and Journals of an Indian Geologist.* London: Thos. de la Rue, 1880.

Bance, A.F. "The Kaspar Hauser Legend and Its Literary Survival." *German Life and Letters* 28, no. 3 (April 1975): 199–210.

Barnard, Alan. "*Orang Outang* and the Definition of Man: The Legacy of Lord Monboddo." In *Fieldwork and Footnotes: Studies in the History of European Anthropology,* edited by H.F. Vermeulen and A. Alvarez Roldán, 95–112. London: Routledge, 1995.

Baron-Cohen, Simon, Helen Tager-Flusberg, and Donald J. Cohen, eds. *Understanding Other Minds: Perspectives from Autism.* Oxford: Oxford University Press, 1993.

Barr, Martin. *Mental Defectives: Their History, Treatment and Training.* Philadelphia: P. Blakiston's Son, 1904.

Bartra, Roger. *Wild Men in the Looking Glass: The Mythic Origins of European Otherness.* Translated by C.T. Berrisford. Ann Arbor: University of Michigan Press, 1994.

– *The Artificial Savage: Modern Myths of the Wild Man.* Translated by C. Follett. Ann Arbor: University of Michigan Press, 1997.

Bayle, Pierre. *Réponse aux questions d'un provincial.* 3d part (1706). In *Œuvres diverses.* Vol. 3, part 2. La Haye: P. Husson, 1727.

Becchi, Egle, and Dominique Julia, eds. *Histoire de l'enfance en Occident*. Vol. 2: *Du XVIIIe siècle à nos jours*. Paris: du Seuil, 1998.

Bedel, Christian-Pierre. *Sent-Sarnin: Balaguièr, Brasc, Combret, Copiac, La Bastida-Solatges, La Sèrra, La Val-Ròca-Cesièira, Martrinh, Montclar, Montfranc, Plasença, Postòmis, Sant-Jòri*. Rodez: Mission Départamentale de la Culture, 1994.

Bendyshe, Thomas. "The History of Anthropology." *Memoirs Read Before the Anthropological Society of London* 1 (1865): 335–458.

Benedict, Ruth. *Patterns of Culture* (1934). 2d ed. Cambridge: Riverside, 1959.

Benichou, Claude, and Claude Blanckaert, eds. *Julien-Joseph Virey: naturaliste et anthropologue*. Paris: Vrin, 1988.

Bentham, Jeremy. *Panopticon: or, the Inspection-House. Containing the Idea of a New Principle of Construction applicable to any Sort of Establishment, in which Persons of any Description are to be kept under Inspection ... In a Series of Letters, Written in the Year 1787 ...* Dublin: Thomas Byrne, 1791.

Benzaquén, Adriana S. "Kamala of Midnapore and Arnold Gesell's *Wolf Child and Human Child*: Reconciling the Extraordinary and the Normal." *History of Psychology* 4, no. 1 (2001): 59–78.

– "Childhood, Identity, and Human Science in the Enlightenment." *History Workshop Journal* 57 (Spring 2004): 34–57.

– "Childhood, the Sciences of Childhood, and the History of Science." In *Multiple Lenses, Multiple Images: Perspectives on the Child across Time, Space and Disciplines*, edited by H. Goelman, S. Marshall, and S. Ross, 14–37. Toronto: University of Toronto Press, 2004.

Bernard, René. *Surdité, surdi-mutité et mutisme dans le Théâtre français*. Paris: Vrin, 1941.

Bernard, René, ed. "Autour du Sauvage de l'Aveyron." *Revue générale de l'enseignement des déficients auditifs* 66, no. 2 (1974): 82–9.

– "Un dossier sur Victor le Sauvage de l'Aveyron à l'Institution des Sourds-Muets de Paris." *Bulletin d'audiophonologie* 7, no. 5 (1977): 33–68.

Bernheimer, Richard. *Wild Men in the Middle Ages: A Study in Art, Sentiment, and Demonology*. Cambridge: Harvard University Press, 1952.

Bettelheim, Bruno. "Feral Children and Autistic Children." *American Journal of Sociology* 64, no. 5 (1959): 455–67.

– *The Empty Fortress: Infantile Autism and the Birth of the Self*. New York: Free Press, 1967.

Bewell, Alan. *Wordsworth and the Enlightenment: Nature, Man, and Society in the Experimental Poetry*. New Haven: Yale University Press, 1989.

Biklen, Douglas. *Communication Unbound: How Facilitated Communication is Challenging Traditional Views of Autism and Ability/Disability*. New York: Teachers College Press, 1993.

Biklen, Douglas, and Donald N. Cardinal, eds. *Contested Words, Contested Science: Unraveling the Facilitated Communication Controversy.* New York: Teachers College Press, 1997.

Binet, Alfred, and Th. Simon, *Mentally Defective Children.* Translated by W.B. Drummond. London: Edward Arnold, 1914.

Birch, Thomas. *The History of the Royal Society of London for Improving of Natural Knowledge, From Its First Rise.* Vol. 1. London: A. Millar, 1756.

Blumenbach, Johann Friedrich. "Vom Homo sapiens *ferus* Linn. und namentlich von Hamelschen *wilden Peter.*" In *Beyträge zur Naturgeschichte.* Vol. 2, 13–14. Göttingen: Heinrich Dieterich, 1811.

– *The Anthropological Treatises of Johann Friedrich Blumenbach.* Edited and translated by T. Bendyshe. London: Longman, 1865.

Bompas, Cecil Henry, ed. and trans. *Folklore of the Santal Parganas* (1909). New Delhi: Ajay, 1981.

Bonnaterre, Pierre-Joseph. *Notice historique sur le sauvage de l'Aveyron et sur quelques autres individus qu'on a trouvé dans les forêts, à différentes époques.* Paris: Vve. Panckouke, 1800. In T. Gineste. *Victor de l'Aveyron,* 180–212.

Bonnet, Charles. *Essai analytique sur les facultés de l'âme.* Copenhagen: Cl. & Ant. Philibert, 1760.

Bory de Saint-Vincent (Jean-Baptiste-Geneviève Marcellin). *L'Homme (*Homo*): Essai zoologique sur le genre humain.* 2d ed. 2 vols. Paris: Rey et Grevier, 1827.

Boswell, James. *The Journal of a Tour to the Hebrides, with Samuel Johnson, LL.D.* London: Henry Baldwin, 1785.

– *The Life of Samuel Johnson, LL.D. Comprehending an Account of His Studies and Numerous Works.* 2 vols. London: Henry Baldwin, for Charles Dilly, 1791.

Bourdieu, Pierre. *Language and Symbolic Power.* Translated by G. Raymond and M. Adamson. Cambridge: Harvard University Press, 1994.

Boyd, William. *From Locke to Montessori: A Critical Account of the Montessori Point of View.* London: George G. Harrap, 1912.

Brauner, Alfred, and Françoise Brauner. "Le 'Sauvage' psychotique de l'Aveyron." *Tribune de l'enfance* 7, no. 61 (1969): 41–50.

– *L'enfant déréel: Histoire des autismes depuis les contes de fées: Fictions littéraires et réalités cliniques.* Toulouse: Privat, 1986.

Broberg, Gunnar. *Homo Sapiens L.: Studier i Carl von Linnés naturuppfattning och människolära.* Stockholm: Almquist & Wiksell, 1975.

– "Homo sapiens: Linnaeus's Classification of Man." In *Linnaeus: The Man and His Work,* edited by T. Frängsmyr, 156–94. Berkeley: University of California Press, 1983.

Broche, François. "Le secret des enfants sauvages." *Miroir de l'histoire* 224 (1968): 48–55.

Brown, Roger. *Words and Things*. Glencoe: Free Press, 1958.

Buffon, Georges-Louis Leclerc de. *Histoire naturelle, générale et particulière*. 15 vols. Paris: Imprimerie royale, 1749–1767.

Burroughs, Edgar Rice. "Tarzan of the Apes: A Romance of the Jungle." *All-Story*, October 1912.

Burton, R.G. "Wolf-Children and Werewolves." *Chambers's Journal* 14, 7th series, no. 698 (12 April 1924): 306–10.

Butler, Samuel. *Hudibras* (1663–1678). With notes and a preface by Zachary Grey. 2 vols. Dublin: A. Reilly, 1744.

Camerarius, Philipp. *Operæ horarvm svbcisivarvm Sive meditationes historicæ avctiores quam antea editæ*. Frankfurt: Egenolphi Emmelij, 1615. Originally published in 1591.

– *The Living Librarie, or, Meditations and Observations Historical, Natural, Moral, Political, and Poetical*. Translated by Iohn Molle. London: Adam Islip, 1621.

Candland, Douglas Keith. *Feral Children and Clever Animals: Reflections on Human Nature*. New York: Oxford University Press, 1993.

Carrey, Normand J. "Itard's 1828 Mémoire on 'Mutism Caused by a Lesion of the Intellectual Functions': A Historical Analysis." *Journal of the American Academy of Child and Adolescent Psychiatry* 34, no. 12 (December 1995): 1,655–61.

Carroll, Michael P. "The Folkloric Origins of Modern 'Animal-Parented Children' Stories." *Journal of Folklore Research* 21, no. 1 (April 1984): 63–85.

Case, Jan, and Charles C. Cleland. "Eminence and Mental Retardation as Determined by Cattell's Space Method." *Mental Retardation* 3, no. 3 (June 1975): 20–1.

Castan, Bruno. *Le babou ou l'enfant sauvage*. Paris: Ges-éditions, 1991.

Certeau, Michel de, Dominique Julia, and Jacques Revel. *Une politique de la langue: La Révolution française et les patois: L'enquête de Grégoire*. Paris: Gallimard, 1975.

Chamberlain, Alexander Francis. *The Child and Childhood in Folk-Thought*. New York: Macmillan, 1896.

Chappey, Jean-Luc. *La Société des Observateurs de l'homme (1799–1804): Des anthropologues au temps de Bonaparte*. Paris: Société des études robespierristes, 2002.

Chapple, Eliot Dismore, and Carleton Stevens Coon. *Principles of Anthropology*. New York: Henry Holt, 1942.

Chatwin, Bruce. "The Quest for the Wolf Children." *Sunday Times Magazine*, 30 July 1978, 10–13.

Chauchard, Paul. *Le langage et la pensée*. Paris: Presses Universitaires de France, 1956.

"Children Suckled by Wolves." *Chambers' Edinburgh Journal* 425, new series (21 February 1852): 122–3.

Cloyd, Emily L. *James Burnett, Lord Monboddo*. Oxford: Clarendon Press, 1972.

Code, Lorraine. *Epistemic Responsibility*. Hanover: University Press of New England, 1987.

Colapinto, John. *As Nature Made Him: The Boy Who Was Raised as a Girl*. New York: Harper Collins, 2000.

Coleridge, Samuel Taylor. *The Notebooks of Samuel Taylor Coleridge*. Edited by K. Coburn. Vol. 1: 1794–1804, text (1957). 2d ed. New Jersey: Princeton University Press, 1980.

– *The Notebooks of Samuel Taylor Coleridge*. Edited by K. Coburn. Vol. 3: 1808–1819, text. New Jersey: Princeton University Press, 1973.

Condillac, Étienne Bonnot, abbé de. *Essai sur l'origine des connoissances humaines, ouvrage où l'on réduit à un seul principe tout ce qui concerne l'entendement humain*. Amsterdam: P. Mortier, 1746.

– *Traité des sensations*. 2 vols. London and Paris: De Bure l'aîné, 1754.

Connor, Bernard. *Evangelium medici: Seu Medicina Mystica; de Suspensis Naturæ Legibus, sive De Miraculis*. London: Richard Wellington, 1697.

– *The History of Poland, In Several Letters to Persons of Quality*. 2 vols. London: J.D. for Dan Brown, 1698.

Copans, Jean, and Jean Jamin, eds. *Aux origines de l'anthropologie française: Les mémoires de la Société des Observateurs de l'homme en l'an VIII*. Paris: Le Sycomore, 1978.

Coulton, G.G., ed. and trans. *From St. Francis to Dante: Translations from the Chronicle of the Franciscan Salimbene (1221–1288)* (1907). 2d ed. Philadelphia: University of Philadelphia Press, 1972.

Cox, Nicholas. *The Gentleman's Recreation*. 2d ed. London: J.C. for N.C., 1677.

Cranefield, Paul F. "Historical Perspectives." In *Prevention and Treatment of Mental Retardation*, edited by I. Philips, 3–14. New York: Basic, 1966.

Crooke, William. *Things Indian: Being Discursive Notes on Various Subjects Connected with India*. London: John Murray, 1906.

Cunningham, D.J. "Anthropology in the Eighteenth Century." *Journal of the Royal Anthropological Institute of Great Britain and Ireland* 38 (1908): 10–35.

Cunningham, Hugh. "Histories of Childhood." *American Historical Review* 103, no. 4 (1998): 1,195–208.

Curtiss, Susan. *Genie: A Psycholinguistic Study of a Modern-Day "Wild Child."* New York: Academic Press, 1977.

– "Dissociations between Language and Cognition: Cases and Implications." *Journal of Autism and Developmental Disorders* 11, no. 1 (March 1981): 15–30.

– "The Development of Human Cerebral Lateralization." In *The Dual Brain: Hemispheric Specialization in Humans*, edited by D.F. Benson and E. Zaidel, 97–116. New York: Guildford, 1985.

– "Abnormal Language Acquisition and Grammar: Evidence for the Modularity of Language." In *Language, Speech and Mind: Studies in Honour of Victoria A. Fromkin,* edited by L.M. Hyman and C.N. Li, 81–102. London: Routledge, 1988.

Curtiss, Susan, Victoria Fromkin, Stephen Krashen, David Rigler, and Marilyn Rigler. "The Linguistic Development of Genie." *Language* 50, no. 3 (September 1974): 528–54.

Dalitz, R.H., and G.C. Stone. "Doctor Bernard Connor: Physician to King Jan III Sobieski and Author of *The History of Poland* (1698)." *Oxford Slavonic Papers* 14 (1981): 14–35.

Darnton, Robert. *The Great Cat Massacre and Other Episodes in French Cultural History.* New York: Vintage, 1984.

Daston, Lorraine, ed. *Biographies of Scientific Objects.* Chicago: University of Chicago Press, 2000.

Davis, Kingsley. "Extreme Social Isolation of a Child." *American Journal of Sociology* 45 (1940): 554–65.

– "Final Note on a Case of Extreme Isolation." *American Journal of Sociology* 52 (1947): 432–7.

La Décade philosophique, littéraire et politique. Paris: au Bureau de la Décade, 1794–1804.

De Pauw, Cornelius. *Recherches philosophiques sur les Americains, ou Mémoires intéressants pour servir à l'Histoire de l'Espèce Humaine.* 2 vols. Berlin: G.J. Decker, 1768 and 1769.

[Defoe, Daniel]. *Mere Nature Delineated: Or, a Body without a Soul. Being Observations upon the Young Forester Lately brought to Town from Germany. With Suitable Applications. Also, A Brief Dissertation upon the Usefulness and Necessity of Fools, whether Political or Natural.* London: T. Warner, 1726.

Delasiauve, Louis-Jean-François. "Le sauvage du Var, par M. le docteur Mesnet." *Journal de médecine mentale* 5 (May–June 1865): 156–63.

– "Le sauvage de l'Aveyron." *Journal de médecine mentale* 5 (July 1865): 197–211.

Delisle de Sales (Jean-Baptiste-Claude Izouard). *De la Philosophie de la nature, ou Traité de morale pour l'espèce humaine, Tiré de la Philosophie et fondé sur la nature.* 3d ed. 6 vols. London, 1778.

Demaison, André. *Le livre des enfants sauvages.* Paris: André Bonne, 1953.

DeMause, Lloyd, ed. *The History of Childhood.* New York: Psychohistory Press, 1974.

– "On Writing Childhood History." *Journal of Psychohistory* 16, no. 2 (Fall 1988): 135–71.

Dennis, Wayne. "The Significance of Feral Man." *American Journal of Psychology* 54 (1941): 425–32.

– "A Further Analysis of Reports of Wild Children." *Child Development* 22, no. 2 (June 1951): 153–8.

Desmond, Adrian J. *The Ape's Reflexion*. New York: Dial, 1979.

The Devil to pay at St. James's: or, a full and true Account of a most horrid and bloody Battle between Madam Faustina and Madam Cuzzoni ... And How the Wild Boy is come to Life again, and has got a Dairy Maid with Child ... London: A. Moore, 1727.

Digby, Kenelm. *Two Treatises. In the One of Which, the Nature of Bodies; In the Other, the Nature of Mans Soule; Is Looked into: In Way of Discovery, of the Immortality of Reasonable Soules*. Paris: Gilles Blaizot, 1644.

Dilich, Wilhelm. *Hessische Chronica*. 2 vols. Cassel, 1605. Facs. reprint (in one vol.). Kassel: Bärenreiter-Verlag, 1961.

Doll, Eugene E. "A Historical Survey of Research and Management of Mental Retardation in the United States." In *Readings on the Exceptional Child: Research and Theory*, edited by E.P. Trapp and P. Himelstein, 21–68. New York: Appleton-Century-Crofts, 1962.

Douglas, Adam. *The Beast Within: Man, Myths and Werewolves*. London: Orion, 1993.

Douthwaite, Julia. "Rewriting the Savage: The Extraordinary Fictions of the 'Wild Girl of Champagne.'" *Eighteenth-Century Studies* 28, no. 2 (1994–95): 163–92.

– "*Homo ferus*: Between Monster and Model." *Eighteenth-Century Life* 20 (May 1997): 176–202.

– *The Wild Girl, Natural Man, and the Monster: Dangerous Experiments in the Age of Enlightenment*. Chicago: University of Chicago Press, 2002.

Duche, D.J., and M. Dugas. "La psychiatrie de l'enfant en France hier et aujourd'hui." *Revue de psychologie appliquée* 36 (1986): 203–17.

Duchet, Michèle. *Anthropologie et histoire au siècle des lumières: Buffon, Voltaire, Rousseau, Helvétius, Diderot*. Paris: François Maspero, 1971.

Ducray-Duminil, François-Guillaume. *Victor, ou L'enfant de la forêt*. 4 vols. Paris: Le Prieur, 1797.

Dunn, Charles W. *The Foundling and the Werwolf: A Literary-Historical Study of Guillaume de Palerne*. Toronto: University of Toronto Press, 1960.

Durand-Sendrail, Béatrice. "*L'Elève de la nature* de Gaspard Guillard de Beaurieu: Un avatar de l'expérience de Psammétique." *Studies on Voltaire and the Eighteenth Century* 346 (1996): 381–4.

Dusselthal Abbey: Count Von Der Recke's Institutions for Destitute Orphans and Jewish Proselytes. Edinburgh: J. Ritchie, 1836.

Edgeworth, Richard Lovell, and Maria Edgeworth. *Practical Education*. 2 vols. London: J. Johnson, 1798.

Elias, Norbert. *The Civilizing Process: The History of Manners and State Formation and Civilization* (1939). Translated by E. Jephcott. New York: Blackwell, 1994.

– *The Norbert Elias Reader: A Biographical Selection*. Edited by J. Goudsblom and S. Mennell. Oxford: Blackwell, 1998.

L'enfant sauvage de l'Aveyron. Rodez: Mission Départementale de la Culture, 1992.

An Enquiry how the Wild Youth, Lately taken in the Woods near Hanover, (and now brought over to England) could be there left, and by what Creature he could be suckled, nursed, and brought up. London: H. Parker, 1726.

Ernct, Sophie. "Un admirable echec." *Les temps modernes* 50, no. 582 (May–June 1995): 151–82.

Esquirol, Jean-Etienne-Dominique. "Idiotisme." In *Dictionnaire des Sciences médicales, par une société des médecins et de chirurgiens*. Vol. 23, 507–24. Paris: C.L.F. Panckoucke, 1818.

– *Des Maladies mentales: Considérées sous les rapports médical, hygiénique et médico-légal*. 2 vols. Paris: J.-B. Baillière, 1838.

Evans, Bergen. "Wolf! Wolf!" *New Republic* 104 (26 May 1941): 734–5.

– *The Natural History of Nonsense*. New York: Alfred A. Knopf, 1946. Reprint. 1953.

Fairfax, John. *Wild Children*. Hermitage, Newbury: Phoenix Press, 1985.

Favazza, Armando R. "Feral and Isolated Children." *British Journal of Medical Psychology* 50, no. 1 (March 1977): 105–11.

Feijoo, Benito Jerónimo. *Teatro crítico universal*. Vol. 6 (1734). New ed. Madrid: Andrés Ortega, 1778.

– *Cartas eruditas y curiosas*. Vol. 3 (1750). New ed. Madrid: Imprenta Real de la Gazeta, 1774.

Fein, Leah Gold. "Clinical Child Psychology: International Perspective." *Journal of Clinical Child Psychology* 5, no. 3 (Winter 1976): 30–5.

Ferguson, Adam. *An Essay on the History of Civil Society*. Edinburgh: A. Millar & T. Caddel, 1767.

Feuerbach, Anselm von. *Caspar Hauser: An Account of an Individual Kept in a Dungeon, Separated from All Communication with the World, from Early Childhood to about the Age of Seventeen*. Translated from the German (1833). In J.A.L. Singh and R.M. Zingg. *Wolf-Children and Feral Man*, 277–356.

Fiedler, Leslie. *Freaks: Myths and Images of the Secret Self*. New York: Simon and Schuster, 1978.

Flatley, Guy. "So Truffaut Decided to Work His Own Miracle." *New York Times*, 27 September 1970, D13.

Foley, John P. "The 'Baboon Boy' of South Africa." *American Journal of Psychology* 53 (January 1940): 128–33.

– "The 'Baboon Boy' of South Africa." *Science* 91, no. 2,360 (22 March 1940): 291–2, and no. 2,374 (28 June 1940): 618–19.

Formey, Jean-Henri-Samuel. *Anti-Emile*. Berlin: Joachim Pauli, 1763.

Formigari, Lia. "Language and Society in the Late Eighteenth Century." *Journal of the History of Ideas* 35, no. 2 (April–June 1974): 275–92.

Forness, Steven R., and Donald L. MacMillan. "The Origins of Behavior Modification with Exceptional Children." *Exceptional Children* 37, no. 2 (October 1970): 93–100.

Forrester, John. "If *p*, Then What? Thinking in Cases." *History of the Human Sciences* 9, no. 3 (1996): 1–25.

Fortean Times. 1973–.

Foucault, Michel. *The Archaeology of Knowledge and the Discourse on Language* (1969). Translated by A.M. Sheridan Smith. New York: Pantheon, 1972.

– ed. *I, Pierre Rivière, Having Slaughtered My Mother, My Sister, and My Brother ... : A Case of Parricide in the 19th Century* (1973). Translated by F. Jellinek. New York: Pantheon, 1975.

– *Discipline and Punish: The Birth of the Prison* (1975). Translated by A. Sheridan. New York: Vintage, 1979.

– *The History of Sexuality*. Vol. 1: *An Introduction* (1976). Translated by R. Hurley. New York: Vintage, 1990.

– "Questions of Method: An Interview with Michel Foucault." *Ideology & Consciousness* 8 (Spring 1981): 3–14.

Foulquier-Lavergne, Paul. "Étude historique et statistique sur le canton de Saint-Sernin." *Mémoires de la Société des letters, sciences et arts de l'Aveyron* 11 (1874–1878): 81–194.

– *Le sauvage de l'Aveyron*. Rodez: Broca, 1875. Reprinted in *L'enfant sauvage de l'Aveyron*, 126–35.

Fox, Christopher, Roy Porter, and Robert Wokler, eds. *Inventing Human Science: Eighteenth-Century Domains*. Berkeley: University of California Press, 1995.

Frazer, James George, ed. and trans. *The* Fasti *of Ovid*. Vol. 2: Commentary on Books 1 and 2. London: Macmillan, 1929.

Freedman, David A., and Stuart L. Brown. "On the Role of Coenesthetic Stimulation in the Development of Psychic Structure." *Psychoanalytic Quarterly* 37, no. 3 (July 1968): 418–38.

Freud, Sigmund. *Civilization and Its Discontents* (1930). Translated by J. Strachey. New York: Norton, 1961.

Friedman, Erwin. "A Historical Note to 'The Wild Boy of Kronstadt.'" *Journal of the History of the Behavioral Sciences* 1 (July 1965): 284.

Frith, Uta. *Autism: Explaining the Enigma*. Oxford: Basil Blackwell, 1989.

Fromkin, Victoria, Stephen Krashen, Susan Curtiss, David Rigler, and Marilyn Rigler. "The Development of Language in Genie: A Case of Language Acquisition beyond the 'Critical Period.'" *Brain and Language* 1 (1974): 81–107.

Fynne, Robert John. *Montessori and Her Inspirers*. London: Longmans, Green, 1924.

Gall, Franz Josef, and Johann Gaspar Spurzheim. *Anatomie et physiologie du système nerveux en géné-ral, et du cerveau en particulier*. 4 vols. Paris: F. Schoell, 1810–1819.

Galton, Francis. "The First Steps towards the Domestication of Animals." *Transactions of the Ethnological Society of London* 3, new series (1865): 122–38.

Gardner, R. Allen, and Beatrix T. Gardner. "Cross-Fostered Chimpanzees: I. Testing Vocabulary." In *Understanding Chimpanzees*, edited by P.G. Heltne and L.A. Marquardt, 220–33. Cambridge: Harvard University Press, 1989.

Garmon, Linda. *Secret of the Wild Child*. Boston: WGBH, 1994. Videocassette.

Garraty, J.A., and M.C. Carnes, eds. *American National Biography*. Vol. 8. New York: Oxford University Press, 1999.

Gayda, M. "A l'avènement de la thérapeutique des psychoses et du polyhandicap de l'enfant: J.-M.-G. Itard (pour le 150ᵉ anniversaire de sa mort)." *Année médicopsychologique* 147, no. 2 (March–April 1989): 187–9.

Gaynor, John F. "The 'Failure' of J.M.G. Itard." *Journal of Special Education* 7, no. 4 (1973): 439–45.

Gayon, Jean, and Jean-Claude Beaune, eds. *Buffon 88*. Paris: Vrin, 1992.

Gayral, Louis, Pierre Chabbert, and Hélène Baillaud-Citeau. "Les premières observations de l'enfant sauvage de Lacaune (dit 'Victor' ou 'Le sauvage de l'Aveyron'): Nouveaux documents." *Annales médico-psychologiques* 130, no. 4 (November 1972): 465–90.

Gemünden, Gerd. "The Enigma of Hermeneutics: The Case of Kaspar Hauser." In *Reading after Foucault: Institutions, Disciplines, and Technologies of the Self in Germany, 1750–1830*, edited by R.S. Leventhal, 127–49. Detroit: Wayne State University Press, 1994.

Gentleman's Magazine. London: E. Cave, 1736–1785.

Gerstein, Mordicai. *Victor: A Novel Based on the Life of the Savage of Aveyron*. New York: Farrar, Straus and Giroux, 1998.

– *The Wild Boy: Based on the True Story of the Wild Boy of Aveyron*. New York: Farrar, Straus and Giroux, 1998.

Gesell, Arnold. "The Biography of a Wolf-Child." *Harper's Magazine* 182 (December 1940 – May 1941): 183–93.

– *Wolf Child and Human Child: Being a Narrative Interpretation of the Life History of Kamala, the Wolf Girl*. New York: Harper and Brothers, 1941.

– "Wolf-Children and Genetic Psychology." *Saturday Review of Literature* 26 (9 January 1943): 14.

– *How a Baby Grows: A Story in Pictures*. New York: Harper, 1945.

Gesell, Arnold, and Catherine S. Amatruda. *Developmental Diagnosis: Normal and Abnormal Child Development, Clinical Methods and Pediatric Applications* (1941). 2d ed. New York: Harper and Row, 1947.

Gesell, Arnold, H. Thompson, and Catherine S. Amatruda. *An Atlas of Infant Behavior: A Systematic Delineation of the Forms and Early Growth of Human Behavior Patterns*. 2 vols. New Haven: Yale University Press, 1934.

Gesell, Arnold, et al. *The First Five Years of Life: A Guide to the Study of the Preschool Child*. New York: Harper, 1940.

Giddens, Anthony. *Sociology*. Cambridge: Polity, 1989.

Giglioli, Enrico. "Ragazzi allevati e conviventi con lupi nell'Hindustan." *Archivio per l'Antropologia e la Etnologia* 12 (1882): 49–54.

Gill, Jerry H. *If a Chimpanzee Could Talk and Other Reflections on Language Acquisition*. Tucson: University of Arizona Press, 1997.

Gineste, Thierry. "La crèche ou le tombeau: L'enfant connu sous le nom de sauvage de l'Aveyron devant ses 'bienfaiteurs' parisiens." *Perspectives psychiatriques* 1, no. 65 (1978): 43–8.

– "Post-scriptum à l'immaculée conception de la pédopsychiatrie: Du sauvage de l'Aveyron au sauvage de la Drôme." *L'evolution psychiatrique* 44, no. 1 (1979): 130–7.

– "A propos de *L'enfant sauvage de l'Aveyron* de Harlan Lane." *L'évolution psychiatrique* 45, no. 1 (1980): 185–90.

– *Victor de l'Aveyron: Dernier enfant sauvage, premier enfant fou* (1981). 2d ed. Paris: Hachette/Pluriel, 1993.

– "Les écrits psychiatriques de J.-M.-G. Itard: A propos d'un manuscrit inédit intitulé Vésanies (1802)." *Annales médico-psychologiques* 147, no. 2 (March–April 1989): 183–6.

– "Jean Marc Gaspard Itard: Psychothérapeute de l'enfant sauvage." In *L'enfant sauvage de l'Aveyron*, 57–68.

– "Naissance de la psychiatrie infantile (destins de l'idiotie, origine des psychoses)." In *Nouvelle histoire de la psychiatrie*, edited by J. Postel and C. Quétel, 387–405. 2d ed. Paris: Dunod, 1994.

Gineste, Thierry, and J. Postel. "J.M.G. Itard et l'enfant connu sous le nom de 'Sauvage de l'Aveyron.'" *Psychiatrie de l'enfant* 23, no. 1 (1980): 251–307.

Ginzburg, Carlo. *The Cheese and the Worms: The Cosmos of a Sixteenth-Century Miller* (1976). Translated by J. and A. Tedeschi. Baltimore: Johns Hopkins University Press, 1980.

– *Clues, Myths, and the Historical Method*. Translated by J. and A.C. Tedeschi. Baltimore: Johns Hopkins University Press, 1989.

– "Microhistory: Two or Three Things That I Know about It." Translated by J. and A.C. Tedeschi. *Critical Inquiry* 20 (Autumn 1993): 10–35.

– "Checking the Evidence: The Judge and the Historian." In *Questions of Evidence: Proof, Practice, and Persuasion across the Disciplines*, edited by J. Chandler, A. Davidson, and H. Harootunian, 290–303. Chicago: University of Chicago Press, 1994.

Ginzburg, Carlo, and Carlo Poni. "The Name and the Game: Unequal Exchange and the Historiographic Marketplace." In *Microhistory and the Lost Peoples of Europe*, edited by E. Muir and G. Ruggiero, translated by E. Branch, 1–10. Baltimore: Johns Hopkins University Press, 1991.

Girard, P.F. "L'histoire véridique de Victor, l'enfant sauvage de l'Aveyron, ou les origines lointaines de la psychiatrie infantile." *Lyon médical* 251, no. 8 (April 1984): 361–7.

Goerke, Heinz. "Linnaeus' German Pupils and Their Significance." In *Linnaeus: Progress and Prospects in Linnaean Research*, edited by G. Broberg, 225–39. Stockholm: Almqvist and Wiksell, 1980.

Goldstein, Jan. *Console and Classify: The French Psychiatric Profession in the Nineteenth Century.* Cambridge: Cambridge University Press, 1987.

Gould, Stephen Jay. *Ontogeny and Phylogeny.* Cambridge: Harvard University Press, 1977.

Graham, Lorraine. "Wild Boys and Idiots: The Beginnings of Special Education." *BC Journal of Special Education* 15, no. 1 (1991): 76–95.

Gramont, Antoine de. "Relation de mon voyage en Pologne." Edited by E. de Clermont-Tonnerre. *Revue de Paris* 29th year, 2, no. 8 (15 April 1922): 698–737.

Greene, Edward L. "Linnaeus as an Evolutionist." *Proceedings of the Washington Academy of Sciences* 11 (31 March 1909): 17–26.

Greene, John C. *The Death of Adam: Evolution and Its Impact on Western Thought* (1959). Ames: University of Iowa Press, 1996.

Groff, Marné Lauritsen. "Jean Marc Gaspard Itard (1775–1838)." *Psychological Clinic* 20, no. 8 (January 1932): 246–56.

Gusdorf, Georges. *Dieu, la nature, l'homme au siècle des lumières.* Vol. 5 of *Les sciences humaines et la pensée occidentale.* Paris: Payot, 1972.

– *La conscience révolutionnaire: Les idéologues.* Vol. 8 of *Les sciences humaines et la pensée occidentale.* Paris: Payot, 1978.

Hacking, Ian. "Making up People." In *Reconstructing Individualism: Autonomy, Individuality, and the Self in Western Thought*, edited by T. Heller et al., 222–36. Stanford: Stanford University Press, 1986.

– *The Taming of Chance.* Cambridge: Cambridge University Press, 1990.

– "The Making and Molding of Child Abuse." *Critical Inquiry* 17 (1991): 253–88.

– "World-Making by Kind-Making: Child Abuse for Example." In *How Classification Works: Nelson Goodman among the Social Sciences*, edited by M. Douglas and D. Hull, 180–238. Edinburgh: Edinburgh University Press, 1992.

– "Historical Epistemology." Informal workshop discussion paper. Graduate workshop on historical epistemology. University of Toronto, 29 October – 3 November 1993.

– "Styles of Scientific Thinking or Reasoning: A New Analytical Tool for Historians and Philosophers of Science." In *Trends in the Historiography of Science*, edited by K. Gavroglu, 31–48. Dordrecht: Kluwer, 1994.

– *Rewriting the Soul: Multiple Personality and the Sciences of Memory.* Princeton: Princeton University Press, 1995.

- "The Looping Effects of Human Kinds." In *Causal Cognition: A Multidisciplinary Debate*, edited by D. Sperber, D. Premack, and A. James Premack, 351–94. Oxford: Clarendon, 1995.
- "Normal People." In *Modes of Thought: Explorations in Culture and Cognition*, edited by D.R. Olson and N. Torrance, 59–71. Cambridge: Cambridge University Press, 1996.
- *The Social Construction of What?* Cambridge: Harvard University Press, 1999.
- *Historical Ontology.* Cambridge: Harvard University Press, 2002.

Halbwachs, Maurice. *Les cadres sociaux de la mémoire* (1925). Paris: Moutin, 1976.
- *On Collective Memory.* Edited and translated by L.A. Coser. Chicago: University of Chicago Press, 1992.

Handke, Peter. *Kaspar* (1967). In *Kaspar and Other Plays*, translated by M. Roloff, 55–140. New York: Farrar, Straus and Giroux, 1969.

Hardyment, Christina. *Dream Babies: Child Care from Locke to Spock.* London: Jonathan Cape, 1983.

Hauser, Kaspar. *Kaspar Hauser Speaks for Himself: Kaspar's Own Writings.* Edited by A. Damico Gibson. Translated by W.B. Forward. Botton Village: Camphill, 1993.

H...t [Hecquet], Madame. *Histoire d'une jeune fille sauvage, Trouvée dans les Bois à l'âge de dix ans.* Paris: N.p., 1755.
- *Histoire d'une jeune fille sauvage trouvée dans les bois à l'age de dix ans.* Edited by F. Tinland. Bordeaux: Ducros, 1970.
- *An Account of a Savage Girl Caught Wild in the Woods of Champagne.* Translated from the French. With a preface, containing several particulars omitted in the original account, by the Hon. Lord Monboddo (1768). Aberdeen: Burnett and Rettie, 1796.

Herder, Johann Gottfried von. *Outlines of a Philosophy of the History of Man* (1784). Translated by T. Churchill. London: J. Johnson, 1800.

Herodotus. *The History of Herodotus.* Translated by G. Rawlinson. Vol. 1. London: J.M. Dent, 1910.

Herzog, Werner. *Every Man for Himself and God against All* (1974, film). In *Screenplays*, translated by Alan Greenberg and Martje Herzog, 97–181. New York: Tanam, 1980.

Heuvelmans, Bernard. *Les bêtes humaines d'Afrique.* Paris: Plon, 1980.

Heuvelmans, Bernard, and Boris F. Porchnev. *L'homme de Néanderthal est toujours vivant.* Paris: Plon, 1974.

Heywood, Colin. *A History of Childhood: Children and Childhood in the West from Medieval to Modern Times.* Cambridge: Polity, 2001.

Histoire de l'Académie royales des sciences. Année M. DCC. III. 2d ed. Paris: Charles-Estienne Hochereau, 1720.

"Histoire d'une jeune fille sauvage, Trouvée dans les bois de la Champagne en 1731." *Magasin pittoresque* 17 (1849): 18–20.

Horigan, Stephen. *Nature and Culture in Western Discourses*. London: Routledge, 1988.

Humphrey, George. "Introduction." In J.-M.-G. Itard. *The Wild Boy of Aveyron*, v–xix.

Hunter, Ian M.L. "Heritage from the Wild Boy of Aveyron." *Early Child Development and Care* 95 (1993): 143–52.

Husband, Timothy. *The Wild Man: Medieval Myth and Symbolism*. New York: Metropolitan Museum of Art, 1980.

Hutton, J.H. "Wolf-Children." *Folk-Lore* 51, no. 1 (March 1940): 9–31.

– "Wolf-Children and Feral Man." *Man* 2, new series, no. 4 (December 1967): 630–1.

"India's 'Wolf-Children' Found in Caves." *Literary Digest* 95, no. 2 (8 October 1927): 54, 56.

Ireland, William W. *The Mental Affections of Children, Idiocy, Imbecility and Insanity*. London: J. & A. Churchill, 1898.

Itard, E.M. [Jean-Marc-Gaspard]. *De l'Éducation d'un homme sauvage, ou des premiers développemens physiques et moraux du jeune sauvage de l'Aveyron*. Paris: Goujon fils, vendémiaire year X [1801].

– trans. and ed. *Hygiène domestique, ou l'art de conserver la santé et de prolonger la vie, Mis à la portée des gens du monde*, by A.F.M. [Anthony Florian Madinger] Willich. 2 vols. Paris: Ducauroy, 1802.

– *Rapport fait à Son Excellence le Ministre de l'Interieur, sur les nouveaux développemens et l'état actuel du sauvage de l'Aveyron*. Paris: Imprimerie impériale, 1807.

Itard, Jean-Marc-Gaspard. "Vésanies." Edited by T. Gineste. *L'évolution psychiatrique* 53, no. 3 (July–September 1988): 573–610.

– *Traité des maladies de l'oreille et de l'audition*. 2d ed. 2 vols. Paris: Méquignon-Marvis fils, 1842.

– *The Wild Boy of Aveyron*. Translated by G. and M. Humphrey (1932). Englewood Cliffs: Prentice-Hall, 1962.

Janer Manila, Gabriel. *La problemàtica educativa dels infants selvàtics: El cas de "Marcos."* Barcelona: Laia, 1979.

– *Marcos, Wild Child of the Sierra Morena*. Translated by D. Bonner. London: Souvenir, 1982.

Jauffret, Louis-François. "Introduction aux Mémoires de la Société des Observateurs de l'homme." In "Le premier programme de l'anthropologie," edited by G. Hervé. *Bulletins et mémoires de la Société d'anthropologie de Paris* 10, 5th series (1909): 476–87.

Joisten, Charles, ed. *Récits et contes populaires de Savoie, recueillis par Charles Joisten dans la Tarentaise*. Paris: Gallimard, 1980.

Jones, Peter E. "Contradictions and Unanswered Questions in the Genie Case: A Fresh Look at the Linguistic Evidence." *Language and Communication* 15, no. 3 (July 1995): 261–80.

Kanner, Leo. "Autistic Disturbances of Affective Contact." *Nervous Child* 2 (1943): 217–50.

– "Itard, Seguin, Howe – Three Pioneers in the Education of Retarded Children." *American Journal of Mental Deficiency* 65 (July 1960): 2–10.

– *A History of the Care and Study of the Mentally Retarded*. Springfield: Charles C. Thomas, 1964.

Kanold, Johann, ed. *Sammlung von Natur- und Medicin-, wie auch hierzu gehörigen Kunst- und Literatur- Geschichten*, or *Breslauer Sammlungen*. January 1718, 546–50, and October 1722, 437–44.

Kant, Immanuel. *Sämtliche Werke*. Edited by G. Hartenstein. Vol. 2. Leipzig: Leopold Voss, 1867.

Kapoor, Surinder Kumar. "Socialization and Feral Children." *Revista Internacional de Sociología* 31, no. 5–6 (January–June 1973): 195–213.

Kellogg, Winthrop N. "Humanizing the Ape." *Psychological Review* 38 (1931): 160–76.

– "More about the 'Wolf Children' of India." *American Journal of Psychology* 43 (1931): 508–9.

– "A Further Note on the 'Wolf Children' of India." *American Journal of Psychology* 46 (1934): 149–50.

Kellogg, Winthrop N., and Luella A. Kellogg. *The Ape and the Child: A Study of Environmental Influence upon Early Behavior* (1933). New York: Hafner, 1967.

Kincaid, James R. *Erotic Innocence: The Culture of Child Molesting*. Durham: Duke University Press, 1998.

Kinneir, John Macdonald. *Journey through Asia Minor, Armenia, and Koordistan in the Years 1813 and 1814; With Remarks on the Marches of Alexander, and Retreat of the Ten Thousand*. London: John Murray, 1818.

Kipling, John Lockwood. *Beast and Man in India: A Popular Sketch of Indian Animals in their Relations with the People* (1904). New Delhi: Inter-India Publications, 1984.

Kipling, Rudyard. *The Jungle Book* (1894 and 1895). New York: Harper, 1994.

Kircher, Athanasius. *China monumentis, qua Sacris qua Profanis, Nec non variis naturæ & artis spectaculis, Aliarumque rerum memorabilium Argumentis illustrata*. Amstelodam: Jacobum à Meurs, 1667.

– *China illustrata*. Translated by C.D. Van Tuyl. Muskogee: Indian University Press, 1987.

Kirk, Samuel A. *Early Education of the Mentally Retarded: An Experimental Study*. Urbana: University of Illinois Press, 1958.

Kitchen, Martin. *Kaspar Hauser: Europe's Child.* New York: Palgrave, 2001.

Knight, William, ed. *Lord Monboddo and Some of His Contemporaries.* New York: E.P. Dutton, 1900.

Krout, Maurice H. *Introduction to Social Psychology.* New York: Harper and Bros., 1942.

Krueger, E.T., and Walter C. Reckless. *Social Psychology.* New York: Longmans, Green, 1931.

"L." "Children Nurtured by Wolves in India." *Notes and Queries* 10, no. 247, 1st series (22 July 1854): 62–5; 5, no. 112, 2d series (20 February 1858): 153; and no. 118 (3 April 1858): 280.

La Mettrie, Julien Offray de. *Histoire naturelle de l'ame, Traduite de l'Anglois de M. Charp, Par feu M. H** de l'Académie des Sciences, &c.* La Haye: Jean Neaulme, 1745.

– *Œuvres philosophiques.* Londres [Berlin]: Jean Nourse, 1751.

Lakoff, George. *Women, Fire, and Dangerous Things: What Categories Reveal about the Mind.* Chicago: University of Chicago Press, 1987.

Lamberts, Frances, and Ted L. Miller. "Itard and Language Pedagogy: A Commentary for Teachers of Children with Special Language Needs." *Language, Speech, and Hearing Services in Schools* 10, no. 4 (October 1979): 203–11.

Landucci, Sergio. *I filosofi e i selvaggi: 1580–1780.* Bari: Laterza, 1972.

Lane, Harlan. *The Wild Boy of Aveyron.* Cambridge: Harvard University Press, 1976.

– *When the Mind Hears: A History of the Deaf.* New York: Random House, 1984.

– *The Mask of Benevolence: Disabling the Deaf Community.* New York: Knopf, 1992.

Lane, Harlan, and Richard Pillard. *The Wild Boy of Burundi: A Study of an Outcast Child.* New York: Random House, 1978.

Le Cat, Claude-Nicolas. *Traité des sens.* New ed. Amsterdam: J. Wetsstein, 1644.

– *A Physical Essay on the Senses.* Translated from the French. London: R. Griffiths, 1750.

Le Loyer, Pierre. *IIII. Ljvres des spectres ov apparitions et visions d'esprits, anges et demons se monstrans sensiblement aux hommes.* Angers: Georges Nepueu, 1586.

– *Discovrs, et histoires des spectres, visions et apparitions des esprits, anges, demons, et ames, se monstrans visibles aux hommes.* Paris: Nicolas Bvon, 1605.

– *A Treatise of Specters or straunge Sights, Visions and Apparitions appearing sensibly vnto men.* London: Val. S. for Matthew Lownes, 1605.

Le Roux, Hughes. *Notes sur la Norvège.* Paris: Calmann Lévy, 1895.

Leary, David E. "Nature, Art, and Imitation: The Wild Boy of Aveyron as a Pivotal Case in the History of Psychology." In *Studies in Eighteenth Century Culture* 13, edited by O.M. Brack, Jr, 155–72. Madison: University of Wisconsin Press, 1984.

Lebrun, Yvan. "Victor of Aveyron: A Reappraisal in Light of More Recent Cases of Feral Speech." *Language Sciences* 2, no. 1 (March 1980): 32–43.

Leibniz, Gottfried Wilhelm. *New Essays on Human Understanding* (1765). Translated and edited by P. Remnant and J. Bennett. Cambridge: Cambridge University Press, 1996.

Lemaistre, J.G., Esq. *A Rough Sketch of Modern Paris; or, Letters on Society, Manners, Public Curiosities, and Amusements, in that Capital, Written During the Last Two Months of 1801 and the First Five of 1802.* 2d ed. London: J. Johnson, 1803.

Lenneberg, Eric H. "The Natural History of Language." In *The Genesis of Language: A Psycholinguistic Approach*, edited by F. Smith and G.A. Miller, 219–52. Cambridge: MIT Press, 1966.

– *Biological Foundations of Language.* New York: Wiley, 1967.

Léonetti, Jean. "Analyse d'un cas d'observation clinique de la communication chez des enfants sauvages." *Sémiotica* 53, no. 1/3 (1985): 259–72.

– "Victor de l'Aveyron: De l'interaction volontaire à la communication comportementale et gestuelle." *La linguistique* 22, no. 2 (1986): 125–31.

– "Victor de l'Aveyron: Échec d'une tentative d'apprentissage du langage parlé." *La linguistique* 23, no. 1 (1987): 137–46.

– "Victor de l'Aveyron: L'apprentissage inachevé du langage écrit." *La linguistique* 26, no. 1 (1990): 115–30.

Leroy, Alphonse. *Médecine maternelle, ou l'art d'élever et de conserver les enfans.* Paris: Mequignon, 1803.

– "Réflexions sur le rapport fait au Ministre de l'intérieur sur le Sauvage de l'Aveyron, avec des observations sur les causes et le mécanisme de l'intelligence, ou Lettre à M. Itard ... au sujet de ce même rapport." *Revue philosophique* 9 (21 March 1807): 513–23.

Leroy, J.-J.-S. *Mémoire sur les travaux qui ont rapport à l'exploitation de la mâture dans les Pyrennées.* London [Paris], 1776.

Leuba, Clarence. *The Natural Man: As Inferred Mainly from Field Studies of Men and Chimpanzees.* Garden City, New York: Doubleday, 1954.

Lévesque, Pierre-Charles. "Notice des travaux de la classe des sciences morales et politiques, pendant le premier trimestre de l'an 10." *Magasin encyclopédique* 7th year, vol. 5, no. 18 (pluviôse year 10 [January–February 1802]): 247–65.

Lévi-Strauss, Claude. *The Elementary Structures of Kinship* (1949). Revised ed. (1967). Translated by J.H. Bell, J.R. von Sturmer, and R. Needham. Boston: Beacon, 1969.

Lewis, D. [David], ed. *Miscellaneous Poems, by Several Hands.* London: J. Watts, 1726.

Lieberman, Lawrence M. "Itard: The Great Problem Solver." *Journal of Learning Disabilities* 15, no. 9 (November 1982): 566–8.

Lindsay, Robert. *The Historie and Cronicles of Scotland, from the Slauchter of King James the First to the Ane Tousande Fyve Hundreith Thrie Scoir Fyftein Zeir.* Edited by Æ.J.G. Mackay. 3 vols. Edinburgh: William Blackwood and Sons, 1899.

Linguist discussion list archives. April 1992 and May 1993. <http://listserv.linguist-list.org/archives/linguist.html> (accessed September 2004).

Linnaeus, Carolus. *Systema naturae per regna tria naturae, secundum classes, ordines, genera, species, cum characteribus, differentiis, synonymis, locis.* 10th ed. Holmiae: Laurentii Salvii, 1758.

– *Anthropomorpha.* Respondent, Christian E. Hoppius (1760). *Amoenitates Academicae.* Vol. 6, 63–76. Holmiae: apud Wetstenium, 1764.

– *Systema naturae per regna tria natura, secundum classes, ordines, genera, species, cum characteribus, differentiis, synonymis, locis.* 12th ed. Holmiae: Laurentii Salvii, 1766.

Locke, John. *An Essay Concerning Humane Understanding.* London: Tho. Basset, 1690.

Lotterie, Florence. "Les Lumières contre le progrès? La naissance de l'idée de perfectibilité." *Dix-huitième siècle* 30 (1998): 383–96.

Lovejoy, Arthur O. *Essays in the History of Ideas.* New York: George Braziller, 1955.

Luynes, Charles Philippe d'Albert, duc de. *Mémoires du Duc de Luynes sur la Cour de Louis XV (1735–1758).* Edited by L. Dussieux and E. Soulié. Vol. 13. Paris: Firmin Didot, 1863.

Macanaz, Melchor Rafael de. "Varias notas al Teatro critico del eruditisimo Feyjoo, á cuya correcion van sujetas por su autor." In *Semanario erudito,* edited by Don Antonio Valladares de Sotomayor. Vol. 8. Madrid: Don Blas Roman, 1788.

MacKenzie, Paul A. "Kaspar Hauser in England: The First Hundred Years." *German Life and Letters* 35, new series, no. 2 (January 1982): 118–37.

Maclean, Charles. *The Wolf Children.* London: Allen Lane, 1977.

Magasin encyclopédique; ou Journal des sciences, des lettres et des arts. Edited by A.-L. Millin. Paris, 1795–1816.

Magny, Claude-Edmond, ed. *Les enfants célèbres.* Paris: Lucien Mazenod, 1949.

Maldinier, Michel. *Lacaune-les-Bains (Des origines à nos jours).* Lacaune: Centre de Recherche de Rieumontagné, 1988.

Malouf, David. *An Imaginary Life.* London: Chatto and Windus, 1978.

Malson, Lucien. *Les enfants sauvages: Mythe et réalité.* Paris: Union Générale d'Éditions, 1964.

– *Wolf Children and the Problem of Human Nature.* Translated by E. Fawcett, P. Ayrton, and J. White. New York: Monthly Review Press, 1972.

Mandelbaum, David G. "Wolf-Child Histories from India." *Journal of Psychology* 17 (1943): 25–44.

The Manifesto of Lord Peter. London: J. Roberts, 1726.

Mannoni, Maud. *The Child, His "Illness," and the Others*. New York: Pantheon, 1970.

Mannoni, Octave. "Itard et son sauvage." *Les temps modernes* 21, no. 233 (October 1965): 647–63.

– "Itard and His Savage." *New Left Review* 74 (July–August 1972): 37–49.

Manuel, Frank E. *The New World of Henri Saint-Simon*. Cambridge: Harvard University Press, 1956.

Maranz, George I. "Raised by a She-bear that Stole her when a Baby." *American Weekly*, 5 September 1937. In R.M. Zingg. "Feral Man and Cases of Extreme Isolation of Individuals," 222–6.

Marchese, Frank J. "The Place of Eugenics in Arnold Gesell's Maturation Theory of Child Development." *Canadian Psychology* 36, no. 2 (May 1995): 89–114.

Marcus, Steven. "The Wild Boy of Nuremberg." Review of *Lost Prince*, by J.M. Masson. *New York Times Book Review*, 31 March 1996, 11–12.

Mason, Marie K. "Learning to Speak after Six and One-Half Years of Silence." *Journal of Speech Disorders* 7, no. 4 (December 1942): 295–304.

Masson, Jeffrey Moussaieff. *The Assault on Truth: Freud's Suppression of the Seduction Theory*. New York: Farrar, Straus and Giroux, 1984.

Masson, Jeffrey Moussaieff, ed. and trans. *Lost Prince: The Unsolved Mystery of Kaspar Hauser*. New York: Free Press, 1996.

Maupertuis, Pierre-Louis Moreau de. *Lettre sur le progrès des sciences* (1752). In *Œuvres*. New ed. Vol. 2, 375–431. Lyon: J.M. Bruyset, 1756.

McCartney, Eugene S. "Greek and Roman Lore of Animal-Nursed Children." *Papers of the Michigan Academy of Science, Arts and Letters* 4, pt. 1. Edited by P.S. Welch and E.S. McCartney, 15–43. New York: Macmillan, 1925.

McDermott, Dennis. "Jean Itard: The First Child and Youth Counsellor." *Journal of Child and Youth Care* 9, no. 1 (1994): 59–71.

McElderry, B.R., Jr. "Boswell in 1790–91: Two Unpublished Comments." *Notes and Queries* 9, no. 7 (July 1962): 266–8.

McNeil, Mary Charles, Edward A. Polloway, and J. David Smith. "Feral and Isolated Children: Historical Review and Analysis." *Education and Training of the Mentally Retarded* 19, no. 1 (February 1984): 70–9.

Mercure de France. December 1731, April 1755.

Métraux, Alexandre. "Victor de l'Aveyron and the Relativist-Essentialist Controversy." In *Contributions to a History of Developmental Psychology: International William T. Preyer Symposium*, edited by G. Eckardt, W.G. Bringmann, and L. Sprung, 101–15. Berlin: Mouton, 1985.

Miller, Lois Mattox. "The Wolf-Girls and the Baboon-Boy: Scientists Study with Interest Reports of Children Said to Have Been Brought Up by Animals in the Wild." *Science News Letter* 38, no. 2 (13 July 1940): 26–9.

Mitchell, Peter. *Introduction to Theory of Mind: Children, Autism and Apes*. London: Arnold, 1997.

Mitra, Sarat Chandra. "On a Wild Boy and a Wild Girl." *Journal of the Anthropological Society of Bombay* 3 (1897): 109–11. In R.M. Zingg. "Feral Man and Cases of Extreme Isolation of Individuals," 220–1.

Modi, Jivanji Jamshedji. "Recorded Instances of Children Having Been Nourished by Wolves and Birds of Prey." *Journal of the Bombay Natural History Society* 4 (1889): 142–7.

Monboddo, James Burnett, Lord. *Of the Origin and Progress of Language*. Vol. 1. 2d ed. Edinburgh: J. Balfour, 1774.

– *Antient Metaphysics*. 6 vols. Vol. 3. *The History and Philosophy of Men*. 1784. Vol. 4. *The History of Man*. 1795. London: T. Cadell, 1779–1799.

Money, John. *The Kaspar Hauser Syndrome of "Psychosocial Dwarfism": Deficient Statural, Intellectual, and Social Growth Induced by Child Abuse*. Buffalo: Prometheus, 1992.

Montagu, M.F. Ashley. *Edward Tyson, MD, FRS 1650–1708 and the Rise of Human and Comparative Anatomy in England: A Study in the History of Science*. Philadelphia: American Philosophical Society, 1943.

– Review of *Wolf-Children and Feral Man*, by J.A.L. Singh and R.M. Zingg. *American Anthropologist* 45, no. 8 (1943): 468–72.

– *Anthropology and Human Nature*. Boston: Porter Sargent, 1957.

Monteil, Amans-Alexis. *Description de l'Aveyron*. 2 vols. Rodez: Imprimerie de Carrère, 1801.

Montesquieu, Charles-Louis de Secondat, baron de la Brède et de. *De l'esprit des loix* (1748). New ed. 2 vols. Edinburgh: G. Hamilton and J. Balfour, 1750.

– *Œuvres complètes*. Edited by D. Oster. Paris: du Seuil, 1964.

Montessori, Maria. *The Montessori Method: Scientific Pedagogy as Applied to Child Education in "The Children's Houses"* (1912). Translated by A.E. George. Cambridge: Robert Bentley, 1965.

Moran, Francis, III. "Between Primates and Primitives: Natural Man as the Missing Link in Rousseau's *Second Discourse*." *Journal of the History of Ideas* 54, no. 1 (January 1993): 37–58.

Moravia, Sergio. *La scienza dell'uomo nel Settecento: con una appendice di testi*. Bari: Laterza, 1970.

– "The Enlightenment and the Sciences of Man." *Studies on Voltaire and the Eighteenth Century* 192 (1980): 1,153–7.

Moreri, Louis. *Le grand dictionaire historique, ou Le mélange curieux de l'histoire sacrée et profane*. Amsterdam: Boom and Van Someren, Pierre Mortier, Henri Desbordes, 1694.

– *The Great Historical, Geographical and Poetical Dictionary, Being A Curious Miscellany of Sacred and Prophane History*. London: Henry Rhodes, 1694.

Morss, John R. "Gesell, Arnold Lucius." In *Biographical Dictionary of Psychology*, edited by N. Sheehy, A.J. Chapman, and W.A. Conroy, 229–31. London: Routledge, 1997.

Müller, Max. "Wolf-Children." *The Academy* 6 (7 November 1874): 512–13.

Murchison, Roderick I., and F. Egerton. "On Wolves Suckling Children." *Annals and Magazine of Natural History, Including Zoology, Botany, and Geology* 8, no. 44, 2d series (August 1851): 153–4.

Nash, Richard. *Wild Enlightenment: The Borders of Human Identity in the Eighteenth Century*. Charlottesville: University of Virginia Press, 2003.

Neilson, H.B. "Wolf-Children." *Badminton Magazine of Sports and Pastimes* 2 (January–June 1896): 249–57.

Newton, Michael. "Bodies without Souls: The Case of Peter the Wild Boy." In *At the Borders of the Human: Beasts, Bodies and Natural Philosophy in the Early Modern Period*, edited by E. Fudge, R. Gilbert, and S. Wiseman, 196–214. Houndmills: Macmillan, 1999.

– *Savage Girls and Wild Boys: A History of Feral Children*. London: Faber and Faber, 2002.

Norton, Rictor. "Peter the Wild Boy." In *Early Eighteenth-Century Newspaper Reports: A Sourcebook*. 28 November 2001. Updated 23 April 2002. <http://www.infopt.demon.co.uk/grub/wildboy.htm> (accessed 2003).

Notes africaines 26 (April 1945): 5–7.

Notes and Queries: A Medium of Inter-Communication for Literary Men, Artists, Antiquaries, Genealogists, etc. 9 April 1853; 22 July 1854; February–April 1858; April–August 1885.

Novak, Maximillian E. "The Wild Man Comes to Tea." In *The Wild Man Within: An Image in Western Thought from the Renaissance to Romanticism*, edited by E. Dudley and M.E. Novak, 183–221. Pittsburgh: University of Pittsburgh Press, 1972.

Ogburn, William Fielding. "The Wolf Boy of Agra." *American Journal of Sociology* 64, no. 5 (March 1959): 449–54.

Ogburn, William Fielding, and Nirmal K. Bose. "On the Trail of the Wolf-Children." *Genetic Psychology Monographs* 60 (1959): 117–93.

"Old Stories Re-told: Wild Boys." *All the Year Round* 18, no. 439 (21 September 1867): 301–6.

O'Malley, C.D., and H.W. Magoun. "Early Concepts of the Anthropomorpha." *Physis* 4 (1962): 39–64.

O'Neal, John C. *The Authority of Experience: Sensationist Theory in the French Enlightenment*. University Park: Pennsylvania State University Press, 1996.

Ornstein, B. "Wilden Menschen in Trikkala." *Zeitschrift für Ethnologie* 23 (1891): 817–18.

Ozment, Steven. *Ancestors: The Loving Family in Old Europe.* Cambridge: Harvard University Press, 2001.

Parr, Samuel. *Bibliotheca Parrianna: A Catalogue of the Library of the Late Reverend and Learned Samuel Parr, LL.D., Curate of Hatton, Prebendary of St. Paul's, &c. &c.* London: John Bohn, 1827.

Paton Walsh, Jill. *Knowledge of Angels.* Boston: Houghton Mifflin, 1994.

"Peter the Wild Boy; and the Savage of Aveyron." *Penny Magazine* 2 (4 May 1833): 170–1.

Petersson, R.T. *Sir Kenelm Digby: The Ornament of England, 1603–1665.* London: Jonathan Cape, 1956.

A Philosophical Survey of Nature: In which the Long Agitated Question Concerning Human Liberty and Necessity, is Endeavoured to be Fully Determined From Incontestable Phaenomena. London: N.p., 1763.

Pichot, Pierre. "French Pioneers in the Field of Mental Deficiency." *American Journal of Mental Deficiency* 53, no. 1 (July 1948): 128–37.

Pinel, Philippe. "Rapport fait à la Société des Observateurs de l'homme sur l'enfant connu sous le nom de Sauvage de l'Aveyron." In "Le sauvage de l'Aveyron devant les observateurs de l'homme," edited by G. Hervé. *Revue anthropologique* 21 (1911): 383–98 and 441–54.

Pistorius, Johann. *Illustrivm vetervm scriptorvm, qvi rervm a Germanis per mvltas ætates gestarvm Historias vel Annales posteris reliqvverunt.* Vol. 1. Frankfurt: Apud hæredes Andræ Wecheli, 1583.

– *Rervm germanicarvm scriptores aliqvot insignes, qvi historiam et res gestas germanorvm medii potissimvm ævi, inde a Carolo M. ad Carolvm V vsqve, per annales litteris consignarunt.* 3d ed. of *Illustrivm vetervm scriptorvm.* Edited by B.G. Struve. Vol. 1. Ratisbonæ: Sumptibus Joannis Conradi Peezii, 1726.

Plancke, René-Charles. *La vie quotidienne au pays de l'enfant sauvage (évocation historique).* Le Mée-sur-Seine: Amattéis, 1989.

Poole, Rebecca. "Uganda's Wild Child." *Sierra* 72 (January–February 1987): 14.

Prasad, Kali. "Ramu – The 'Wolf-Boy' of Lucknow: A Legend Investigated." *Illustrated London News* (27 February 1954): 328.

Procopius. *History of the Wars.* Translated by H.B. Dewing. Cambridge: Harvard University Press, 1924.

Purchas, Samuel. *Purchas His Pilgrimage. Or Relations of the World and the Religions Observed in all Ages and Places discouered, from the Creation unto this present.* London: William Stansby for Henrie Fetherstone, 1613.

Racault, Jean-Michel. "Le motif de 'l'enfant de la nature' dans la littérature du XVIIIe siècle, ou la recréation expérimentale de l'origine." In *Primitivisme et mythes des origines dans la France des Lumières, 1680–1820,* edited by C. Grell and C. Michel, 101–17. Paris: Presses de l'Université de Paris-Sorbonne, 1989.

Racine, Louis. *Œuvres de Louis Racine*. Vols. 2 and 6. Paris: Le Normant, 1808.

Rauber, August Antinous. *Homo sapiens ferus oder die Zustände der Vewilderten und ihre Bedeutung für Wissenschaft, Politik und Schule* (1885). 2d ed. Leipzig: Julius Brehse, 1888.

Reboul, Robert-Marie, ed. *Les cartons d'un ancien bibliothécaire de Marseille. Variétés bio-bibliographiques, historiques et scientifiques*. Draguignan: C. et A. Latil, 1875.

"Réflexions sur le *Sauvage de l'Aveyron*, et sur ce qu'on appelle en général, par rapport à l'homme, l'état de nature." *Décade philosophique, littéraire et politique* 27, no. 1 (October 1800): 8–18.

Régaldo, Marc. *Un milieu intellectuel: La Décade philosophique (1794–1807)*. 4 vols. Lille: Atelier Reproduction des Thèses Université Lille III, 1976.

Rigler, David. Letter to the editor of the *New York Times Book Review*, 13 June 1993, 35.

Ritson, Joseph. *An Essay on Abstinence from Animal Food, as a Moral Duty*. London: Richard Phillips, 1802.

Robinet, Jean-Baptiste. *Considérations philosophiques de la gradation naturelle des formes de l'être, ou Les essais de la nature qui apprend à faire l'homme*. Paris: Charles Saillant, 1768.

Robinson, Mary. *The Poetical Works of the Late Mrs. Mary Robinson: Including Many Pieces Never Before Published*. 3 vols. London: Richard Phillips, 1806.

Roger, Jacques. *Buffon: A Life in Natural History*. Translated by S.L. Bonnefoi. Edited by L. Pearce Williams. Ithaca: Cornell University Press, 1997.

Roland, Marie-Jeanne (Manon). *Lettres de Madame Roland. Nouvelle série, 1767–1780*. 2 vols. Edited by C. Perroud. Paris: Imprimerie Nationale, 1913.

Rosch, Eleanor. "Principles of Categorization." In *Cognition and Categorization*, edited by E. Rosch and B.B. Lloyd, 27–48. Hillsdale: Lawrench Erlbaum, 1978.

Rose, Nikolas. *The Psychological Complex: Psychology, Politics and Society in England, 1869–1939*. London: Routledge and Kegan Paul, 1985.

Rosenfeld, Sophia. *A Revolution in Language: The Problem of Signs in Late Eighteenth-Century France*. Stanford: Stanford University Press, 2001.

Ross, Alexander. *Arcana Microcosmi: or, The hid secrets of man's body discovered; In an Anatomical Duel between Aristotle and Galen concerning the Parts thereof: As also, by a Discovery of the strange and marveilous Diseases, Symptomes & Accidents of Man's Body*. London: Tho. Newcomb, 1652.

Rousseau, Jean-Jacques. *Discours sur l'origine et les fondemens de l'inégalité parmi les hommes*. Amsterdam: Marc Michel Rey, 1755.

– *Du contract social; ou, Principes du droit politique*. Amsterdam: Marc Michel Rey, 1762.

- *Discourse on the Origin and Foundations of Inequality among Men.* In *The Basic Political Writings*, edited and translated by D.A. Cress, 23–109. Indianapolis: Hackett, 1987.

Routh, Donald K., and Victoria del Barrio. "European Roots of the First Psychology Clinic in North America." *European Psychologist* 1, no. 1 (March 1996): 44–50.

Ruch, Floyd L. *Psychology and Life.* 3d ed. Chicago: Scott, Foresman and Company, 1948.

Rudolphi, Karl Asmund. *Grundriss der Physiologie.* Vol. 1. Berlin: Ferdinand Dümmler, 1821.

Rymer, Russ. "A Silent Childhood." *New Yorker* (13 April 1992): 41–81, and (20 April 1992): 43–77.

- *Genie: A Scientific Tragedy.* New York: HarperPerennial, 1993.

Rzaczynski, Gabriel. *Historia naturalis curiosa Regni Poloniae.* Sandomiriae: Typis Collegii Soc. Jesu, 1721.

Saint-Simon, Claude-Henri de. *Mémoire sur la science de l'homme* (1813; 1858). In *Œuvres de Saint-Simon.* Vol. 11. Paris: E. Dentu, 1876.

Sampath, Ursula. *Kaspar Hauser: A Modern Metaphor.* Columbia: Camden House, 1991.

Sarason, Seymour B. *Psychological Problems in Mental Deficiency.* New York: Harper and Brothers, 1949.

- *Psychological Problems in Mental Deficiency.* 3d ed. New York: Harper and Row, 1959.

Sargent, S. Stansfeld. *Social Psychology: An Integrative Interpretation.* New York: Ronald, 1950.

Saussure, César de. *A Foreign View of England in the Reigns of George I. & George II: The Letters of Monsieur César de Saussure to His Family.* Translated and edited by Madame Van Muyden. New York: E.P. Dutton, 1902.

Schiebinger, Londa. *Nature's Body: Gender in the Making of Modern Science.* Boston: Beacon, 1993.

Schøsler, Jørn. *John Locke et les philosophes français: La critique des idées innées en France au dix-huitième siècle. Studies on Voltaire and the Eighteenth Century* 353. Oxford: Voltaire Foundation, 1997.

Schreber, Johann Christian Daniel. *Die Saugthiere in Abbildungen nach der Natur mit Beschreibungen.* Vol. 1. Erlangen: Wolfgang Walther, 1775.

Science News Letter. March and April 1941.

Séguin, Édouard. *Traitement Moral, hygiène et éducation des idiots et des autres enfants arriérés.* Paris: J.B. Baillière, 1846.

- "Origin of the Treatment and Training of Idiots." *American Journal of Education* 2 (1856): 145–52.

– *Idiocy: And Its Treatment by the Physiological Method* (1866). New York: Teachers' College, Columbia University, 1907. In Disability History Museum. <http://www.disabilitymuseum.org> (accessed 2003–04).

Sehr, Peter. *Kaspar Hauser* (film). 1994.

Shakespeare, William. *The Winter's Tale*. Edited by F. Kermode. New York: New American Library, 1988.

Shattuck, Roger. "How Much Nature, How Much Nurture?" Review of *The Wild Boy of Aveyron*, by H. Lane. *New York Times Book Review* (16 May 1976): 27–32.

– *The Forbidden Experiment: The Story of the Wild Boy of Aveyron* (1980). New York: Kodansha, 1994.

Shengold, Leonard. "Kaspar Hauser and Soul Murder: A Study of Deprivation." *International Review of Psycho-Analysis* 5 (1978): 457–76.

Shuttleworth, G.E. *Mentally-Deficient Children: Their Treatment and Training.* London: H.K. Lewis, 1895.

Sicard, Roch-Ambroise. "Chapitre préliminaire d'un ouvrage sur l'art d'instruire les sourd-muets." *Magasin encyclopédique* 1st year, vol. 3, no. 9 (year 3 [1795]): 30–50.

– *Cours d'instruction d'un sourd-muet de naissance, pour servir à l'éducation des sourds-muets, Et qui peut être utile à celle de ceux qui entendent et qui parlent.* Paris: Le Clere, 1800.

– *Théorie des signes pour servir d'introduction à l'étude des langues, ou le sens des mots, au lieu d'être défini, est mis en action* (1808). 2d ed. 2 vols. Paris: Roret, 1823.

Sieveking, Paul. "News from the Wild Frontiers." *Fortean Times* 45 (Winter 1985): 45.

– "Feral News." *Fortean Times* 49 (Winter 1987): 12.

– "Forteana." *New Statesman and Society* 4, no. 169 (20 September 1991): 55.

– "Wild Things." *Fortean Times* 161 (August 2002). <http://www.forteantimes.com/articles/161_feralkids.shtml> (accessed 13 August 2004).

Sigaud-Lafond, Joseph Aigan. *Dictionnaire des merveilles de la nature.* 2 vols. Paris: Rue et Hotel Serpente, 1781.

Silberstein, Richard M., and Helen Irwin. "Jean-Marc-Gaspard Itard and the Savage of Aveyron: An Unsolved Diagnostic Problem in Child Psychiatry." *Journal of the American Academy of Child Psychiatry* 1 (1962): 314–22.

Simon, Nicole. "Kaspar Hauser's Recovery and Autopsy: A Perspective on Neurological and Sociological Requirements for Language Development." *Journal of Autism and Childhood Schizophrenia* 8, no. 2 (1978): 209–17.

Singh, J.A.L., and Robert M. Zingg. *Wolf-Children and Feral Man.* New York: Harper, 1942.

[Sleeman, William Henry] An Indian Official. *An Account of Wolves Nurturing Children in their Dens.* Plymouth: Jenkin Thomas, 1852.

Sleeman, William Henry. *A Journey through the Kingdom of Oude, in 1849–1850.* 2 vols. London: Richard Bentley, 1858.

Small, Maurice H. "On Some Psychical Relations of Society and Solitude." *Pedagogical Seminary* 7 (1900): 13–69.

Smith, Gilbert N. "Wolves Nursing Children." *Notes and Queries* (9 April 1853): 355.

Smith, Marian W. "Wild Children and the Principle of Reinforcement." *Child Development* 25, no. 2 (June 1954): 115–23.

Smith, Roger. *The Fontana History of the Human Sciences.* London: Fontana, 1997.

Soda, Marcelle Marie. "Biography of the Wild Child." PhD thesis, Saint Louis University, 1982.

Sotomayor, Don Antonio Valladares de. "Nota del editor." In *Semanario erudito.* Vol. 7, 1–11. Madrid: Don Blas Roman, 1788.

Spangenberg, August Gottlieb. *The Life of Nicolas Lewis, Count of Zinzendorf and Pottendorf.* 2 vols. Translated by L.T. Nyberg. Bath: T. Mills and S. Hazard, 1773.

Squires, Paul C. "'Wolf Children' of India." *American Journal of Psychology* 38 (1927): 313–15.

Stark, Werner. *Antecedents of the Social Bond. The Phylogeny of Sociality.* Vol. 1 of *The Social Bond: An Investigation into the Bases of Law-Abidingness.* New York: Fordham University Press, 1976.

Staum, Martin. *Minerva's Message: Stabilizing the French Revolution.* Montreal: McGill-Queen's University Press, 1996.

Steedman, Carolyn. *Childhood, Culture and Class in Britain: Margaret McMillan, 1860–1931.* London: Virago, 1990.

– *Strange Dislocations: Childhood and the Idea of Human Interiority, 1780–1930.* Cambridge: Harvard University Press, 1995.

Stockwell, George Archie. "Wolf-Children." *Lippincott' Monthly Magazine* 61 (January–June 1898): 117–24.

Stone, Michael H. "Mesmer and His Followers: The Beginnings of Sympathetic Treatment of Childhood Emotional Disorders." *History of Childhood Quarterly: The Journal of Psychohistory* 1, no. 4 (Spring 1974): 659–79.

Stratton, G.M. "Jungle Children." *Proceedings of the Western Psychological Association* (21–23 June 1932): 596–7.

Sułek, Antoni. "The Experiment of Psammetichus: Fact, Fiction, and Model to Follow." *Journal of the History of Ideas* 50, no. 4 (1989): 645–51.

Swain, Gladys. *Dialogue avec l'insensé: Essais d'histoire de la psychiatrie.* Paris: Gallimard, 1994.

Swift, Jonathan. *The Correspondence of Jonathan Swift.* Edited by H. Williams. Vol. 3. Oxford: Clarendon, 1963.

[Swift, Jonathan and/or John Arbuthnot]. *It cannot Rain but it Pours, or, London strow'd with Rarities. Being, An Account of the Arrival of a White Bear ... And Lastly, Of the wonderful Wild Man that was nursed in the Woods of Germany by a Wild Beast, hunted and taken in Toyls; how he behaveth himself like a dumb Creature, and is a Christian like one of us, being call'd Peter; and how he was brought to Court all in Green, to the great Astonishment of the Quality and Gentry.* London: J. Roberts, 1726.

- *The Most Wonderful Wonder that ever appear'd to the Wonder of the British Nation. Being, An Account of the Travels of Mynheer Veteranus, thro' the Woods of Germany: And an Account of his taking a most monstrous She Bear, who had nurs'd up the Wild Boy: Their Landing at the Tower; Their Reception at Court; The Daily Visits they receive from Multitudes of all Ranks and Orders of both Sexes. With a Dialogue between the Old She Bear and her Foster Son.* London: A. More, 1726.

"Syria: Triumph of Civilization." *Time* (9 September 1946): 34.

Tennant, C.M. [Catherine Mary]. *Peter the Wild Boy.* New York: Harper and Brothers, 1939.

Terrall, Mary. *The Man Who Flattened the Earth: Maupertuis and the Sciences in the Enlightenment.* Chicago: University of Chicago Press, 2002.

Thelen, Esther, and Karen E. Adolph. "Arnold L. Gesell: The Paradox of Nature and Culture." *Developmental Psychology* 28, no. 3 (May 1992): 368–80.

Thomas, Keith. *Man and the Natural World: A History of the Modern Sensibility.* New York: Pantheon, 1983.

Thornton, Percy M. *Harrow School and its Surroundings.* London: W.H. Allen & Co., 1885.

Tiedemann, Dietrich. "Beobachtungen über die Entwickelung der Seelenfähigkeiten bei Kindern." *Hessische Beiträge zur Gelehrsamkeit und Kunst* 2 and 3 (1787). Reprinted as *Beobachtungen über die Entwickelung der Seelenfähigkeiten bei Kindern. Mit Einleitung, sowie mit einem Litteraturverzeichnis zur Kinderpsychologie.* Edited by Chr. Ufer. Altenburg: Druck und Verlag von Oskar Bonde, 1897.

- "Tiedemann's Observations on the Development of the Mental Faculties of Children." Edited and translated by C. Murchison and S. Langer. *Pedagogical Seminary and Journal of Genetic Psychology* 34, no. 2 (June 1927): 205–30.

Tinker, Chauncey B. *Nature's Simple Plan: A Phase of Radical Thought in the Mid-Eighteenth Century.* Princeton: Princeton University Press, 1922.

Tinland, Franck. *L'Homme sauvage: Homo ferus et Homo sylvestris, de l'animal à l'homme.* Paris: Payot, 1968.

Todorov, Tzvetan. *The Conquest of America: The Question of the Other* (1982). Translated by R. Howard. New York: HarperCollins, 1984.

- *The Morals of History* (1991). Translated by A. Waters. Minneapolis: University of Minnesota Press, 1995.

- *Les abus de la mémoire.* Paris: Arléa, 1995.

– *Imperfect Garden: The Legacy of Humanism* (1998). Translated by C. Cosman. Princeton: Princeton University Press, 2002.

Tourneux, Maurice, ed. *Correspondance littéraire, philosophique et critique par Grimm, Diderot, Raynal, Meister, etc.* Vol. 2. Paris: Garnier, 1877.

Tredgold, A.F. *Mental Deficiency (Amentia).* 4th ed. New York: William Good, 1922.

Tredgold, Roger F., and Kenneth Soddy, eds. *Tredgold's Textbook of Mental Deficiency (Subnormality).* 10th ed. Baltimore: Williams and Wilkins, 1963.

Trent, James W. *Inventing the Feeble Mind: A History of Mental Retardation in the United States.* Berkeley: University of California Press, 1994.

Trevarthen, Colwyn, Kenneth Aitken, Despina Papoudi, and Jacqueline Robarts. *Children with Autism: Diagnosis and Interventions to Meet Their Needs.* London: Jessica Kingsley Publishers, 1996.

Truffaut, François. *L'enfant sauvage. Aesculape* 53, no. 1 (1970): 2–64, and no. 2 (1970): 2–47.

– *L'enfant sauvage* (film). 1969.

– *Truffaut par Truffaut.* Edited by D. Rabourdin. Paris: Chêne, 1985.

Tulp, Nicolaas. *Observationes medicæ.* New ed. Amsterdam: Apud Danielem Elsevirium, 1672.

Tylor, Edward Burnet. "Wild Men and Beast-Children." *Anthropological Review* 1 (1863): 21–32.

Verlaine, Paul. "Je suis venu, calme orphelin" (1873). In *Œuvres poétiques complètes,* edited by Y.-G. Le Dantec and J. Borel, 279. Paris: Gallimard, 1962.

Verri, Antonio. *Lord Monboddo: Dalla Metafisica all'Antropologia.* Ravenna: Longo, 1975.

"La vie de Sidi Mohamed avec les autruches pendant dix ans. La scène est passée dans l'Assaba la dangereuse, d'après moi Beyboune (Développement rédigé par M. Beyboune, d'après M. Sidi Mohamed Ould Sidia Ould Mohamed, fraction Taguat)." *Notes africaines* 26 (April 1945): 4–5.

Virey, Julien-Joseph. "Questions de Physiologie et de Métaphysique. L'Instinct dépend-il de la sensibilité vitale et de l'organisation? et les philosophes doivent-ils nier à l'homme, l'instinct qu'ont les animaux?" *Magasin encyclopédique* 5th year, no. 19 (ventôse year 8 [February 1800]): 341–52.

– *Histoire naturelle du genre humaine, Ou Recherches sur ses principaux Fondemens physiques et moraux ... On y a joint une dissertation sur le sauvage, de l'Aveyron.* 2 vols. Paris: F. Dufart, year 9 [1801].

– "Homme sauvage." In *Nouveau dictionnaire d'histoire naturelle, appliquée aux Arts, à l'Agriculture, à l'Économie rurale et domestique, à la Médecine, etc.* New ed. Vol. 15, 260–70. Paris: Deterville, 1817.

Vivitur Ingenio: Being a Collection Of Elegant, Moral, Satirical, and Comical Thoughts, on Various Subjects: As, Love and Gallantry, Poetry and Politicks, Religion and History, &c. London: J. Roberts, 1726.

Voltaire (François-Marie Arouet). "Poëme sur la loi naturelle" (1756). In *Œuvres complètes de Voltaire.* Vol. 2, 498–506. Paris: Furne, 1835.

– *La Philosophie de l'histoire* (1765). Edited by J.H. Brumfitt. *Studies on Voltaire and the Eighteenth Century* 28. Oxford: Voltaire Foundation, 1963.

Wairy, Louis-Constant. *Mémoires de Constant, premier valet de chambre de l'empereur, sur la vie privée de Napoléon, sa famille et sa cour.* 6 vols. Paris: Ladvocat, 1830.

Wallin, J.E. Wallace. *Children with Mental and Physical Handicaps.* New York: Prentice Hall, 1949.

Ward, Andrew. "FeralChildren.com." <http://www.feralchildren.com> (accessed 2003–04).

Warren, Dawson. *The Journal of a British Chaplain in Paris during the Peace Negotiations of 1801–2. From the Unpublished MS. of the Revd. Dawson Warren, M.A., unofficially attached to the Diplomatic Mission of Mr. Francis James Jackson.* Edited by A.M. Broadley. London: Chapman and Hall, 1913.

Warren, S.A. "Letter from an Editor." *Mental Retardation* 15, no. 2 (April 1977): 2.

Wassermann, Jakob. *Caspar Hauser* (1908). Translated by C. Newton. New York: Carroll and Graf, 1985.

Watson, Goodwin. "Life History of the Wolf Girl." *Saturday Review of Literature* 24 (19 July 1941): 15.

Weber, Eugen. *Peasants into Frenchmen: The Modernization of Rural France, 1870–1914.* Stanford: Stanford University Press, 1976.

Webster, John. *The Displaying of Supposed Witchcraft. Wherein is affirmed that there are many sorts of Deceivers and Impostors, and Divers persons under a passive Delusion of Melancholy and Fancy. But that there is a Corporeal League made betwixt the Devil and the Witch, Or that he sucks on the Witches Body, has Carnal Copulation, or that Witches are turned into Cats, Dogs, raise Tempests, or the like, is utterly denied and disproved.* London: J.M., 1677.

Weichhold, G.M., J.E. Bark, W. Korte, W. Eisenmenger, and K.M. Sullivan. "DNA Analysis in the Case of Kaspar Hauser." *International Journal of Legal Medicine* 111, no. 6 (1998): 287–91.

Weiner, Dora B. *The Citizen-Patient in Revolutionary and Imperial Paris.* Baltimore: Johns Hopkins University Press, 1993.

Weiss, Harry B. *A Book about Chapbooks: The People's Literature of Bygone Times* (1942). Hatboro: Folklore, 1969.

Wicke, Jennifer. "Koko's Necklace: The Wild Child as Subject." *Critical Quarterly* 30, no. 1 (Spring 1988): 113–27.

Wilmot, Catherine. *An Irish Peer on the Continent (1801–1803): Being a Narrative of the Tour of Stephen, 2d Earl Mount Cashell, through France, Italy, etc.* Edited by T.U. Sadleir. London: Williams and Norgate, 1920.

Wilson, Henry and James Caulfield. *The Book of Wonderful Characters: Memoirs and Anecdotes of Remarkable and Eccentric Persons in All Ages and Countries.* London: John Camden Hotten, 1869.

Wing, John. "Kanner's Syndrome: A Historical Introduction." In *Early Childhood Autism: Clinical, Educational and Social Aspects,* edited by L. Wing, 2d ed., 3–14. Oxford: Pergamon, 1976.

Wing, John K., and Lorna Wing. "A Clinical Interpretation of Remedial Teaching." In *Early Childhood Autism: Clinical, Educational and Social Aspects,* edited by J.K. Wing, 185–203. Oxford: Pergamon, 1966.

Wittgenstein, Ludwig. *Philosophical Investigations.* Translated by G.E.M. Anscombe. Oxford: B. Blackwell, 1953.

Wokler, Robert. "Tyson and Buffon on the Orang-utan." *Studies on Voltaire and the Eighteenth Century* 155 (1976): 2,301–19.

– "The Ape Debates in Enlightenment Anthropology." *Studies on Voltaire and the Eighteenth Century* 192 (1980): 1,164–75.

"Wolf-Children." *Chambers' Edinburgh Journal* 446, new series (17 July 1852): 33–6.

"Wolf-Children." *Chambers's Journal* 19, 4th series, no. 977 (16 September 1882): 597–9.

"Wolf Children of India." *Living Age* 332, no. 4,307 (1 June 1927): 1,021–2.

"Wolf Girls." *Time* (1 November 1926): 25.

"Wolf Nurses in India." *Harper's New Monthly Magazine* 9, no. 50 (July 1854): 199–201.

Wolff, Christian. *Psychologia rationalis* (1734). Edited by Jean École. Vol. 6 of *Gesammelte Werke.* Hildesheim: Georg Olms, 1972.

Wood, Ernest. "The Wild Boy of Aveyron ('Itard's Syndrome'?)." *Nursing Mirror and Midwives Journal* 140, no. 18 (1 May 1975): 61–3.

Wood, Paul B. "The Science of Man." In *Cultures of Natural History,* edited by N. Jardine, J.A. Secord, and E.C. Spary, 197–210. Cambridge: Cambridge University Press, 1996.

Yolen, Jane. *Children of the Wolf.* New York: Viking, 1984.

Young, Kimball. *Sociology: A Study of Society and Culture.* New York: American Book Company, 1942.

Yousef, Nancy. "Savage or Solitary? The Wild Child and Rousseau's Man of Nature." *Journal of the History of Ideas* 62, no. 2 (2001): 245–63.

Zimmermann, Eberhard August G. *Zoologie géographique. Premier article L'Homme.* Cassel: de l'Imprimerie française, 1784.

Zingg, Robert M. "More about the 'Baboon Boy' of South Africa." *American Journal of Psychology* 53 (1940): 455–62.

– "Feral Man and Extreme Cases of Isolation." *American Journal of Psychology* 53 (October 1940): 487–517.

– "India's Wolf-Children: Two Human Infants Reared by Wolves." *Scientific American* (March 1941): 135–7.

– "The Wolf Child." *The New Republic* 104 (30 June 1941): 892.

– "Feral Man and Cases of Extreme Isolation of Individuals." In J.A.L. Singh and R.M. Zingg. *Wolf-Children and Feral Man*, 131–276.

Zusne, Leonard. *Biographical Dictionary of Psychology*. Westport: Greenwood, 1984.